0030991

KU-160-550

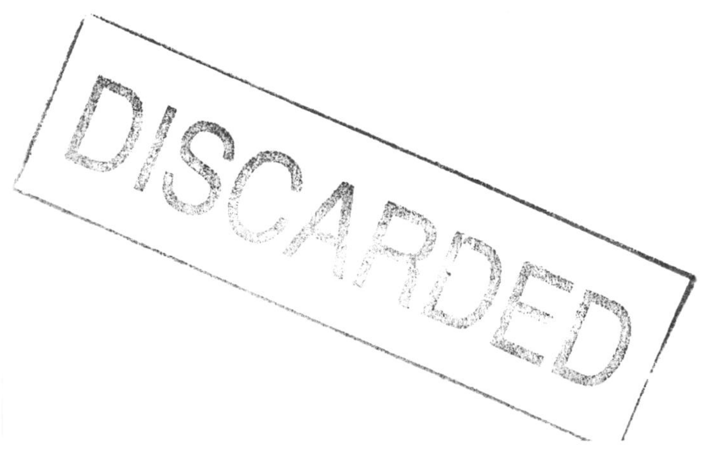
DISCARDED

International Review of RESEARCH IN MENTAL RETARDATION

VOLUME 22

Board of Associate Editors

International Review of RESEARCH IN MENTAL RETARDATION

EDITED BY

LARAINE MASTERS GLIDDEN

DEPARTMENT OF PSYCHOLOGY
ST. MARY'S COLLEGE OF MARYLAND
ST. MARY'S CITY, MARYLAND

VOLUME 22

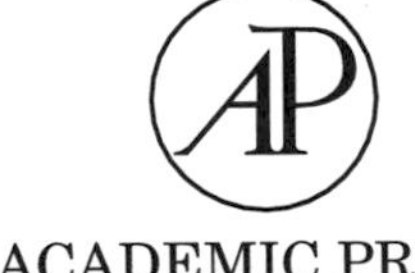

ACADEMIC PRESS
A Division of Harcourt Brace & Company
San Diego London Boston
New York Sydney Tokyo Toronto

This book is printed on acid-free paper. 

Academic Press
a division of Harcourt Brace & Company
525 B Street, Suite 1900, San Diego, California 92101-4495, USA
http://www.apnet.com

Academic Press
24-28 Oval Road, London NW1 7DX, UK
http://www.hbuk.co.uk/ap/

International Standard Book Number: 0-12-366222-2

PRINTED IN THE UNITED STATES OF AMERICA
99 00 01 02 03 04 BB 9 8 7 6 5 4 3 2 1

Contents

The Nature and Long-Term Implications of Early Developmental Delays: A Summary of Evidence from Two Longitudinal Studies

Ronald Gallimore, Barbara K. Keogh, and Lucinda P. Bernheimer

Savant Syndrome

Ted Nettelbeck and Robyn Young

The Cost-Efficiency of Supported Employment Programs: A Review of the Literature

Robert E. Cimera and Frank R. Rusch

Decision Making and Mental Retardation

Linda Hickson and Ishita Khemka

"The Child That Was Meant?" or "Punishment for Sin?": Religion, Ethnicity, and Families with Children with Disabilities

Laraine Masters Glidden, Jeannette Rogers-Dulan, and Amy E. Hill

Contributors

Numbers in parentheses indicate the pages on which the authors' contributions begin.

Arthur J. Baroody (51), *College of Education, University of Illinois at Urbana-Champaign, Champaign, Illinois 61820*

Lucinda P. Bernheimer (105), *Department of Psychiatry, University of California, Los Angeles, Los Angeles, California 90095*

Robert E. Cimera[1] (175), *Institute on Research on Disability and Human Development, University of Illinois at Chicago, Chicago, Illinois 60608*

Elisabeth M. Dykens (1), *Neuropsychiatric Institute, University of California, Los Angeles, Los Angeles, California 90024*

Ronald Gallimore (105), *Department of Psychiatry, University of California, Los Angeles, Los Angeles, California 90095*

Laraine Masters Glidden (267), *Department of Psychology, St. Mary's College of Maryland, St. Mary's City, Maryland 20686*

Linda Hickson (227), *Center for Opportunities and Outcomes for People with Disabilities, Teachers College, Columbia University, New York, New York 10027*

Amy E. Hill (267), *Department of Psychology, St. Mary's College of Maryland, St. Mary's City, Maryland 20686*

Robert M. Hodapp (27), *Graduate School of Education and Information Studies, University of California, Los Angeles, Los Angeles, California 90095*

Barbara K. Keogh (105), *Department of Psychiatry, University of California, Los Angeles, Los Angeles, California 90095*

[1]Current address: Department of Curriculum Instruction and Educational Psychology, Loyola University of Chicago, 1041 Ridge Road, Wilmette, IL 60091

Ishita Khemka (227), *Center for Opportunities and Outcomes for People with Disabilities, Teachers College, Columbia University, New York, New York 10027*

Ted Nettelbeck (137), *Department of Psychiatry, University of Adelaide, Adelaide 5001, South Australia*

Jeannette Rogers-Dulan (267), *School of Education, La Sierra University, Riverside, California 92515*

Frank R. Rusch (175), *College of Education, University of Illinois at Urbana-Champaign, Champaign, Illinois 61820*

Robyn Young (137), *Department of Psychology, Flinders University of South Australia, Adelaide 5001, South Australia*

Preface

It is both a delight and an honor to write this first preface as the new editor of the International Review of Research in Mental Retardation. I was just beginning to do research in psychology when volume 1 of the *Review* was published in 1966. A few years later when I entered the field of mental retardation, I looked on each issue as a guidepost, and read all chapters with interest, and a few with unbridled enthusiasm, sometimes coupled with critical intent. When I was invited to write a chapter ("Semantic Processing, Semantic Memory, and Recall," volume 13, 1985), I did so with the knowledge that my work would reach a wide and appropriate audience. Moreover, when I was invited to assume the editorship I accepted with honor, humility, and dedication. I was honored to have been selected; humble in the realization that the two previous editors, Norman Ellis and Norman Bray, had elevated and maintained this serial to an unequivocally eminent position in the field of mental retardation. I dedicated myself to doing whatever I could to keep it that way.

It was in that context that I continued the practice of a Board of Associate Editors, selected to represent diversity in the field and to provide support and counsel, helping both to solicit manuscripts and to review them. They have been indispensable as I have worked on this volume, and I thank them individually and collectively. I also thank the following individuals who are not on the Board who were willing to devote their time to provide knowledgeable and timely reviews of chapters submitted for this volume. Without their wisdom and hard work, this volume would be less valuable than it is: Leonard Abbeduto, Jan Blacher, J. P. Das, Penny Hauser-Cram, Judith Palfrey, Steven Reiss, Robert Stromer, Carol Thornton, Donald Treffert, Paul Wehman, and Michael Wehmeyer.

The current volume follows in the tradition of previous ones in that it is eclectic, with chapters that are both summative and seminal. Chapter topics range across the entire field of mental retardation, with focus on specific genetic and behavioral syndromes; academic and cognitive functioning in children and adults; and issues relating to family adjustment and supported employment. Methodologies are also varied. Longitudinal designs, traditional experimental techniques, and cost-benefit analyses are utilized in different chapters. Throughout, authors attend to past research, their own and that of others, to summarize their fields and develop recommendations for future work.

In the first chapter, Elisabeth Dykens examines the direct effects on personality and psychopathology of six genetic conditions—fragile-X, Prader-Willi, Down syndrome, Williams syndrome, 5p-syndrome, and Smith-Magenis syndrome. She outlines both the advantages and challenges of studying phenotypes, and she argues persuasively that more investigators should undertake the necessary collaborations between geneticists and behavioral scientists that are required. In the second chapter, Robert Hodapp also focuses on genetic syndromes, but on their indirect effects—how etiology-specific behaviors can consistently, and therefore, predictably evoke (and sometimes, provoke!) responses from persons and other environmental agents. He provides numerous examples from research findings involving a variety of genetic syndromes.

In Chapter 3, Arthur Baroody examines the very different, but equally important, domain of mathematical functioning in children with mental retardation. Anchoring this work on mathematical learning of children with mental retardation firmly in the mathematical learning of typically developing children, he reviews several decades of research (with reference to earlier work as appropriate) on three critical elements of basic mathematical knowledge: counting, number, and addition. He also discusses the specific implications of the research in mathematical learning on such important cognitive and behavioral issues as adaptive expertise, informal knowledge, and active learning. This chapter should be of interest not only to researchers, but also to teachers of children with mental retardation, for whom there are specific recommendations regarding instructional strategies and techniques.

Longitudinal research, as we all know, is extraordinarily valuable, but also difficult to do and expensive in time and other resources. That makes the chapter by Ronald Gallimore, Barbara Keogh, and Lucinda Bernheimer particularly noteworthy because they examine the results of two different longitudinal studies and what they have to tell us about the long-term functioning of children with early developmental delays. In both Project REACH and Project CHILD, children with unspecified but measurable developmental delays were recruited when they were 3–4 years old, and followed over time for at least 3 years. In both studies, results indicated that the early developmental delays did predict later cognitive delays, even to 11 years of age for some of the children. Obviously, this work is of interest to both developmental theorists and interventionists.

Normally, those of us in the field of mental retardation focus on what persons with intellectual deficiencies cannot do. In their fascinating chapter, "Savant Syndrome," Ted Nettelbeck and Robyn Young take a quite different perspective: They focus on the skills that persons with mental retardation display at or above a level expected of persons without mental retardation. In a comprehensive 20-year review of the literature, they summarize what we know about skills that involve memory and those that involve talent, such as musical ability and artistic ability. They also address the implications of the existence of savant performance for models of intellectual growth and functioning, concluding that savant skills are rather automatic, developed by practice, and essentially unintelligent.

Of course, most adults with mental retardation do not have savant skills. They do, however, frequently have other skills, ones that help them seek and obtain employment. This employment, although sometimes competitive, often must be supported in a variety of ways. This support can be justified from a humanitarian point of view, but in chapter 6, Robert Cimera and Frank Rusch present an economic analysis. They examine the cost-efficiency of supported employment programs through an extensive review of the literature, comparing supported employment with sheltered workshops. They explore the issue from three different perspectives: the worker, the taxpayer, and the society. They conclude that, in general, from an economic perspective, supported employment is a better investment than are sheltered workshops.

Linda Hickson and Ishita Khemka also focus on adults with mental retardation in their chapter on decision making. Recognizing that the opportunities for societal integration also pose challenges for persons with limited cognitive skills, they approach their experimental paradigms with an ecologically valid orientation. Their emphasis is on interpersonal decision making and how it can influence domains such as workplace conduct; child care and parenting; sexual, physical, and verbal abuse; and peer relations. They point out that most available research in this area has emphasized cognitive factors of decision making and has ignored motivational and emotional factors. They describe some of their own work that does include these neglected factors, and propose a framework that integrates the cognitive, motivational, and emotional processes. This framework is likely to prove useful to other investigators, and it will not be surprising to see it generate a larger body of work that informs us about how people with mental retardation handle interpersonal situations.

The concluding chapter also extends research in mental retardation beyond its usual boundaries. Laraine Masters Glidden, Jeannette Rogers-Dulan, and Amy Hill claim that although there is an extensive research literature on how families adjust to rearing a child with mental retardation, investigators have generally neglected the influence of culture, ethnicity, and religion in their research on adjustment. They examine the influence of religiousness in both African-American and Latino families and conclude that for both groups there is some evidence that religiousness is a source of support. They are careful, however, to point out that it may also be a source of difficulty, as indicated in the eponymous question, "punishment for sin?" Using case examples, they caution about the need for contextualizing families within their culture and ethnicity in order to avoid inappropriate generalizations from one cultural/ethnic group to another.

Laraine Masters Glidden

Direct Effects of Genetic Mental Retardation Syndromes: Maladaptive Behavior and Psychopathology

ELISABETH M. DYKENS

NEUROPSYCHIATRIC INSTITUTE
UNIVERSITY OF CALIFORNIA, LOS ANGELES
LOS ANGELES, CALIFORNIA

Sparked by revolutionary advances in the Human Genome Project, researchers are increasingly concerned with how genetic diseases are manifest at the genetic, physical, behavioral, and developmental levels. Yet for many reasons, research on genetic syndromes has trickled into the field of mental retardation at a relatively slow pace (Dykens, 1996). Even so, syndromic findings have already had a profound impact on the developmental disability field, especially in the area of psychopathology.

Most work on mental retardation syndromes focuses on so-called direct behavioral effects, or the ways in which a genetic diagnosis predisposes persons to show certain behaviors relative to those without the diagnosis. This chapter focuses on many of the complexities involved in studying direct effects, otherwise known as behavioral phenotypes. These complexities include defining and measuring phenotypes; assessing genetic and psychosocial sources of within-syndrome behavioral variability; and examining unique versus shared behaviors across syndromes.

In contrast, syndromes are also characterized by so-called indirect effects, or how syndrome-specific behaviors elicit reactions from others, such as parents, siblings, peers, and teachers. Less researched than direct effects, work on indirect effects assesses how different syndromic phenotypes set the stage for different types of interactions with others. As described by Hodapp (1997) elsewhere, and in his chapter in this volume, indirect effects are primarily concerned with the person's effects on others, and the person–environment transactions that are elicited by various behavioral phenotypes.

INTERNATIONAL REVIEW OF RESEARCH IN MENTAL RETARDATION, Vol. 22
0074-7750/99 $30.00

To briefly illustrate these two approaches, consider possible direct and indirect effects of children with Down syndrome. As described later in this chapter, direct effects include a controversial but persistent personality stereotype involving a pleasant and charming demeanor, as well as fewer and less severe maladaptive behaviors relative to other children with mental retardation. As discussed in Hodapp's chapter on indirect effects, these features, in turn, may be associated with less family stress, fewer sibling concerns, and more family harmony and cohesion.

In short, then, the two complementary chapters in this volume on direct and indirect effects both clarify and expand key assumptions about behavioral phenotypes. But work on behavioral phenotypes is actually at its beginning stages, and researchers within this growing speciality often struggle with basic conceptual, definitional, and measurement issues. This chapter on direct effects takes up many of these issues, with particular reference to within- and between-syndromic differences, logistical and attitudinal challenges to phenotypic research, and the importance of phenotypic work for furthering our understandings of gene–brain–behavior relationships. Hodapp's subsequent chapter on indirect effects further expands phenotypic work, showing how different behavioral phenotypes shape interactions with others. Although child effects on adults or peers are increasingly studied in other fields, such as developmental psychology, this approach has yet to be applied to people with genetic mental retardation syndromes. The two chapters on direct and indirect effects show both the problems and promise in conducting research on specific genetic mental retardation syndromes.

I. DIRECT EFFECTS: PSYCHOPATHOLOGY AS EXAMPLE

Phenotypic research should examine the profiles and developmental trajectories of a broad range of behavior, including domains such as cognition, achievement, speech, language, personality, adaptive skills, and social competence (Dykens, 1995). Yet most studies on direct effects focus on maladaptive behavior or psychopathology, in part because of the clinical urgency associated with these problems. I primarily use psychopathology in various syndromes as examples of direct effects of genetic mental retardation syndromes.

Before considering psychopathology in people with syndromes, however, some background information is necessary about maladaptive behavior in people with mental retardation in general. Relative to the general population, people with mental retardation are twice as likely to suffer from psychiatric disorders or significant psychopathology. It is now well appreciated that people with mental retardation show the full range of psychiatric disease, as well as a host of maladaptive behaviors rarely seen in the general population, such as stereotypies and self-injury. These problems are the leading culprits for failed residential, educational, and vocational placements, and they often lead people with mental retardation to need more restrictive levels of care.

In all this work, however, researchers have yet to decipher why people with mental retardation are at increased risk for psychopathology in the first place. In the absence of any well-proven theory, workers have hypothesized many reasonable explanations for the co-occurrence of mental retardation and psychiatric dysfunction, often referred to as dual diagnosis. In the most comprehensive hypothesis to date, Matson and Sevin (1994) propose a biopsychosocial theory of dual diagnosis. In this model, psychopathology is attributed to a confluence of factors, including limited skills in cognitive, adaptive, social, linguistic, and memory functioning; organic problems such as neurologic and genetic abnormalities, epilepsy, biochemical and sensory impairments; aberrant patterns of learning and behavioral reinforcement, such as learned helplessness and social deprivation; aberrant personality styles; psychosocial stressors; heightened family stress; de-institutionalization; and societal stigma. Although comprehensive, it is unclear the exact role that each of these risk factors plays in the development of psychopathology.

In this chapter, I propose that examining genetic etiology of mental retardation is an important first step in sorting out the relative importance of the many risk factors for psychopathology. Differentiating genetic from psychosocial risk factors is a particularly promising strategy as it takes advantage of recent and dramatic breakthroughs in molecular genetics and the Human Genome Project. Over 750 known genetic causes of mental retardation have now been identified (Opitz, 1996), and more accurate diagnostic procedures for both new and previously known syndromes will result in more and more people being diagnosed with genetic syndromes in the years ahead. Indeed, prevalence studies suggest that genetic syndromes may already account for 40 to 50% of people with developmental delay (e.g., Matilanen, Airaksinen, Monen, Launiala, & Kaariainen, 1995). Further, mental retardation syndromes have been pivotal to the discoveries of new mechanisms of human disease, leading to revolutionary advances in the genetics field.

Despite these remarkable accomplishments, however, genetic etiology has yet to be widely studied by behavioral researchers in the mental retardation field. In particular, most behavioral and dual diagnosis researchers use subject groups with heterogeneous etiologies (Dykens, 1995, 1996; Hodapp & Dykens, 1994). Thus, persons with known syndromes or other organic causes for their delay are mixed together in the same group, along with subjects with unknown etiologies. Subsequent behavioral data are then analyzed by age, IQ, level of impairment, gender, or residential status (see Borthwick-Duffy, 1994, for a review).

To show this, I reviewed Aman's (1991) comprehensive bibliography of articles published between 1970 and 1990 on behavioral and emotional problems in people with mental retardation. Over this 20-year period, only 11% of the articles (41 out of 375) were devoted to people with specific genetic syndromes. Most of these syndrome-specific studies were on Down syndrome (n = 24), leaving just a handful of studies on people with all other genetic disorders. The majority of articles (89%) used heterogeneous subjects and did not examine etiology at all. These very same percentages were seen as well in a review of psychopathology articles from 1990 to 1995 (Dykens, 1996).

It makes it hard, if not impossible, to sort out genetic from psychosocial risk factors for psychopathology if 90% of dual diagnosis studies simply ignore the genetic etiology of their participants. One way to advance a greater understanding of psychopathology is to examine groups of people with discrete genetic disorders. Although rare relative to mixed groups, syndrome-specific studies to date find strong associations between genetic syndromes and distinctive patterns of psychopathology.

This chapter reviews maladaptive and psychiatric features in six of these syndromes, including fragile X syndrome, Williams syndrome, Prader-Willi syndrome, Down syndrome, 5p- syndrome, and Smith-Magenis syndrome. Although not representative of all 750 or so syndromes, these disorders have rich or growing databases, and demonstrate both the advantages and problems in conducting phenotypic research. Findings from these syndromes also hold much promise for identifying specific genetic, brain, and biochemical pathways to psychiatric problems in people with or without mental retardation.

After the syndrome review, I discuss broader considerations in conducting phenotypic research, including how to define a behavioral phenotype, to appreciate individual differences within syndromes, and to compare similarities and differences between syndromes. Throughout, I specify advantages of a syndrome-specific approach to dual diagnosis research, including how phenotypic data further our understandings of gene–brain–behavior relationships and psychiatric disease, inform treatment and intervention, and lead to a more precise science of mental retardation. Challenges to the work are then discussed. Some challenges rest in the work itself, such as sampling people with rare conditions, and selecting specific syndromes and behavioral domains for study. Yet a bigger challenge concerns researchers themselves. Here I and others often encounter indifferent or antagonistic attitudes about genetic diagnoses from social scientists and advocates, as well as a reluctance for social scientists to collaborate with geneticists. I conclude with recommendations for overcoming these obstacles, to the benefit of researchers in both fields.

II. SYNDROME REVIEW

A. Fragile X Syndrome

1. OVERVIEW

Fragile X syndrome, the most common inherited cause of mental retardation, results in a wide range of learning and behavioral problems, with males being more often and severely affected than females (see Dykens, Hodapp, & Leckman, 1994, for a review). The recently discovered fragile X gene (FMR-1) represents a newly identified type of human disease, caused by an amplification (or excessive repetition) of three nucleotide sequences (CGG) that make up DNA. Above a certain threshold of these triplet repeats (about 200), people are fully affected with the syndrome. Below that number (and above the normal threshold of 50), they show premutations. Persons with premutations may be affected or unaffected carriers of the syndrome, depending on the mode of inheritance and other genetic factors. As many as 1 in 259 women in the general population may carry the premutation, with 1 in 4,000 males and 1 in 2,500 females being fully affected with the syndrome (see Hagerman, 1996, for a review).

2. PERSONALITY/PSYCHOPATHOLOGY

Many fully affected males with fragile X syndrome show autistic-like symptoms such as language delay, echolalia, stereotypies, self-injurious behavior, perseveration, poor eye contact, and tactile defensiveness. Not surprisingly, then, early workers tried to link fragile X syndrome to autism, spurred on by the possibility of a common genetic cause of autism. Yet highly variable prevalence rates resulted from this work, due primarily to discrepancies in diagnostic criteria for autism (see Dykens & Volkmar, 1997, for a review).

This flurry of research faded as new studies emerged suggesting that instead of autism per se, many males showed a willingness to interact with others coupled with social and performance anxiety and mutual gaze aversion (e.g., Cohen, Viteze, Sudhalter, Jenkins, & Brown, 1989). Controlled studies and meta-analyses now suggest that only about 5% of fragile X males have full-blown autistic disorder (Einfeld, Molony & Hall, 1989; Fisch, 1992). Instead, the majority of affected males can be placed on a spectrum of social anxiety, shyness, avoidance, and gaze aversion. While some of these boys have anxiety disorders (Bregman, Leckman, & Ort, 1988) or pervasive developmental disorder—not otherwise specified (PDD-NOS) (Reiss & Freund, 1990), others may simply show slow-to-warm temperament styles, including shyness or social withdrawal (Kerby & Dawson, 1994).

Similarly, many females with fragile X syndrome show variable levels of social dysfunction, primarily shyness, gaze aversion, and social anxiety. Many of these women meet clinical criteria for schizotypal disorder, showing interpersonal discomfort and difficulties in communication and social relationships. Fully affected women (with CGG repeats in excess of 200) are more likely to have schizotypal disorder or schizotypal features than women with a premutation (with 50 to 200 repeats), or appropriately matched non-fragile X control women (Freund, Reiss, Hagerman, & Vinogradov, 1992; Sobesky, Porter, Pennington, & Hagerman, 1995). Although shyness is thus a central feature of the fragile X behavioral phenotype, affected females may also show increased risks of depression, even as compared to non-fragile X mothers of developmentally delayed children (Freund et al., 1992; Reiss, Hagerman, Vinogradov, Abrams, & King, 1988).

In addition to these difficulties, attention deficit-hyperactivity disorder (ADHD) is seen in the vast majority of clinic-referred boys and girls with fragile X syndrome (Bregman et al., 1988; Hagerman, 1996). ADHD symptoms are higher among fragile X boys relative to control subjects (Baumgardner, Reiss, Freund, & Abrams, 1995), and although hyperactivity may diminish with age, inattention seems to persist even with advancing age (Dykens, Hodapp, & Leckman, 1994). Girls with fragile X syndrome have lower prevalence rates of ADHD relative to fragile X boys, but higher rates relative to the general population (Lachiewicz, 1992). Many girls suffer more from inattention than hyperactivity. Among adults, problems in attending and in sustaining effort have been found in the neuropsychological profiles of women who carry the FMR-1 gene, which may contribute to problems in math, abstract reasoning, and planning (e.g., Mazzocco, Hagerman, Cronister-Silverman, & Pennington, 1992).

Fragile X syndrome thus involves vulnerabilities toward shyness, gaze aversion, social anxiety, avoidant disorders, schizotypal disorder, ADHD, PDD-NOS, and more rarely, autistic disorder. These difficulties vary in severity, but are typically found in persons across the IQ spectrum, from those with moderate mental retardation to those with mild learning disabilities.

B. Prader-Willi Syndrome

1. OVERVIEW

First identified 41 years ago, Prader-Willi syndrome affects about 1 in 15,000 births, and is best known for its food-related characteristics. Whereas babies invariably show hypotonia, and pronounced feeding-sucking difficulties, young children between 2 to 6 years of age develop hyperphagia and food-seeking behavior such as food foraging and hoarding (see Dykens & Cassidy, 1996, for a review). Hyperphagia is likely associated with a hypothalamic abnormality resulting in a lack of satiety (Holland, Treasure, Coskeran, & Dallow, 1995; Swaab, Purba, & Hofman, 1995). Food preoccupations are life-long, and without prolonged dietary management, affected individuals invariably become obese. Indeed, complications of obesity remain the leading cause of death in this syndrome.

Prader-Willi syndrome is the first known human disease to show the effects of genomic imprinting, or the idea that genes are modified and expressed differently depending on whether they are inherited from the mother or the father. About 70% of Prader-Willi syndrome cases are caused by a paternally derived deletion on the long arm of chromosome 15. Remaining cases are attributed to maternal uniparental disomy (UPD) of chromosome 15, in which both members of the chromosome 15 pair come from the mother. In either etiology, there is absence of the paternally-derived contribution to this specific region of the genome. When missing information in this same region of chromosome 15 is maternally derived, it results in a completely different and more severe developmental disorder, Angelman's syndrome.

2. PERSONALITY/PSYCHOPATHOLOGY

Although people with Prader-Willi syndrome invariably obsess about food, a remarkably high proportion of persons also show non-food obsessions and compulsive behaviors (Dykens, Leckman, & Cassidy, 1996). These non-food symptoms include skin-picking, hoarding, needing to tell, ask, or say things, and having concerns with symmetry, exactness, ordering, arranging, cleanliness, and sameness in daily routine. Often these symptoms are associated with distress or adaptive impairment, suggesting marked risks of obsessive-compulsive disorder (OCD) in this population (Dykens et al., 1996). Indeed, we estimate that OCD is many more times likely in people with Prader-Willi syndrome than in the general population of people with mental retardation.

In addition, even as compared to others with mental retardation, children and adults with Prader-Willi syndrome show high rates of temper tantrums, aggression, stubbornness, underactivity, excessive daytime sleepiness, and emotional lability (Dykens & Kasari, 1997). Coupled with food seeking, these impulsive behaviors often lead people with Prader-Willi syndrome to need more restrictive levels of care than would be predicted by their mild levels of mental retardation.

Psychopathology may be associated with the individual's genetic variant of Prader-Willi syndrome. Preliminary findings from ongoing work suggest some behavioral differences between Prader-Willi syndrome cases due to paternal deletion versus maternal UPD. Cases with deletions may show lower IQs, especially verbal IQs, and more frequent or severe problem behaviors, such as skin-picking, hoarding, temper tantrums, overeating, and social withdrawal (Dykens, Cassidy, & King, 1999). Although a dampening of symptom severity is suggested in many UPD cases, we also observe occasional cases of more severe problems in UPD, primarily autistic-like features and relatively low IQs.

Many people with Prader-Willi syndrome are at increased risk for OCD, impulse control, and affective disorders. Yet even those who do not meet diagnostic criteria for these full-blown psychiatric disorders often show salient maladaptive behaviors that interfere with optimal adaptive functioning. Future research is needed to clarify if psychiatric disorders of maladaptive behaviors differ across those with paternal deletions versus maternal UPD.

C. Down Syndrome

1. OVERVIEW

Down syndrome, the most common chromosomal cause of mental retardation, affects about 1 in 800 births, and increased risks of trisomy 21 are seen among women with advanced maternal age. Down syndrome enjoys more behavioral research than all other mental retardation syndromes combined (Hodapp, 1996).

2. PERSONALITY/PSYCHOPATHOLOGY

Persistent personality stereotypes depict persons with Down syndrome as cheerful, friendly, eager to please and affectionate—the so-called Prince Charming syndrome. Some findings, however, call this stereotype into question. Many mothers, for example, describe their children with Down syndrome as having a wide range of personality features (Rogers, 1987), and the temperaments of some children with Down syndrome are active, distractible, and difficult (Ganiban, Wagner, & Cicchetti, 1990). Further, some studies find that Down syndrome children are no easier to rear than children with other types of disabilities (Cahill & Glidden, 1996; Glidden & Cahill, 1998). Still, fathers often spontaneously remark on their child's sociability (Hornby, 1995), and the temperaments of many children with Down syndrome have been described as easygoing (Ganiban et al., 1990). Even with these equivocal findings, the personality stereotype persists, with parents and researchers alike often remarking that children and adults with Down syndrome are extraordinarily charming and eager to please.

Yet these endearing features do not necessarily protect these same individuals from showing behavioral problems such as stubbornness, defiance, aggressive behavior, and psychopathology. Children with Down syndrome have elevated behavioral problems relative to their siblings without developmental delay (Gath & Gumley, 1986; Pueschel, Bernier, & Pezzullo, 1991). About 13 to 15% of children with Down syndrome appear to have significant behavioral difficulties. Prevalence estimates are higher and more variable in studies of children and adolescents, ranging from 18 to 38% (Gath & Gumley, 1986; Meyers & Pueschel, 1991). Primary problems include disruptive disorders such as ADHD, oppositional and conduct disorders, and occasionally, anxiety disorders.

In contrast to the "externalizing" disorders of childhood, adults with Down syndrome are particularly vulnerable to depressive disorders (e.g., Collacott, Cooper, & McGrother, 1992; Meyers & Pueschel, 1991). Depression in Down syndrome is often characterized by passivity, apathy, withdrawal and mutism, and several cases of major depressive disorder have now been well described (e.g., Dosen & Petry, 1993). Prevalence estimates of affective disorders among adults with Down syndrome range from 6 to 11% (Collacott et al., 1992; Meyers & Pueschel, 1991), many times higher than the 1 to 3% rates seen in the general population of persons with mental retardation (Lund, 1985).

It is not yet known why adults with Down syndrome appear vulnerable to depression. One hypothesis implicates dementia. Almost all persons with Down syndrome over age 35 to 40 show neuropathological signs of Alzheimer's disease (Zigman, Schupf, Zigman, & Silverman, 1993). Yet not all adults with Down syndrome develop the behavioral correlates of Alzheimer-type dementia, and the risk for doing so dramatically increases with advancing age. Some researchers find rates of dementia as high as 55% in persons aged 40 to 50 years, and 75% in persons aged 60 years and older (Lai & Williams, 1989). Collectively, however, most studies suggest that less than 50% of adults aged 50 years or more show symptoms of dementia (Zigman et al., 1993).

Thus, while only a relatively small number of children with Down syndrome show disruptive behavior or other disorders, adults with Down syndrome are at considerable risk for depression and dementia. Aside from these two disorders, the overall rate of psychiatric illness in the population of persons with Down syndrome is low relative to other groups of persons with mental retardation (Collacott et al., 1992; Dykens & Kasari, 1997; Girzenko, Cvejic, Vida, & Sayegh, 1991). While sociable, charming personalities may be associated with lower rates of psychopathology, the interplay between personality and psychopathology has not yet been studied in children or adults with Down syndrome.

D. Williams Syndrome

1. OVERVIEW

First identified in 1961, Williams syndrome is caused by a microdeletion on one of the chromosome 7's that includes the gene for elastin, a protein that provides strength and elasticity to certain tissues such as the heart, skin, blood vessels, and lungs (Ewart et al., 1994). Affecting about 1 in 20,000 births, persons with Williams syndrome often show hyperacusis, hypercalcemia, neuromuskeletal and renal abnormalities, and characteristic facial features described as elfin-like, cute, and appealing (see Pober & Dykens, 1996, for a review). People with Williams syndrome also typically show cardiovascular disease, especially supravalvular aortic stenosis, and these problems are likely associated with elastin insufficiency.

Williams syndrome is perhaps best known for its cognitive-linguistic profile. Many people with Williams syndrome show pronounced weaknesses in perceptual and visual-spatial functioning. Despite these difficulties, however, they often do well on facial recognition tasks. Significant, relative strengths are often seen in expressive language, including vocabulary, syntax, semantics, and prosody (e.g., Reilly, Klima, & Bellugi, 1990; Udwin & Yule, 1990). But not all persons with Williams syndrome show these linguistic strengths, and the representativeness of this profile is now open to considerable debate (Karmiloff-Smith et al., 1997).

2. PERSONALITY/PSYCHOPATHOLOGY

In contrast to work on cognitive-linguistic profiles, studies have yet to fully examine the personality or psychiatric features of people with Williams syndrome. Early descriptions of people with Williams syndrome hinted at a "classic" Williams syndrome personality, described as pleasant, unusually friendly, affectionate, loquacious, engaging, and interpersonally sensitive and charming (e.g., Dilts,

Morris, & Leonard, 1990). Such qualities may change over the course of development, with adults being more withdrawn and less overly friendly than children (Gosch & Pankau, 1997).

Recent findings from our ongoing work on Williams syndrome expand these observations. Using the Reiss Personality Profiles (Reiss & Havercamp, 1998), we find that relative to controls, adolescents and adults with Williams syndrome are more likely to approach others, to draw attention to themselves, and to empathize with the positive and negative feelings of others (Dykens & Rosner, in press). At the same time, however, these subjects did not fare well making or keeping friends, and were often dangerously indiscriminate in their relating to others.

Indeed, although sociability in Williams syndrome has generally been viewed as a strength, these features also seem to reflect the type of social disinhibition that is characteristic of people who are anxious, impulsive, and overly aroused. Not surprisingly, salient problems in Williams syndrome include hyperactivity and inattentiveness, and a proneness for ADHD that may diminish with age (Gosch & Pankau, 1997; Pober & Dykens, 1996). Generalized anxiety, worry, and perseverative thinking are also commonly seen (e.g., Einfeld, Tonge, & Florio, 1997), and people with Williams syndrome appear to show unusually high levels of fears and phobias (Dykens, 1999). Relative to suitably matched controls, fears in persons with Williams syndrome are more frequent, wide-ranging, and severe, and they are also associated with impaired social-adaptive adjustment (Dykens, 1999). In addition to anxiety and fears, some young adults with Williams syndrome struggle with depression, sadness, and low self-esteem (Pober & Dykens, 1996).

Sociable personalities and strengths in facial recognition tasks suggest a low probability of psychiatric disorders in the Williams syndrome population involving an inability to read social cues, such as autism or PDD-NOS (see Dykens & Volkmar, 1997, for a review). It is unknown how cognitive-linguistic or personality profiles might mediate the expression of other difficulties associated with Williams syndrome, including anxiety, fears, depression, inattention, and hyperactivity.

E. 5p- Syndrome

1. OVERVIEW

First described 33 years ago, 5p- syndrome occurs in only 1 in 50,000 births, and typically results in early hypotonia, severe levels of mental retardation, motor and language delays, microcephaly, and prominent epicanthal folds. More distinctive to 5p- syndrome is the infantile, high-pitched, cat-like cry for which the syndrome was initially named. About 90% of cases with 5p- syndromes are caused by a de novo deletion on the short arm of chromosome 5; most of the remaining 10% of cases are associated with translocations. The critical region for 5p- syndrome is localized to 5p15 (Overhauser et al., 1994). Recent advances pinpoint the syndrome's cat-like cry to 5p15.3, with remaining clinical features of the syndrome associated with deletions at 5p15.2 (Gersh et al., 1995).

Early reports of institutionalized individuals with 5p- syndrome cast a rather bleak prognostic view of this syndrome. More recent surveys with noninstitutionalized children find much more variability in outcome, with many individuals learning to walk, engage in self-help skills, and communicate via speech, signs, or communicative aids (Carlin, 1990; Wilkins, Brown, Nance, & Wolf, 1983).

2. PERSONALITY/PSYCHOPATHOLOGY

Examining maladaptive behavior, Dykens and Clarke (1997) found that hyperactivity was the most striking problem in a sample of 146 individuals with 5p- syndrome aged 4 to 40 years. Seen in up to 85% of the group, hyperactivity was pervasive across males and females, children and adults, those with relatively high versus low adaptive levels, and those with translocations versus deletions. Further, hyperactivity was significantly elevated in persons with 5p- syndrome relative to two other comparison groups of subjects with mixed etiologies.

Persons with 5p- syndrome also appear vulnerable to other problems, with 50 to 70% of the Dykens and Clarke (1997) sample showing aggression, temper tantrums, self-injurious behavior, general irritability, and stereotyped movements. Many of these problems were inversely correlated with cognitive-adaptive level.

Unlike early work that depicted most persons with 5p- syndrome as profoundly withdrawn, we observed withdrawal and autistic-like symptoms primarily in subjects with translocations as opposed to deletions. Controlling for the lower cognitive-adaptive level of the translocation group, those with translocations were more withdrawn, isolative, unresponsive to others, and difficult to reach, with fewer communicative gestures or responses to others. In contrast, those with deletions are often described as quite social; they readily approach peers and adults, often try to engage others, and seemingly show joint attention.

Though behavioral studies in 5p- syndrome are just underway, next steps need to build on these findings by relating hyperactivity and other salient problems to the size and location of the deletion on chromosome 5p. Early reports hinted that larger deletion sizes correlated with more severe levels of delay (Wilkins et al., 1983), yet this finding has yet to be replicated, with some individuals showing large deletion sizes and only mild levels of cognitive or language delay (Church et al., 1995; Smith, Field, Murray, & Nelson, 1990). Expanding such genotype–phenotype studies to include maladaptive behavior may shed further light on these contradictory findings.

F. Smith–Magenis Syndrome

1. OVERVIEW

Although currently an underdiagnosed condition, Smith-Magenis syndrome is a recently delineated disorder that may affect as many as 1 in 25,000 births (Smith,

Dykens, & Greenberg, 1998a). Caused by interstitial deletions at 17p11.2, many genes are now mapped to this region, though none explain the syndrome's complex physical or behavioral phenotype (see Chen et al., 1996, for a review). Physically, people with Smith-Magenis syndrome show craniofacial abnormalities such as a flat midface, prominent forehead, a broad nasal bridge, and flat head shape; short hands and stature; visual problems (e.g., strabismus, myopia); a hoarse voice; and speech delay with or without hearing loss (see Greenberg et al., 1996, for a review). Many of these features are subtle in childhood, and become more distinctive with advancing age. Most people with Smith-Magenis syndrome show moderate mental retardation, with relative weaknesses in short-term memory (Dykens, Finucance, & Gayley, 1996).

2. PERSONALITY/PSYCHOPATHOLOGY

Although behavior has yet to be as widely studied, findings to date suggest unusual and distinctive maladaptive features. Examining 35 children and adolescents with Smith-Magenis syndrome, Dykens and Smith (1998) found extraordinarily high rates of temper tantrums, attention seeking, property destruction, aggression, hyperactivity, distractibility, toileting difficulties, self-injurious behaviors, and sleep disturbance. These multiple problems were elevated relative to two other matched comparison groups of subjects, with all but four Smith-Magenis subjects showing clinically elevated maladaptive behavior scores. In addition to high severity and frequency ratings, youngsters with Smith-Magenis syndrome showed a wide variety of self-injurious behaviors: self-biting and hitting; head banging; and less commonly, toe and finger nail yanking; and inserting foreign objects into bodily openings. Self-injurious behaviors are likely related to clinical signs of neuropathy, seen in up to 75% of those with this syndrome (Greenberg et al., 1996).

Stereotypies were also unusual, with about half the sample showing a previously described "upper body spasmodic squeeze," or self-hug, seen especially when persons are excited or happy (see also Finucane, Konar, Haas-Givler, Kurtz, & Scott, 1994). The most frequent stereotypies involved the mouth in some way; placing fingers or objects in the mouth, nail biting, teeth grinding, and a sequential hand-licking and page-flipping behavior. This "lick-and-flip" behavior was observed as well with remarkable consistency in a separate sample of subjects during their cognitive test sessions (Dykens et al., 1996). All these behaviors seem oral variants of bodily insertion tendencies.

Sleep disturbances are also striking in the Smith-Magenis syndrome population, with many people showing difficulties falling asleep, frequent and prolonged night-time awakenings, excessive daytime sleepiness, and reduced or absent REM sleep (see Smith, Dykens, & Greenberg, 1998b, for a review). Sleep disturbance emerged as the strongest predictor of maladaptive behavior in our study of 35 subjects. Overall sleep disturbance, especially snoring and labored nocturnal breathing, were highly related to aggressive, acting out behaviors and attentional problems (Dykens & Smith, 1998). Importantly, increased daytime nap length was associated with decreased aggressive and attentional problems.

Consistent with all these findings, families and professionals alike report that maladaptive behavior in Smith-Magenis syndrome is extraordinarily disruptive and hard to manage; indeed, these behaviors are the single best predictor of family stress (Hodapp, Fidler, & Smith, 1998). Although further work is needed, people with this syndrome appear at risk for ADHD, anxiety disorders, sleep disturbance, and stereotypic movement disorder, with or without a self-injurious component.

G. Summary

Across all six syndromes, we find heightened vulnerabilities toward specific types of psychopathologies (see Table I). As shown in the review, some problems are shared across syndromes, such as hyperactivity, while others seem relatively unique, such as hyperphagia in Prader-Willi syndrome or self-hugs in Smith-Magenis syndrome. Further, not every person with these six or any other syndrome may show the disorder's characteristic behaviors. I now discuss what these between- and within-syndrome similarities and differences mean for the study of behavioral phenotypes in general.

III. CHALLENGES AND ADVANTAGES TO PHENOTYPIC WORK

A. Defining a Behavioral Phenotype

One obstacle to more syndrome-based research may stem from inconsistencies in the definition of a behavioral phenotype. Some workers define behavioral phe-

TABLE I

SUMMARY OF SALIENT MALADAPTIVE BEHAVIORS IN SIX SYNDROMES

Syndrome	Behaviors
Fragile X	Inattention, hyperactivity, gaze avoidance, social anxiety, shyness, perseveration, stereotypies, self-injury, depression (females)
Williams	Anxiety, inattention, hyperactivity, fears, depression, indiscriminate relating, social disinhibition, overly friendly, sensitive, empathic
Prader-Willi	Hyperphagia, anxiety, obsessive-compulsive symptoms, perseveration, skin picking, lability, depression, tantrums
Down	Inattention, noncompliance, overactivity, stubbornness; depression and dementia in adults
5p-	Hyperactivity, inattention, self-injury, stereotypies, infantile high-pitched, cat-like cry
Smith-Magenis	Inattention, hyperactivity, aggression, attention seeking, temper tantrums, self-injury, sleep disturbance, self-hugging

notypes in absolute terms, proposing that a behavioral phenotype only exists when a unique behavior occurs in every case of a genetic disorder (Flynt & Yule, 1994). In this model, for example, every person with Smith-Magenis syndrome needs to show nail yanking or bodily insertions. In contrast, however, we view phenotypes in probabilistic terms, or as the "heightened probability of likelihood that people with a given syndrome will exhibit certain behavioral or developmental sequelae relative to those without the syndrome" (Dykens, 1995, p. 523). Casting behavioral phenotypes as a probability provides researchers with several promising avenues for future research.

B. Within-Syndrome Variability

As behavioral phenotypes involve a probability, not every individual with a given syndrome will show that syndrome's characteristic behavioral profile. Nor will each individual show that behavior to the same extent or level of severity, or at the same point in development. Just as only 57% of infants with Down syndrome show that disorder's characteristic epicanthal folds, so too will individuals with the same syndrome differ in their behaviors. Indeed, that a specific behavior characterizes a given syndrome means only that significantly more of that behavior is noted compared to a mixed or nonspecific group (Dykens, 1995; Einfeld & Hall, 1994; Rosen, 1993).

Identifying genetic and psychosocial sources of within-syndrome variability is perhaps one of the most exciting tasks facing phenotypic researchers in the years ahead. Why, for example, does the severity of hyperphagia differ across people with Prader-Willi syndrome? Why don't all children with 5p- syndrome have an infantile, cat-like cry? Why are some women with fragile X syndrome more shy and socially avoidant than others? Answering these and similar questions will involve untangling a complicated mix of genetic versus psychosocial factors. Yet remarkable strides have already been made in many syndromes.

C. Gene–Brain–Behavior Relationships

Ongoing work in several syndromes is fast uncovering promising new ties between molecular genetic status and brain and behavioral functioning. In this vein, fragile X syndrome leads the way. Many of the previously reviewed behavioral features in people with fragile X syndrome are a function of number of CGG repeats, and a cascade of subsequent effects. The number of repeats relates to the degree that the FMR1 gene is methylated and subsequently silenced, or blocked from transcription and translation. This, in turn, impacts the amount of FMR1 protein (FMR1P) produced, and the range of clinical expression in fragile X syndrome is associated with the amount of FMR1P. Fully affected, fully methylated males have no FMR1P, whereas high-functioning males, though rare, have some FMR1P (e.g.,

Merenstein, Sobesky, & Taylor, 1996). In females, only one X chromosome carries the FMR1 gene, while the other produces some FMR1P. Because all females have one X chromosome that is randomly inactivated in all cells, the degree of involvement in fragile X females is related to the ratio of normally active X chromosomes to the total active plus inactive X chromosomes. About half of fully affected females thus show mild to moderate mental retardation, whereas half have average IQs. But even among those with average intelligence, up to 80% may show emotional features such as shyness, odd communication, lability, and social anxiety, as well as specific problems in planning, memory, and attention (e.g., Mazzocco, Pennington, & Hagerman, 1993; Sobesky et al., 1995). Neuroimaging studies link performance on some of these cognitive tasks to the size of the posterior vermis, which is smaller in males and females with fragile X syndrome relative to controls (Mostofsky et al., 1998).

New insights into gene–behavior relations are also being made in other syndromes. In Williams syndrome, a candidate gene, LIM-kinase1 (LIM K1) has now been identified that may account for deficits in spatial cognition often shown by people with this syndrome (Frangiskakis et al., 1996). This finding complements previous work showing that the deletion of the elastin gene on chromosome 7 is responsible for the cardiac involvements often seen in people with Williams syndrome, specifically supravalvular stenosis (Ewart et al., 1994).

In 5p- syndrome, the infantile cat-like cry was once considered diagnostic of the syndrome. Recent advances, however, localize the cat-like cry to 5p15.3, with remaining clinical features of the syndrome associated with deletions at 5p15.2 (Gersh et al., 1995). People can thus show the cognitive, behavioral, and physical features of "*cri-du-chat*" syndrome, without ever having the infantile cat-like cry. Ongoing work is examining how the size and location of deleted material might relate to the severity of clinical expression.

In Prader-Willi syndrome, differences are now being found between those with paternal deletions versus maternal UPD. Physically, those with deletions may have a more typical facial appearance, and those with maternal UPD may have higher birthweights, a later age of diagnosis, shorter course of gavage feeding in infancy, and a later onset of hyperphagia (see Dykens et al., 1999, for a review). Behaviorally, we find that those with deletions may have lower IQs, especially verbal IQs, as well as more frequent or severe problems such as skin picking, hoarding, overeating, nail biting, sulking, and withdrawal. A handful of persons with UPD, however, seem to show more severe problems than their counterparts in either genetic group, with low IQs and autistic-like symptoms. Although a dampening of symptom severity in UPD cases is suggested, future work may reveal two subgroups of those with UPD: the majority who show a milder behavioral expression, and the relatively few who show more severe clinical involvements.

Across these and other syndromes, the ambitious task of future researchers is to better link genes to brain and to behavior. In Williams syndrome, for example, how are deleted or mutated genes adjacent to the elastin gene associated with the unusual personality or cognitive profiles seen in this disorder? In Prader-Willi syndrome, are there differences in the structure or function of the hypothalamus or other brain regions in persons with deletions as opposed to UPD that might be associated with subtle differences in hyperphagia or compulsivity across these genetic subgroups? Exciting interdisciplinary work has yet to be done, and behavioral researchers have considerable expertise to offer toward this effort.

D. Psychosocial and Other Sources of Within-Syndrome Variability

In addition to genetic correlates, behavior may vary within syndromes as a function of subject variables such as age or IQ, or larger contextual variables, such as family functioning. These sources of within-syndrome variability may be both similar and different across syndrome. In Prader-Willi syndrome, dramatic age-related changes in food ideation and eating occurs in young childhood, due to the onset of hyperphagia in the preschool years. Age is also significant in Down syndrome, where advancing age in children and adolescents may be associated with increased depressive affect (Dykens & Kasari, 1997).

Although IQ in 5p- syndrome emerges as a significant, negative correlate of self-injury, impulsivity, and stereotypies (Dykens & Clarke, 1997), IQ appears unrelated to behavioral dysfunction in children or adults with Prader-Willi syndrome (Dykens & Cassidy, 1995). Degree of obesity may prove a unique correlate of certain difficulties in adults with Prader-Willi syndrome, with lower weights associated with heightened anxiety, distorted thinking, and depression (Dykens & Cassidy, 1995).

In addition to subject variables, family and other social interactions may also prove to be important correlates of within-syndrome differences. For example, maladaptive behaviors are strong predictors of family stress in Prader-Willi, Smith-Magenis, and 5p- syndromes, and levels of stress are high in these families relative to families of offspring with Down syndrome or other types of developmental delay (Hodapp, Dykens, & Massino, 1997; Hodapp, Fidler, & Smith, 1998; Hodapp, Wijma, & Massino, 1997). Yet the causal direction of these relations are uncertain. As syndromic behaviors unfold over time, they may create family stress, and parental and sibling responses to these behaviors may serve to alter some of these behavioral predispositions and expressions. Furthermore, certain parental coping styles may help alleviate stress associated with even highly disturbing or hard-to-manage syndromic behaviors. Thus, differences in family stress and coping styles are likely associated with variable expressions of syndromic behavior within and across syndromes in ways that are only now starting to be explored (Hodapp, this volume).

E. Between-Syndrome Similarities and Differences

In addition to work on within-syndrome variability, a second line of work that stems from a probabilistic view of phenotypes involves total versus partial specificity. The goal of many behavioral phenotype studies is to discover the unique behaviors of a given etiology. Indeed, sometimes there appears to be a one-to-one correspondence, such that a particular behavior appears unique to one and only one genetic etiology. Although speculative, as comparative studies have yet to be done, examples of potentially unique syndromic behaviors include hyperphagia in Prader-Willi syndrome (Dykens & Cassidy, 1996), hand wringing in Rett syndrome (Van Acker, 1991), self-mutilation in Lesch-Nyan syndrome (Anderson & Ernst, 1994), self-hugging in Smith-Magenis syndrome (Finucane et al., 1994), and the infantile cat-cry in 5p- (*cri du chat*) syndrome (Gersh et al., 1995).

It is more often the case, however, that syndromic behaviors are not unique. Instead, as shown in the syndrome review, different genetic etiologies may share a propensity for a particular behavior. We call this situation "partial specificity," and it occurs when two or more different syndromes share a predisposition to a particular outcome (Hodapp, 1997). Although totally specific behaviors may exist, research to date suggests that many syndromes are partially specific in their effects (see Table II). Such thinking follows the developmental psychopathology principle of "equifinality," the idea that, when considering psychiatric disorders, many roads lead to a single outcome (Cicchetti, 1990). Or, as Opitz (1985) notes, "the causes are many, but the final common developmental pathways are few" (p. 9).

Partial specificity often shows itself in the maladaptive behaviors and psychopathologies common to different genetic syndromes. In partial specificity, a specific etiological group more often shows a particular behavior or psychiatric diagnosis compared to mixed or nonspecific groups, but the behavior or diagnosis also occurs in more than one syndrome. For example, hyperactivity and inattention are salient in people with fragile X syndrome (Bregman et al., 1988), Williams syndrome (Pober & Dykens, 1996), and 5p- syndrome (Dykens & Clarke, 1997), even as hyperactivity is less often seen in mixed groups or in oth-

TABLE II
ILLUSTRATION OF TOTAL AND PARTIAL SPECIFICITY

Total		
Prader-Willi syndrome	→	hyperphagia
5p- syndrome	→	infantile cat-like cry
Partial		
Fragile X syndrome	→	hyperactivity, inattention
Williams syndrome	→	hyperactivity, inattention
5p-syndrome	→	hyperactivity, inattention

er genetic disorders (e.g., Prader-Willi syndrome; Dykens & Kasari, 1997). Similarly, children with Prader-Willi syndrome and Down syndrome share a propensity for "stubborness" and "inattention," yet at the same time are different in their rates of obsessive-compulsive behavior (Dykens & Kasari, 1997).

Future research may reveal shifts from total to partial specificity in some syndromes, or from partial to total specificity in others. To illustrate the latter possibility, adolescents and young adults with Williams and Prader-Willi syndromes both show high levels of global anxiety, worry, and perseverative thinking, suggesting a shared or partial behavioral effect (Dykens & Rosner, in press). Yet on closer examination, anxiety in Williams syndrome is associated with unusually high rates of specific fears and phobias (Dykens, 1999), suggesting a possible unique effect. In contrast, anxiety in Prader-Willi syndrome is best associated with obsessive-compulsive symptoms (Dykens, Leckman, & Cassidy, 1996). These findings underscore the need for future phenotypic studies to become more refined, to move from global to more fine-tuned descriptors of maladaptive and other behaviors (Dykens & Rosner, in press).

Indeed, if the field is ever to ascertain which behaviors are totally specific and which partially specific, more detailed studies are needed that compare maladaptive behavior across various etiological groups. Between-syndrome studies have important implications for work on mechanisms associated with behavioral phenotypes. Both totally and partially specific effects will be of interest in the search for causal mechanisms. By identifying totally specific effects, researchers will be able to hone in on a single pathway, for example, how the lack of imprinted paternal contribution to the Prader-Willi critical region on chromosome 15 (via paternal deletion or maternal UPD) may lead to hyperphagia. Conversely, evidence that two or more etiologies lead to a certain behavior may indicate that researchers need to examine commonalities: What protein has not been produced, or what other mechanism disrupted, that leads to a single outcome across two or more conditions?

Alternatively, between-syndrome similarities may shed new light on problems that have multiple gene loci. For example, behavior genetic studies now suggest that ADHD in the general population is associated with multiple genetic contributions. Mental retardation syndromes may provide new, alternative clues to understanding these multiple associations. What are the implications of hyperactivity in both individuals with fragile X syndrome and animal models of this disorder (Willems, Reyniers, & Oostra, 1995) for links between the X chromosome and some cases of ADHD in the general population? Can the salient hyperactivity in 5p- syndrome provide new insights to the function of a dopamine transporter gene, DAT1, which is located on the tip of chromosome 5 and strongly implicated in ADHD (Gill, Daly, Heron, Hawi, & Fitzgerald, 1997)? And if a gene can be identified in Williams syndrome that accounts for this syndrome's attention deficits, what might this discovery mean for the genetics of ADHD in those without

Williams syndrome? Although answers to these questions are presently unknown, both total and partial specificity should eventually aid in the search for the mechanisms leading to psychopathology in people with and without mental retardation.

F. The Treatment Advantage

For most syndromes, it will take many years before questions are resolved involving within-syndrome variability and total versus partial specificity. In the meantime, data on behavioral phenotypes can be put to immediate good use in the treatment and intervention arena. Behavioral phenotypes guide treatment priorities, providing novel adaptations to more standard clinical care.

Consider, for example, the increased risk of non-food compulsivity in people with Prader-Willi syndrome. This vulnerability suggests that many people with Prader-Willi syndrome need particular help getting "unstuck"; these people may particularly benefit from environmental or pharmacologic interventions to help them transition from one thought or activity to the next (e.g., Dykens & Hodapp, 1997). While many people with developmental disabilities need help with transitions, this seems particularly true in Prader-Willi syndrome.

In another example, the sociability and keen interests in others shown by many people with Williams syndrome may be particularly well suited to group therapies, social skills training, and use of the team or buddy systems at school or work. Further, to the extent that verbal comprehension and expressivity are indeed strengths, they may help the person with Williams syndrome to accurately express their thoughts and feelings in individual or group therapy. Without supports and training, however, the sociability in Williams syndrome may lead to increased risks of impulsivity, exploitation, and abuse (Dykens & Hodapp, 1997).

In contrast, people with fragile X syndrome are prone to shyness, gaze aversion, distractibility, and social anxieties, and are likely to respond best to individualized approaches that minimize interpersonal demands and that facilitate attention. Many people learn best, for example, with individualized learning or tasks; minimal auditory or visual distractors at home, school, or work; and a reduced flow of people through work and living settings. Many females also benefit from psychotherapy, and from at-home supports, especially when mothers are mildly affected with the syndrome, or have multiple children affected with the disorder (Dykens & Hodapp, 1997).

Not every syndrome is apt to show striking behavioral profiles, and some syndromes will thus provide more novel directions to intervention or therapy than others. Even so, a syndromic diagnosis in and of itself brings to the forefront many issues of concern. How, for example, does having a specific syndrome affect a person's sense of self? What is the affected individual's understanding of his or her syndrome, and does the person harbor misconceptions about the syndrome? Some people with Prader-Willi syndrome, for example, believe that their syndrome will go away if they achieve their ideal weight, and are disappointed when their adjustment difficulties do not disappear along with their body fat.

In a related way, syndromic diagnoses need to be examined in the context of the family system. In addition to the relief that many families experience in having a known genetic cause for their child's delay, many families also receive genetic diagnoses with a sense of guilt or pessimism. Couples may struggle with having "caused" their child's syndrome, and feel that because the cause is genetic, the prognosis is more guarded. Syndromic diagnoses and their resultant behavioral phenotypes can thus inform and direct treatment in highly specific ways, or they can bring up more general issues of therapeutic concern.

IV. TOWARD INCREASED PHENOTYPIC WORK

Given the many advantages to science and treatment, why don't more behavioral workers engage in phenotypic research? Even today, just 10% of behavioral articles in mental retardation examine specific syndromic groups, and approximately half of these studies are on Down syndrome (Dykens, 1996; Hodapp & Dykens, 1994). We first consider logistical obstacles to phenotypic work, then obstacles related to researchers themselves.

Relative to groups of people with rare genetic disorders, mixed etiologic groups are easy to find and use. Often these heterogenous samples are conveniently recruited from local schools or community programs. In contrast, it is more difficult to assemble an appropriately sized sample of people with the same, rare genetic disorder. Faced with this challenge, some researchers establish speciality clinics that attract a particular patient population, whereas others work with syndrome-specific parent groups to recruit study participants. Either way, one risks ascertainment bias; clinic samples may have more behavioral or medical problems than nonreferred persons, and parent groups often attract motivated, middle to high socioeconomic status families. Though a blending of subjects across clinics and parent groups is often helpful, future phenotypic researchers need to do a much better job recruiting subjects from the population at large.

Second, how do researchers decide which of the 750 or more different mental retardation syndromes to study? Syndromes attract researchers when they have intriguing genetic underpinnings or particular scientific promise. Behavioral studies in fragile X syndrome, for example, have increased dramatically in recent years. Behavioral research in other syndromes may be driven by clinical necessity, as in Lesch-Nyan syndrome or Smith-Magenis syndrome, or simply by the availability of subjects, as in the highly prevalent Down syndrome. Yet what of the hundreds of syndromes that are less genetically understood, or less clinically involved, or less prevalent? We know precious little about the vast majority of most of these conditions. One wonders how many of these unexplored syndromes have behavioral or developmental phenotypes just as compelling as fragile X syndrome, Down syndrome, or other well-described conditions.

Another logistical challenge involves selecting behavioral domains for study. Though each behavioral researcher brings his or her own area of expertise to the work, these areas may not necessarily coincide with a particular syndrome's most salient, intriguing, or unique feature. Preliminary work in relatively unexplored syndromes may thus need to cast a rather broad behavioral net, screening across several domains such as cognition, speech/language, social adaptation, social skills, maladaptive behavior, and psychopathology. Subsequent follow-up studies can then target unusual profiles, trajectories, or behaviors.

A final complication to phenotypic work concerns development. Different behaviors will become more apparent at some ages than at others. Hyperphagia in Prader-Willi syndrome, for example, has its onset between 2 and 6 years of age, dramatically affecting the young child's cognitive and behavioral schema in ways that we have yet to fully appreciate. Further, males with fragile X syndrome show particular developmental trajectories in both cognition and adaptive behavior involving a plateau in mental age and decline in standard scores that occurs in late childhood or early adolescence (Dykens, Ort, et al., 1996; Dykens, Hodapp, & Leckman, 1994). These trajectories differ from patterns of development in Down syndrome, where many children show slowed development in their earliest years, followed by alternating periods of growth and slowing in cognition, grammatical skills, and adaptive behavior (Dykens, Hodapp, & Evans, 1994; Hodapp, 1996). All these examples underscore the importance of adopting a strong developmental orientation in future research on behavioral phenotypes.

Logistical challenges to phenotypic work are relatively easy to overcome. We find more enduring obstacles to syndrome-based work in researchers themselves. Phenotypic research is inherently collaborative, requiring input from geneticists on one hand, and psychologists and other behavioral researchers on the other. Yet for a variety of reasons, behavioral researchers are often reluctant to collaborate with geneticists. Some of these reasons are rooted in outdated attitudes about genetics or syndromes held by behavioral workers: feelings that syndromes are too rare to bother with; that genetic diagnoses lead to further stigma; and that syndromes have few significant behavioral effects (Dykens, 1995, 1996; Hodapp & Dykens, 1994). Beyond these attitudes, it is hard for both behavioral researchers and geneticists to learn the technical languages, jargon, and basic concepts of another field. Behavioral researches and geneticists also have different journals, different standards of training and research excellence, and they travel in different professional circles. We recently identified differences between behavioral and genetic workers as mental retardation's "two cultures" of behavioral research (Hodapp & Dykens, 1994).

Phenotypic work asks that researchers in both "cultures" take professional risks, stumble about in a new language, and learn enough of the rudiments of another field to be able to engage in "cross-cultural" projects and conversations. Doing so leads to a more precise science of mental retardation, which advances knowledge of phenotypes and gene–brain–behavior relationships in general, and of psychopathology and dual diagnosis in particular.

As demonstrated throughout this chapter, people with genetic syndromes vary in their proneness to psychopathology, including both the type and severity of maladaptive behavior or psychiatric disorder. Although syndrome-specific, dual diagnosis studies are rare relative to mixed groups, this chapter highlighted several syndromes that hold particular promise for understanding psychopathology in people with and without mental retardation. Future work in these and other well-defined syndromes can ultimately help differentiate genetic from psychosocial risk factors for psychopathology, as well as create immediate benefits for more fine-tuned interventions and treatments. Although behavioral phenotype studies cannot untangle all the reasons why people with mental retardation are at increased risk for psychopathology, this line of work is a clearly a step in the right direction.

REFERENCES

Aman, M. G. (1991). *Working bibliography on behavioral and emotional disorders and assessment instruments in mental retardation.* Rockville, MD: U.S. Department of Health and Human Services.

Anderson, L. T., & Ernst, M. (1994). Self-injury in Lesch-Nyhan disease. *Journal of Autism and Developmental Disorders, 24,* 67–81.

Baumgardner, T. L., Reiss, A. L., Freund, L. S., & Abrams, M. T. (1995). Specification of the neurobehavioral phenotypes in males with fragile X syndrome. *Pediatrics, 95,* 744–752.

Borthwick-Duffy, S. A. (1994). Epidemiology and prevalence of psychopathology in people with mental retardation. *Journal of Consulting and Clinical Psychology, 62,* 17–27.

Bregman, J. D., Leckman, J. F., & Ort, S. I. (1988). Fragile X syndrome: Genetic predisposition to psychopathology. *Journal of Autism and Developmental Disorders, 18,* 343–354.

Cahill, B. M., & Glidden, L. M. (1996). Influence of child diagnosis on family and parental functioning: Down syndrome versus other disabilities. *American Journal on Mental Retardation, 101,* 149–160.

Carlin, M. E. (1990). The improved prognosis in cri-du-chat (5p-) syndrome. In W. T. Fraser (Ed.), *Proceedings of the 8th Congress of the International Association of the Scientific Study of Mental Deficiency* (pp. 64–73). Edinburgh, UK: Blackwell.

Chen, K. S., Potocki, L., & Lupski, J. R. (1996). The Smith-Magenis syndrome [del(17)p11.2]: Clinical review and molecular advances. *Mental Retardation and Developmental Disability Research Reviews, 2,* 122–129.

Church, D. M., Bengtsson, U., Nielsen, K. V., Wasmuth, J. J., & Neihubr, E. (1995). Molecular definition of deletions of different segments of distal 5p that result in distinct phenotypic features. *American Journal of Human Genetics, 56,* 1162–1772.

Cicchetti, D. (1990). A historical perspective on the discipline of developmental psychopathology. In J. Rolf, A. S. Masten, D. Cicchetti, K. H. Neuchterlein, & S. Weintraub (Eds.), *Risk and protective factors in the development of psychopathology* (pp. 2–28). New York: Cambridge University Press.

Cohen, I. L., Vietze, P. M., Sudhalter, V., Jenkins, E. C., & Brown, W. T. (1989). Parent-child dyadic gaze patterns in fragile X males and in non-fragile X males with autistic disorder. *Journal of Child Psychology and Psychiatry, 30,* 845–856.

Collacott, R. A., Cooper, S. A., & McGrother, C. (1992). Differential rates of psychiatric disorders in adults with Down's syndrome compared with other mentally handicapped adults. *British Journal of Psychiatry, 161*, 671–674.

Dilts, C. V., Morris, C. A., & Leonard, C. O. (1990). Hypothesis for development of a behavioral phenotype in Williams syndrome. *American Journal of Medical Genetics, 6*, 126–131.

Dosen, A., & Petry, D. (1993). Treatment of depression in persons with mental retardation. In R. J. Fletcher & A. Dosen (Eds.), *Mental health aspects of mental retardation: Progress in assessment and treatment* (pp. 242–260). New York: Lexington.

Dykens, E. M. (1995). Measuring behavioral phenotypes: Provocations from the "new genetics". *American Journal on Mental Retardation, 99*, 522–532.

Dykens, E. M. (1996). DNA meets DSM: The growing importance of genetic syndromes in dual diagnosis. *Mental Retardation, 34*, 125–127.

Dykens, E. M. (1999). *Anxiety and fears in Williams syndrome.* Submitted for publication.

Dykens, E. M., & Cassidy, S. B. (1995). Correlates of maladaptive behavior in children and adults with Prader-Willi syndrome. *Neuropsychiatric Genetics, 69*, 546–549.

Dykens, E. M., & Cassidy, S. B. (1996). Prader-Willi syndrome: Genetic, behavioral and treatment issues. *Child and Adolescent Psychiatric Clinics of North America, 5*, 913–928.

Dykens, E. M., Cassidy, S. B., & King, B. H. (1999). Maladaptive behavior differences in Prader-Willi syndrome associated with paternal deletion versus maternal uniparental disomy. *American Journal on Mental Retardation, 104*, 67–77.

Dykens, E. M., & Clarke, D. J. (1997). Correlates of maladaptive behavior in individuals with 5p- (cri du chat) syndrome. *Developmental Medicine and Child Neurology, 75*, 752–756.

Dykens, E. M., Finucane, B. M., & Gayley, C. (1996). Cognitive and behavioral profiles in persons with Smith-Magenis syndrome. *Journal of Autism and Developmental Disorders, 27*, 203–211.

Dykens, E. M., & Hodapp, R. M. (1997). Treatment issues in genetic mental retardation syndromes. *Professional Psychology: Research and Practice, 28*, 263–270.

Dykens, E. M., Hodapp, R. M., & Evans, D. W. (1994). Profiles and development of adaptive behavior in children with Down syndrome. *American Journal on Mental Retardation, 98*, 675–687.

Dykens, E. M., Hodapp, R. M., & Leckman, J. F. (1994). *Behavior and development in fragile X syndrome.* Thousand Oaks, CA: Sage.

Dykens, E. M., & Kasari, C. (1997). Maladaptive behavior in children with Prader-Willi syndrome, Down syndrome, and non-specific mental retardation. *American Journal on Mental Retardation, 102*, 228–237.

Dykens, E. M., Leckman, J. F., & Cassidy, S. B. (1996). Obsessions and compulsions in Prader-Willi syndrome. *Journal of Child Psychology and Psychiatry, 37*, 995–1002.

Dykens, E. M., Ort, S. I., Cohen, I., Finucane, B. M., Freund, L., Hagerman, R. J., Iachiewicz, A. M., Reiss, A., & Spiridigliozzi, G. (1996). Trajectories of adaptive behavior in males with fragile X syndrome: Multicenter studies. *Journal of Autism and Developmental Disorders, 26*, 287–301.

Dykens, E. M., & Rosner, B. A. (in press). Refining behavioral phenotypes: Personality-Motivation in Prader-Willi and Williams syndromes. *American Journal on Mental Retardation.*

Dykens, E. M., & Smith, A. C. M. (1998). Distinctiveness and correlates of maladaptive behavior in children and adolescents with Smith-Magenis syndrome. *Journal of Intellectual Disability Research, 42*, 481–489.

Dykens, E. M., & Volkmar, F. R. (1997). Medical conditions associated with autism. In D. J. Cohen & F. R. Volkmar (Eds.), *Handbook of autism and pervasive developmental disorders* (2nd ed., pp. 388–407). New York: John Wiley.

Einfeld, S. L., Tonge, B. J., & Florio, T. (1997). Behavioral and emotional disturbance in individuals with Williams syndrome. *American Journal on Mental Retardation, 102*, 45–53.

Einfeld, S. L., & Hall, W. (1994). When is a behavioral phenotype not a phenotype? *Developmental Medicine and Child Neurology, 36*, 467–470.

Einfeld, S. L., Molony, H., & Hall, W. (1989). Autism is not associated with the fragile X syndrome. *American Journal of Medical Genetics, 19, 34*, 187–193.

Ewart, A. K., Morris, C. A., Atkinson, D., Jin, W., Sternes, K., Spallone, P., Stock, A. D., Leppart, M., & Keating, M. (1994). Hemizygosity at the elastin locus in a developmental disorders, Williams syndrome. *Nature Genetics, 5*, 11–16.

Finucane, B. M., Konar, D., Haas-Givler, B., Kurtz, M. D., & Scott, L. I. (1994). The spasmodic upper-body squeeze: A characteristic behavior in Smith-Magenis syndrome. *Developmental Medicine and Child Neurology, 36*, 78–83.

Fisch, G. S. (1992). Is autism associated with the fragile X syndrome? *American Journal of Medical Genetics, 43*, 47–55.

Flint, J., & Yule, W. (1994). Behavioral phenotypes. In M. Rutter, E. Taylor, & L. Hersov (Eds.), *Child and adolescent psychiatry: Modern approaches* (3rd ed., pp. 666–687). London: Blackwell Science.

Frangiskasis, J. M., Ewart, A. K., Morris, C. A., Mervis, C. B., Bertrand, J., Robinson, B. F., Klein, B. P., et al. (1996). Lim-kinase1 hemizygosity implicated in impaired visuospatial constructive cognition. *Cell, 86*, 59–69.

Freund, L., Reiss, A. L., Hagerman, R. J., & Vinogradov, S. (1992). Chromosome fragility and psychopathology in obligate female carriers of the fragile X chromosome. *Archives of General Psychiatry, 49*, 54–60.

Ganiban, J., Wagner, S., & Cicchetti, D. (1990). Temperament and Down syndrome. In D. Cicchetti & M. Beeghly (Eds.), *Children with Down syndrome: A developmental perspective* (pp. 63–100). New York: Cambridge University Press.

Gath, A., & Gumley, D. (1986). Behavior problems in retarded children with special reference to Down's syndrome. *British Journal of Psychiatry, 149*, 156–151.

Gersh, M., Goodart, S. A., Pasztor, L. M., Harris, D. J., Weiss, L., & Overhauser, J. (1995). Evidence for a distinct region causing a cat-like cry in patients with 5p deletions. *American Journal of Human Genetics, 56*, 1404–10.

Gill, M., Daly, G., Heron, S., Hawi, Z., & Fitzgerald, M. (1997). Confirmation of association between attention deficit hyperactivity disorder and a dopamine transporter polymorphism. *Molecular Psychiatry, 2*, 311–313.

Glidden, L. M., & Cahill, B. M. (1998). Successful adoption of children with Down syndrome and other developmental disabilities. *Adoption Quarterly, 1*, 27–43.

Gosch, A., & Pankau, R. (1997). Personality characteristics and behavior problems in individuals of different ages with Williams syndrome. *Developmental Medicine and Child Neurology, 39*, 527–533.

Greenberg, F., Lewis, R. A., Potocki, L., Glaze, D., Parke, J., Killian, J., Murphy, M. A., Williamson, D., Brown, F., Dutton, R., McCluggage, C. M., Friedman, E., Sulek, M., & Lupski, J. R. (1996). Multi-disciplinary clinical study of Smith-Magenis syndrome (deletion 17p11.2). *American Journal of Medical Genetics, 62*, 247–254.

Grizenko, N., Cvejic, H., Vida, S., & Sayegh, L. (1991). Behavior problems in the mentally retarded. *Canadian Journal of Psychiatry, 36*, 712–717.

Hagerman, R. J. (1996). Fragile X syndrome. *Child and Adolescent Psychiatric Clinics of North America, 5*, 895–912.

Hodapp, R. M. (1996). Down syndrome: Developmental, psychiatric, and management issues. *Child and Adolescent Psychiatric Clinics of North America, 5*, 881–894.

Hodapp, R. M. (1997). Direct and indirect behavioral effects of different genetic disordes of mental retardation. *American Journal on Mental Retardation, 102*, 67–79.

Hodapp, R. M., & Dykens, E. M. (1994). Mental retardation's two cultures of behavioral research. *American Journal on Mental Retardation, 98*, 675–687.

Hodapp, R. M., Dykens, E. M., & Massino, L. L. (1997). Families of children with Prader-Willi syndrome: Stress-support and relations to child characteristics. *Journal of Autism and Developmental Disorders*, *27*, 11–24.

Hodapp, R. M., Fidler, D., & Smith, A. C. M. (1998). Family stress in children with Smith-Magenis syndrome. *Journal of Intellectual Disability Research*, *42*, 331–340.

Hodapp, R. M., Wijma, C. A., & Massino, L. L. (1997). Families of children with 5p- (cri du chat) syndrome: Familial stress and sibling reactions. *Developmental Medicine and Child Neurology*, *39*, 757–761.

Holland, A. J., Treasure, J., Coskeran, P., & Dallow, J. (1995). Characteristics of the eating disorder in Prader-Willi syndrome: Implications for treatment. *Journal of Intellectual Disability Research*, *39*, 373–381.

Hornby, G. (1995). Fathers' views of the effects on their families of children with Down syndrome. *Journal of Child and Family Studies*, *4*, 103–117.

Karmiloff-Smith, A., Grant, J., Berthoud, J., Davies, M., Howline, P., & Udwin, O. (1997). Language and Williams syndrome: How intact is "intact"? *Child Development*, *68*, 246–262.

Kerby, D. S., & Dawson, B. (1994). Autistic features, personality, and adaptive behavior in males with the fragile X syndrome and no autism. *America Journal on Mental Retardation*, *98*, 455–462.

Lachiewicz, A. M. (1992). Abnormal behavior of young girls with fragile X syndrome. *American Journal of Medical Genetics*, *43*, 72–77.

Lai, F., & Williams, R. S. (1989). A prospective study of Alzheimer disease in Down syndrome. *Archives of Neurology*, *46*, 849–853.

Matson, J., & Sevin, J. A. (1994). Theories of dual diagnosis in mental retardation. *Journal of Consulting and Clinical Psychology*, *62*, 6–16.

Matilanen, R., Airaksinen, E., Monen, T., Launiala, K., & Kaariainen, R. (1995). A population based study on the causes of mild and severe mental retardation. *Acta Paediatrica*, *84*, 261–266.

Mazzocco, M. M., Hagerman, R. J., Cronister-Silverman, A., & Pennington, B. F. (1992). Specific frontal lobe deficits among women with the fragile X gene. *Journal of the American Academy of Child and Adolescent Psychiatry*, *31*, 1141–1148.

Mazzocco, M. M., Pennington, B. F., & Hagerman, R. J. (1993). The neurocognitive phenotype of female carriers of fragile X: Additional evidence for specificity. *Journal of Developmental and Behavioral Pediatrics*, *14*, 328–335.

Merenstein, S. A., Sobesky, W. E., & Taylor, A. K. (1996). Molecular-clinical correlations in males with an expanded FMR1 mutation. *American Journal of Medical Genetics*, *64*, 388–394.

Meyers, B. A., & Pueschel, S. M. (1991). Psychiatric disorders in persons with Down syndrome. *The Journal of Nervous and Mental Disease*, *179*, 609–613.

Mostofsky, S. H., Mazzocco, M. M., Aakalu, G., Warsofsky, I. S., Denckla, M. B., & Reiss, A. L. (1998). Decreased cerebellar posterior vermis size in fragile X syndrome: Correlation with neurocognitive performance. *Neurology*, *50*, 121–130.

Opitz, J. (1985). Editorial comment: The developmental field concept. *American Journal of Medical Genetics*, *21*, 1–11.

Opitz, J. (1996, March). *Historiography of the causal analysis of mental retardation.* Speech to the 29th Annual Gatlinburg Conference on Research and Theory in Mental Retardation, Gatlinburg, TN.

Overhauser, J., Huang, X., Gersh, M., Wilson, W., McMahon, J., Bengtsson, U., Rojas, K., Meyer, M., & Wasmuth, J. J. (1994). Molecular and phenotypic mapping of the short arm of chromosome 5: Sublocalization of the critical region for the cri-du-chat syndrome. *Human Molecular Genetics*, *3*, 247–252.

Pober, B. R., & Dykens, E. M. (1996). Williams syndrome: An overview of medical, cognitive and behavioral features. *Child and Adolescent Psychiatric Clinics of North America*, *5*, 929–944.

Pueschel, S. M., Bernier, J. C., & Pezzullo, J. C. (1991). Behavioral observations in children with Down's syndrome. *Journal of Mental Deficiency Research*, *35*, 502–511.

Reilly, J., Klima, E. S., & Bellugi, U. (1990). Once more with feeling: Affect and language in atypical populations. *Development and Psychopathology, 2*, 367–391.

Reiss, A. L., & Freund, L. (1990). Fragile X syndrome, DSM-III-R and autism. *Journal of the American Academy of Child and Adolescent Psychiatry, 29*, 885–891.

Reiss, A. L., Hagerman, R. J., Vinogradov, S., Abrams, M., & King, R. J. (1988). Psychiatric disability in female carriers of the fragile X chromosome. *Archives of General Psychiatry, 45*, 697–705.

Reiss, S., & Havercamp, S. (1998). Toward a comprehensive assessment of fundamental motivation: Factor structure of the Reiss profile. *Psychological Assessment, 10*, 97–106.

Rogers, C. (1987). Maternal support for the Down's syndrome personality stereotype: The effect of direct experience on the condition. *Journal of Mental deficiency Research, 31*, 271–278.

Rosen, M. (1993). In search of the behavioral phenotype: A methodological note. *Mental Retardation, 31*, 177–178.

Smith, A. C. M., Dykens, E. M., & Greenberg, F. (1998a). The behavioral phenotype of Smith-Magenis syndrome. *American Journal of Medical Genetics, 81*, 179–185.

Smith, A. C. M., Dykens, E. M., & Greenberg, F. (1998b). Sleep disturbance in Smith-Magenis Syndrome. *American Journal of Medical Genetics, 81*, 186–191.

Smith, A., Field, B., Murray, R., & Nelson, J. (1990). Two cases of cri-du-chat syndrome with mild phenotypic expression but with different six 5p deletion. *Journal of Pediatric Child Health, 28*, 152–154.

Sobesky, W. E., Porter, D., Pennington, B. F., & Hagerman, R. J. (1995). Dimensions of shyness in fragile X females. *Developmental Brain Dysfunction, 8*, 280–292.

Swaab, P. F., Purba, J. S., & Hofman, M. A. (1995). Alterations in the hypothalamic paraventricular nucleus and its oxytocin neurons (putative satiety cells) in Prader-Willi Syndrome: A study of 5 cases. *Journal of Clinical Endocrinology and Metabolism, 80*, 573–579.

Udwin, O., & Yule, W. (1990). Expressive language of children with Williams syndrome. *American Journal of Medical Genetics, 6*, 108–114.

Van Acker, R. (1991). Rett syndrome: A review of current knowledge. *Journal of Autism and Developmental Disabilities, 21*, 381–406.

Wilkins, L. E., Brown, J. A., Nance, W. E., & Wolf, B. (1983). Clinical heterogeneity in 80 home-reared children with cri-du-chat syndrome. *Journal of Pediatrics, 102*, 528–533.

Willems, P. J., Reyniers, E., & Oostra, B. A. (1995). An animal model for fragile X syndrome. *Mental Retardation and Developmental Disabilities Research Reviews, 1*, 298–302.

Zigman, W. B., Schupf, N., Zigman, A., & Silverman, W. (1993). Aging and Alzheimer disease in people with mental retardation. *International Review of Research in Mental Retardation, 19*, 41–70.

Indirect Effects of Genetic Mental Retardation Disorders: Theoretical and Methodological Issues

ROBERT M. HODAPP

GRADUATE SCHOOL OF EDUCATION AND INFORMATION STUDIES
UNIVERSITY OF CALIFORNIA, LOS ANGELES
LOS ANGELES, CALIFORNIA

Spurred by work in the "new genetics," mental retardation workers are beginning to appreciate the effects of different genetic disorders on behavior (see Dykens, this volume). We thus see a thriving Society for the Study of Behavioral Phenotypes in Great Britain (O'Brien, 1993), as well as a recent focus on Mental Retardation and Genetics at the 1996 National Institute of Mental Health Gatlinburg Conference on Mental Retardation and Developmental Disabilities. Although such behavioral work is only now beginning, a movement is growing to link new genetic findings to behavior in different genetic disorders of mental retardation.

For the most part, these behavioral studies have focused on the direct effects of different mental retardation syndromes. The term *direct effects* refers to the ways in which a specific genetic disorder predisposes individuals to one or more of a syndrome's characteristic behaviors. Granted, the child's environment and context both influence behavior—and genetic influences only "play themselves out" in particular contexts and environments. Nevertheless, a genetic anomaly sets in motion a chain of events that predisposes individuals to display particular behaviors. Although discussed more fully both later in this chapter and in Dykens's chapter in this volume, genetic disorders' direct influence on behavior comprises a lively area of research in the field of mental retardation (O'Brien & Yule, 1995).

Less often discussed are genetic disorders' indirect effects, or how etiology-specific behaviors elicit specific reactions from parents, siblings, friends, or others. If different genetic disorders predispose individuals to show particular behaviors, might not others in the surrounding environment behave differently toward persons with one versus another genetic disorder? Such an interactional focus is now

INTERNATIONAL REVIEW OF RESEARCH IN
MENTAL RETARDATION, Vol. 22
0074-7750/99 $30.00

common in studies of child psychology and developmental psychopathology (Dunn, 1997). To date, however, this focus has been lacking in studies of children with different genetic causes of mental retardation.

In this chapter I examine these indirect effects of different genetic mental retardation disorders. But before considering the evidence for such indirect effects, two preliminary issues must be addressed. The first concerns a brief mention of direct effects, a topic that is discussed in more detail by Dykens (this volume). The second concerns the nature of interactional or child effects on adults, and how developmental and clinical psychologists have come to appreciate such effects when considering a variety of children.

I. UNDERSTANDING THE WORKINGS OF DIRECT EFFECTS

Direct effects—also called a genetic disorder's behavioral phenotype—must be considered within the context of two issues, total versus partial specificity, and within-group differences. By focusing on these two issues, we also gain some preliminary understandings into how indirect effects may operate.

A. Total versus Partial Specificity

In earlier discussions of behavioral phenotypes, workers emphasized the possibly unique behaviors found in one versus another syndrome. Hence we see studies of hyperphagia in Prader-Willi syndrome (Dykens & Cassidy, 1996), extreme self-mutilation in Lesch-Nyan syndrome (Anderson & Ernst, 1994), and the cat-cry in 5p- (cri-du-chat) syndrome (Carlin, 1990). In each instance, the behavior in question seems unique to one and only one genetic disorder.

Although such totally specific direct effects do sometimes occur, most syndromes show what might be called "partial specificity" for most behaviors (Hodapp, 1997). Partial specificity occurs when a behavior is more often present in a particular syndrome, but is not unique to that syndrome. To take a simple example, children with 5p- syndrome and boys with fragile X syndrome are both prone to show attention deficit-hyperactivity disorder (ADHD) more often than children with mental retardation in general, or compared to other genetic disorders of mental retardation (e.g., Dykens & Clarke, 1997; Dykens, Hodapp, & Leckman, 1994). Thus, hyperactivity is found in both 5p- and in fragile X syndrome: it is unique to neither.

Such considerations are relevant to both direct and indirect effects of genetic disorders of mental retardation. In terms of direct effects, findings of both unique and partial specificity suggest separate (for total specificity) and shared (for partial specificity) pathways from gene to protein to brain structures to behavior. In addition, totally versus partially specific direct effects may provide clues to the workings of indirect effects. In essence, parents, siblings, friends, and teachers react to the behaviors of children with one or another genetic disorder. If so, the surrounding interpersonal environments may be similar or different in their reactions to individuals with different syndromes of mental retardation. For example, if the child's hyperactivity elicits particular emotional or behavioral responses from parents, then one would expect similar parental reactions to children with either fragile X syndrome or 5p- syndrome.

B. Within-Group Differences

A second characteristic of behavioral phenotypes is that few phenotypic behaviors are observed in every single person who has a particular disorder. For example, even though the large majority of individuals with Prader-Willi syndrome show hyperphagia, an occasional person with the syndrome does not. In essence, a behavioral phenotype is best thought of as "the heightened probability or likelihood that people with a given syndrome will exhibit certain behavioral and developmental sequelae relative to those without the syndrome" (Dykens, 1995, p. 523).

In this sense, genetic disorders predispose individuals toward certain behaviors. Having such predispositions, many affected individuals show the disorder's "characteristic" behaviors, but not everyone does. Just as family history predisposes typically developing individuals to high blood pressure or obesity, these outcomes are probabilistic, not determined. Moreover, one can sometimes avoid high blood pressure or obesity through changing one's lifestyle. So too are behavioral phenotypes appropriately conceptualized in a group rather than an individual way: Groups with a particular disorder will more likely show the syndrome's behaviors than other groups without that disorder.

Within-group heterogeneity also relates to indirect effects. If, for example, not every child with Prader-Willi syndrome shows hyperphagia, or not every child with 5p- syndrome is hyperactive, then the reactions of others might also differ for different individuals who have the same genetic disorder. Even if every person with a particular disorder were to display a particular behavior, individuals would still vary in the degree to which they showed that behavior, in the age at which the behavior first came about, and in how the behavior changed with age. Partly as a result of such within-syndrome differences from one individual to the next, reactions from the person's interpersonal environment will also vary. In short, just as individuals with a certain etiology differ in when, if, and the degree to which they show particular, etiology-specific behaviors, so too will there be corresponding differences in the timing and degree of reactions to that behavior by others.

Some behaviors characterizing syndromes, then, are unique and others are shared by other genetic disorders, and not every person with a genetic disorder exhibits that disorder's behaviors. These two ideas underlie our discussions of indirect effects of genetic disorders of mental retardation. But before discussing such indirect effects—or how children with different genetic disorders affect their surrounding interpersonal environments—we first need to describe in more detail the larger question of how children affect adults.

II. CONCEPTUALIZING INDIRECT EFFECTS

Within developmental psychology and psychopathology, two strands have recently converged on the importance of child effects on adults. After discussing these two strands, conduct disorder is provided as one example of the ways in which children influence reactions from their surrounding interpersonal environments.

A. Interactions and Evocative Environments

Thirty years ago, Richard Q. Bell (1968) introduced the idea of interactionism. Simply put, Bell reacted against the field's overemphasis on the idea that, in socializing their children, the sole or predominant influences went from parents to children. In an article entitled "A re-examination of direction of effects in studies of socialization," Bell presented the competing idea that children also strongly influence their parents' behaviors. Studies of mother–child and father–child interaction, of peer relations, and of other types of interactions all arose following Bell's influential writings.

Partly due to its beginnings as a reaction against socialization studies, most interactional work has examined how children affect adults. Such effects arise in a variety of ways. Parents seem influenced by the nature, level, and tempo of their children's behaviors. Examining interactions between mothers and their 3-month-old infants, Brazelton, Koslowski, and Main (1974) noted that such face-to-face games involve back-and-forth behavioral reactions by both mother and infant. Although in some sense mothers lead the games, infants pace interactions due to their own behaviors and underlying abilities to respond to information. Mothers then match their behaviors to the pace of their infant (Hodapp & Mueller, 1982). Thus, if the infant becomes overstimulated, mothers decrease their behaviors or even break off the face-to-face interaction altogether. As a result of mother-and-child mutual control over each other, dyads behave in synchrony one with the other.

In addition to reacting to the child's behavior, adults also react to many status variables of their children. Even after the most minimal of contact after birth, for example, adults differently describe male versus female newborns, simply based on their perceptions of gender roles and behaviors (Rubin, Provenzano, & Luria, 1974). In essence, it is not only the child's behaviors per se that influence adults, but adults' own perceptions and reactions. As Bell (1979) noted, parent–child interactions involve a "thinking parent" as well as an active, thinking child.

A second view of child effects comes from behavior genetics. Scarr (1993) described three senses of interactions between genes (i.e., child) and environment. In the first instance, one can envision a passive child and an active environment. To some extent, children (especially when younger) are somewhat passive recipients of their parents' decisions to place them in day care, to move to a new house or town, or to introduce them to new playmates.

A second type of child–environment interaction reverses the equation, this time focusing on an active child and a passive environment. Especially in later childhood, one sees how adolescents increasingly choose their friends, their interests, and their activities. As adolescents become older, their decisions gain increasing weight, until as adults they themselves will choose with whom, where, and how they will live their lives.

But it is a third sense of the environment that is most interesting in terms of genetic disorders' indirect effects. As various studies have shown, children also elicit their own environments. To take several extreme examples, why is it that certain children—and not others—within a family become targets of child abuse? Most studies show that abused children are more likely to be born prematurely, to have disabilities such as mental retardation and hyperactivity, or to have temperamental characteristics such as irritability, fussiness, and dependency (see Pianta, Egeland, & Erickson, 1990, for a review). Granted, the vast majority of children who are premature, retarded, or who have difficult temperaments are not abused. Nevertheless, certain child characteristics increase the odds of abuse.

Conversely, consider children at risk because they have grown up in chaotic, impoverished, or otherwise unstable households. In Werner's (1993) long-term study of children on the island of Kauai, she found that many of these children adjusted well by early adulthood. But resilient adults showed several personal characteristics along the way: even as toddlers, these resilient children were more likely to exhibit a positive social orientation and to be alert and autonomous. During grade school, teachers reported that these children got along well with peers, and as high schoolers, these children developed a positive self-concept and an internal locus of control.

B. The Example of Conduct Disorder

But the most intriguing of these child elicitation effects on adults may relate to conduct disorder. As defined by the *Diagnostic and Statistical Manual of Mental Disorders, 4th ed.* (*DSM-IV*) (American Psychiatric Association, 1994), conduct disorder involves "a repetitive and persistent pattern of behavior in which the basic rights of others or major age-appropriate societal norms or rules are violated" (p. 85). For many years, researchers puzzled over its causes, with three possibilities predominating: parental environment (marital discord, poor discipline); factors residing in the child (e.g., temperament); and reciprocal effects arising from the ongoing interactions between parental environment and child factors.

Although parental environments contribute to a child's conduct disorder (see Loeber & Stouthamer-Loeber, 1986, for a review), existing child characteristics and ongoing parent–child interactions also play a role. As concerns child effects, children who have from early on been fussy, whiny, less adaptable to change, and strong-willed—the constellation called "difficult temperament"—are much more likely to show conduct disorder at later ages. Loeber, Stouthamer-Loeber, and Green (1991) found that those children rated difficult when in preschool were more likely to become delinquents as adolescents; in the same way, the child's "troublesome" behaviors as rated by teachers and peers at ages 8 to 10 years significantly predict later delinquency (West & Farrington, 1973).

These child characteristics, in turn, elicit particular reactions from the surrounding interpersonal environment. In a study designed to show the effects of problem behaviors on parental control techniques, Brunk and Henggeler (1984) trained two 10-year-old children to exhibit oppositional versus socially withdrawn behaviors with a set of women, all of whom were mothers raising their own children. Over a short interaction playing a board game, adults behaved differently based on the child's overall pattern of behavior. If the child confederate was generally acting in a socially withdrawn manner, any of the child's noncompliant behaviors evoked more indirect commands (20.4% of time) than when in the conduct-disordered condition (5.8%). Conversely, when the child confederate was noncompliant in the conduct-disordered versus withdrawn condition, adults more often provided discipline (23.7 vs. 4.7%) and commands (19.1 vs. 6.8%).

Adult reactions to child behaviors can also be shown over longer periods. Consider the effects of a child's early temperament on conduct disorder. Using a longitudinal path analysis, Olweus (1980) showed that mothers of boys who were aggressive and strong-willed during infancy become more permissive of their child's aggression, which led to their boys' further aggression as time went on. Similarly, conduct-disordered children react differently to punishment than do nonconduct-disordered children. Whereas normal children suppress their hostile and aggressive behaviors in response to parental physical and verbal punishment, children with conduct disorders are about twice as likely as nonconduct-disordered children to persist in their problem behaviors after punishment (Patterson, 1976). As Lytton (1990) noted, "The evidence essentially shows that child effects are operating that then elicit parental reactions, which will in turn have further effects on the child's development; the child effects, though primary, therefore enter into a system of reciprocal relations" (pp. 683–684).

In summarizing research on child effects in both typical and atypical children, then, we see that children affect parents in a variety of ways. Based on their child's behaviors and status characteristics (e.g., gender), parents behave differently. In some cases, such back-and-forth behavioral interactions exacerbate conduct disorder or other child problems.

III. INDIRECT EFFECTS IN MENTAL RETARDATION

When considering the relationship between children and their environments within the mental retardation field, most work has focused on Scarr's first two types of child–environment relations. Many studies demonstrate ways that an active environment changes behavior in children with mental retardation. Studies illustrate how behavior modification, token economies, and other techniques change, teach, chain together, shape, extinguish, or in other ways modify behaviors of the individual with mental retardation. For the most part, children with retardation are considered passive or reactive recipients of such interventions.

The second sense of child–environment relations, that of the active child and the passive environment, is also represented in mental retardation work. Here the best examples come from the field's renewed interest in choice—in the person with mental retardation choosing one or another option from the environment. When considering genetic mental retardation disorders as well, certain etiology-specific skills and behaviors have also generally been considered as primarily due to the active child (and passive environment). Thus, many children with Prader-Willi syndrome show interests in puzzles; an interest in puzzles is even included as one of the syndrome's criteria for clinical diagnosis (Holm et al., 1993). Similarly, many children with Williams syndrome are thought to be especially musical (cf. Pober & Dykens, 1996). In considering the development of most such behaviors, clinicians and researchers have generally relegated the environment to a lesser, almost nonexistent role.

Although these first two types of child–environment relations can be found in mental retardation, the most interesting perspective concerns the evocative effects of different genetic disorders on surrounding environments. Such evocative effects can be divided into those adult behaviors and reactions that seem common in response to most children with mental retardation, and those that may be more specific to children with one versus another type of retardation due to etiology-related behaviors or characteristics.

A. Child Effects on Others: General Findings

General reactions can be seen in response to heterogeneous groups of children with disabilities. Consider the effects of children with severe and profound levels of mental retardation. In one article discussing interactions between such children and their parents, Zirpoli and Bell (1987) extended an earlier view of lower- and upper-limit control (Bell & Harper, 1977). That is, parents faced with an unresponsive child stimulate their children more in an attempt to help the child become more active and engaged. Conversely, parents soothe and calm their overactive children.

In the case of children with severe-profound mental retardation, parents may be more prone to high levels of stimulation and directiveness towards their less responsive children (Marfo, Dedrick, & Barbour, 1998). Such highly directive interactive styles may be due, in part, to the child's less responsive role compared to mental age-matched nonretarded children. At the same time—and in line with Bell's (1979) thinking parent—parents may also behave in accordance with their own emotional reactions and perceptions concerning what their child needs (Hodapp, 1988). In short, the child's behavior and the parent's reaction to both the child's behavior and condition may lead parents to become more active and directive in mother–infant interactions.

Parental behaviors may, however, become more complicated as they react to several recently highlighted characteristics of young children with disabilities. One such characteristic involves behavioral cues that are less clear and specific. For example, Walden (1996) asked three groups of adults—parents of children with disabilities, parents of typical children, and nonparents—to rate where delayed versus nondelayed toddlers were looking during mother–child videotaped interactions of dyads unknown to them. Adult judges were asked to decide if the child was looking toward versus away from the mother.

Results indicated that adults more often misjudged where children were looking when the child had disabilities. Such differences mainly occurred when examining the child's looks to the mother's face (as opposed to looks away or to the mother's body): particularly for this type of child look, adults were extremely accurate in judging nonretarded children and less accurate when judging children with disabilities. Furthermore, within the disabled group, more unclear looking occurred in children with Down syndrome versus with mixed etiologies. Conceptualizing looking behavior within Goldberg's (1977) notion of the "readability" of young children, Walden (1996) noted that young children with disabilities—particularly those with Down syndrome—are particularly difficult to decode.

Consider, too, the issue of achieving developmental milestones. Zirpoli and Bell (1987) noted that parents of typically developing children are reinforced by their child's achievements; conversely, parents of children with severe disabilities may become depressed by their children's lack of progress. But other findings complicate this story. For example, Dunst (1988, 1990) found that infants and toddlers with Down syndrome are much more likely to show developmental regressions from one month to the next. Whereas children with Down syndrome regressed on approximately 17.5% of tasks across seven Piagetian domains, typically developing infants regressed on approximately 7% of Piagetian tasks, a ratio 2.5 to 1 (see also Wishart, 1995). Although we do not know how often children with other types of mental retardation show regressions in development from one month to the next, the unclear achievement of many early milestones may be especially problematic for parents. Not only are their children developing more slowly and providing less clear behavioral cues as they develop, but even the hard-won gains that do occur seem more fragile and transitory.

B. Child Effects on Others: Specific Findings

As lower responsiveness, unclear cues, and developmental regressions are common to many children with disabilities, adult reactions might be considered as more general responses to children with mental retardation, not to any specific genetic disorders per se. In contrast, we now turn to adult reactions to those child characteristics that are specific to one or a few genetic disorders of mental retardation.

Most such studies focus on children with Down syndrome. Indeed, Down syndrome is probably the sole disorder in which a literature exists concerning parents, families, siblings, and peers (Hodapp, 1996). It should also be noted that many of these studies are merely suggestive—some studies have no comparison groups, some compare families of children with Down syndrome to families of same-aged typically developing children, others compare to same age or mental age children with mental retardation of mixed etiologies. Because of the primitive state of the art, we are limited to this set of studies in Down syndrome when overviewing the indirect effects of different genetic disorders of mental retardation.

1. PARENTS

A first issue concerns the presence and effects on parents of a "Down syndrome personality." Admittedly, this issue is controversial. Many parents and researchers object to the possibility that children with Down syndrome are more likely to be pleasant, cheerful, and socially oriented. They fear that such talk leads to dangerous stereotypes. Although such concerns are genuine, we return to one of the original tenets of behavioral phenotypes, that no behavior that is "characteristic" of a particular etiological group occurs in every person with that disorder.

Conscious of the dangers of stereotyping individuals with Down syndrome, what is the evidence for or against a Down syndrome personality? This idea, originally suggested by J. Langdon Down, may have undergone its most interesting test in a study designed to refute its existence. Wishart and Johnston (1990) asked parents, teachers, and students to rate children's personalities on 23 items specifically chosen to tap into the "stereotypical" personality of persons with Down syndrome. Adults with more (versus less) experience with children with the disorder rated items lower; mothers, too, scored relatively lower when asked to report on a typical child with Down syndrome. But when asked to rate the personality of their own child with Down syndrome, these mothers scored significantly higher than all other groups. On a scale ranging from 1 (lowest) to 5 (highest), mothers averaged

4.22 points per item when rating their own child. While teachers and students may not think that persons with Down syndrome show a particular personality—and mothers do not when considering children with Down syndrome in the abstract—mothers highly endorse many elements of this personality when rating their own children with Down syndrome.

Parents, in turn, seem to appreciate such personalities in their children. In a series of interviews with fathers of 7- to 14-year-old children with Down syndrome, a full 46% commented on their children's cheerful personalities (this was fathers' most common spontaneous comment; Hornby, 1995). In addition, nearly one-third of fathers referred to their children as being lovable, and nearly a quarter described their children as sociable or friendly. Similarly in Carr's (1995) 20-year longitudinal study, parents described over half of the children with Down syndrome as "affectionate," "lovable," "nice," and "gets on well with people."

Although neither Hornby (1995) nor Carr (1995) compared parental perceptions of children with Down syndrome to perceptions of children with mixed (or other) etiologies, other studies do show positive parental reactions to their children with Down syndrome. Noh, Dumas, Wolf, and Fisman (1989) compared parents of children with autism, conduct disorder, and Down syndrome to a typically developing control group on Abidin's Parenting Stress Index (PSI). Compared to the nondisabled group, parents of all three disabled groups showed some areas of high stress. On most every domain, however, parents of children with Down syndrome scored lowest among the three disabled groups. Furthermore, when considering the degree to which the child is reinforcing to parents, parents of children with Down syndrome considered their children as more reinforcing that all three contrast groups, even compared to parents of nondisabled children. Granted, parents of children with Down syndrome do experience their children as less attractive, intelligent, and appropriate—one should not conclude that parents experience no problems or are immune from the challenges of parenting a child with disabilities. Yet at the same time, parents of children with Down syndrome "see their children as happier and as a greater source of positive reinforcement than the parents of normal children" (p. 460). In short, even in the face of increased parental stress, parents of children with Down syndrome react positively to their children's (perceived) pleasant personalities.

2. FAMILIES

Families, too, seem to react positively to their children with Down syndrome. Here the research compares families of children with Down syndrome to families of children with mixed etiologies of mental retardation or with other disabilities (e.g., autism, emotional disorder). In most every case, families of children with Down syndrome show lower levels of stress and better coping than families of same-aged children with other disorders.

To give a few examples, when compared to children with autism and to children with unidentified mental retardation, parents of children with Down syndrome exhibit significantly lower amounts of stress (Holroyd & McArthur, 1976; Kasari & Sigman, 1997; Sanders & Morgan, 1997; Seltzer, Krauss, & Tsunematsu, 1993). In a study that classified families of children with mental retardation into varying types, a full 66% of the "cohesive-harmonious" families—the most intact family type—were composed of families of children with Down syndrome (Mink, Nihira, & Myers, 1983). Compared to mothers of children with other disabilities, mothers of children with Down syndrome even report experiencing greater support from friends and the greater community (Erikson & Upshure, 1989).

This advantage to families of children with Down syndrome occurs across a range of ages and relative to a variety of contrast groups; it is also found in most, but not all (e.g., Cahill & Glidden, 1996), studies. The above-mentioned studies examined families of persons with mental retardation who ranged from below 2 years (Erikson & Upshure, 1989) through 25 years of age (Seltzer et al., 1993). Some studies compared individuals with Down syndrome to other groups with retardation, and some to groups of children with autism. In one study (Thomas & Olsen, 1993), researchers began by considering families of adolescents with Down syndrome as "problem families," akin to two groups of families of adolescents with emotional disturbance. As the study progressed, however, these researchers—finding no group differences—combined their "normal" and Down syndrome families into a single control group, concluding that families of children with Down syndrome were not really problem families after all.

Again, however, due to many methodological shortcomings, these findings must be considered cautiously (Glidden & Cahill, 1998). For example, many studies compare families of children with Down syndrome to families of children with autism (e.g., Rodrigue, Morgan, & Geffken, 1990). The excessive behavior problems of children with autism may inappropriately skew findings in favor of families of children with Down syndrome. Other studies adopt group matching versus the more strict case-by-case matching of study families. Finally, parents of children with Down syndrome tend to be older and, possibly, more mature and financially well off (Cahill & Glidden, 1996). Unfortunately, at present no study adequately takes into account *both* parent–family and child characteristics when examining the effects of different etiologies on parent and family functioning. Thus, although the preponderence of evidence supports the better functioning of families of children with Down syndrome versus those of children with other disabilities (including autism, mixed mental retardation, or "disabilities" in general), one must remain cautious.

3. SIBLINGS

Such a possible Down syndrome advantage may also extend to siblings. In two large-scale studies, siblings were found to have few interpersonal problems with their brothers or sisters with Down syndrome (Byrne, Cunningham, & Sloper, 1988;

Carr, 1995). Comparing quarrels in sibling dyads when the index child (Down syndrome versus typically developing) was 11 years of age, Carr (1995) found that 37% of the Down syndrome siblings had no quarrels and 44% had some quarrels; these compare to 18% with no quarrels and 54% with some quarrels among control siblings. As Carr (1995) notes, "the picture is then of quite harmonious relationships between the young people with Down's syndrome and their sibs" (p. 122).

So too may siblings of children with Down syndrome cope better than siblings of other children with other etiologies of mental retardation. In a recent study, we compared older siblings of children with Down syndrome to age- and gender-matched siblings of children with 5p- syndrome (Wijma & Hodapp, 1998). As expected, siblings of children with 5p- syndrome displayed more concerns in a variety of areas. These siblings showed more interpersonal concerns such as "I don't want to bother my parents with my worries" and "I wish that my parents would spend less time with my brother/sister." Compared to same-aged older siblings of children with Down syndrome, siblings of children with 5p- also showed more concerns about intrapersonal issues such as "I feel sad about my brother's/sister's disability" or "I wish that there were something that I could do about my brother's /sister's disability." Just as parents and families seem affected differently by children with different types of mental retardation, so too are these children's older siblings affected differently than older siblings of children with 5p- syndrome.

At this point, then, the evidence is suggestive—not conclusive—that children with Down syndrome elicit more positive reactions from parents, families, and siblings. Most but not all studies show such a "Down syndrome advantage," and the advantage may exist in some areas but not others—for example, in the parents being reinforced by their child's perceived personalities but still experiencing fair amounts of stress in other areas. Finally, few studies examine in depth all of the variables at play, including child characteristics such as the child's personality, IQ, language abilities, adaptive and maladaptive behaviors as well as parent–family characteristics such as parent age, education and marital status, family composition and socioeconomic status (SES). In essence, then, while most studies show that children with Down syndrome elicit better reactions from families, parents, and siblings, why such a Down syndrome advantage exists remains unsolved.

C. The Possible Mechanisms of Indirect Effects

When considering why children with Down syndrome appear to elicit more positive reactions from parents, families, and siblings, several possibilities arise. First, children with Down syndrome may benefit from a variety of factors that surround but are not intrinsic to the syndrome. Down syndrome is the best known and most prevalent genetic-chromosomal disorder of mental retardation. It is also a disorder upon which much medical and behavioral work has been performed; there is even a fair amount of interactional and family work (Hodapp, 1995). Partly as a result of its prevalence, early diagnosis, and familiarity to most people in our society, more parent groups have also arisen. These groups may provide parents with more support and information compared to parents of children with other disabilities.

A second "non-child" explanation relates to the age of parents. Since the risks of having an infant with Down syndrome rise dramatically with advanced maternal age, a higher percentage of mothers of children with the syndrome may be more mature, better off financially, and more experienced in the parenting role. In one of the few studies not finding a Down syndrome advantage, older maternal age and higher SES were cited as possible reasons why most studies find that these parents generally adjust better than parents of children with other disabilities (Cahill & Glidden, 1996).

Although cultural familiarity and more mature mothers may partly account for the Down syndrome advantage, the indirect effects of Down syndrome may also be partly explained by three differences in the children themselves. For each of these three characteristics, preliminary evidence suggests that parents, families, and siblings react differently.

1. SOCIABILITY AND ORIENTATION TOWARD OTHERS

Although seemingly obvious, we all enjoy the company of others who are sociable and pleasant. Werner's resilient children displayed a positive social orientation even as toddlers, and interactions between siblings and peers also seem helped when a child is friendly and outgoing. Conversely, reviewing the sibling literature, Stoneman (1998) observes that sibling dyads show more conflicted relationships when one sibling is highly active and emotional. Children with Down syndrome may thus engender less conflict from siblings and be more rewarding to parents due to their engaging and socially oriented personalities.

2. RELATIVE LACK OF PSYCHOPATHOLOGY

A related issue concerns lower levels of psychopathology in most children with Down syndrome. Although percentages of children with Down syndrome who have psychiatric disturbance range from 15 to 38% (Hodapp, 1996), such percentages are generally lower than those found in same-aged children with mixed etiologies (Dykens, 1996). Furthermore, those maladaptive behaviors that do exist generally involve conduct, attentional, and "generally disruptive" behaviors (Gath & Gumley, 1986; Meyers & Pueschel, 1991). In contrast, children with Down syndrome rarely display more severe psychiatric problems. Psychosis in individuals with Down syndrome is relatively rare, with only about 20 cases of co-occurring Down syndrome and autism reported in the literature (Dykens & Volkmar, 1997).

This difference in psychopathology may partly account for differences in sibling relations among Down syndrome and 5p- groups (Wijma & Hodapp, 1998). Children with Down syndrome show relatively low levels—and children with 5p- syndrome extremely high levels—of severe psychopathology (Dykens & Clarke, 1997; Dykens & Kasari, 1997). In our study, children with 5p- syndrome scored higher on measures of hyperactivity, irritability, and stereotypies. Particularly when the child with mental retardation was above 6 years of age, older siblings experienced increasing difficulties when their younger brother or sister showed increasing behavior problems.

This connection between behavior problems and others' reactions has also been found for parents. In studies of parents of children with Prader-Willi syndrome (Hodapp, Dykens, & Masino, 1997), 5p- (cri-du-chat) syndrome (Hodapp, Wijma, & Masino, 1997), and Smith-Magenis syndrome (Hodapp, Fidler, & Smith, 1998), the best predictor of parent stress was the child's degree of behavior problems. Neither other aspects of the child (age, sex, IQ) nor of the parents or family (education, SES, number or type of supporters) related as strongly to heightened stress levels. When children exhibited higher amounts of behavior problems, parents felt more stressed.

3. APPEARANCE

A final possible explanation for the Down syndrome advantage concerns the facial appearance of these children. To date, most studies of facial appearance have focused on the presence of facial disfigurement. For instance, Wasserman and Allen (1987) examined mother–child interactions between mothers and their toddlers with physical disabilities, serious illness (and born prematurely), and typical children. They found that mothers of children in both disabled groups were more likely to ignore their two-year-olds, but that the finding was most striking in dyads in which the child showed a facial anomaly.

But faces can be examined in other ways as well. One important aspect may be the degree to which a person's face seems immature or "babylike." Just as adults react in characteristic ways to an infant's appearance, there may be a similar reaction to faces that retain infant-like cranio-facial features throughout development. This "baby face overgeneralization" yields positive reactions to "individuals whose appearance merely resembles" a baby in some way (Zebrowitz, 1997, p. 56). Across numerous studies, observers attribute higher ratings of warmth, weakness, and naiveté to pictures of adult faces with baby-like features (Zebrowitz & Montepare, 1992). These features lead others to perceive individuals as dependent and to foster warm, protective responses (Zebrowitz, Kendall-Tackett, & Fafel, 1991).

What characterizes a baby-faced appearance? From Zebrowitz's studies, faces considered baby-like (and which elicit protective responses) include those that have larger eyes relative to the face; a small, concave nose with a sunken bridge; redder lips that are proportionately smaller than adults'; a larger forehead and shorter chin, resulting in lower vertical placement of features on the face; and fuller cheeks and rounder chin, resulting in a rounder face (Berry & McArthur, 1986). Notably, individuals with Down syndrome have many of these baby-like facial features. Compared to age- and sex-matched typically developing children, Allanson, O'Hara, Farkas, and Nair (1993) find that Down syndrome faces characteristically show the following:

1. Striking negative nasal protrusion (akin to Zebrowitz's "sunken bridge")
2. Reduced ear length (i.e., "smaller features")
3. Reduced mouth width (i.e., "smaller mouth")
4. Head length shorter than width (i.e., "rounder face")
5. Lower facial width (i.e., "lower placement of features on the face")

In addition, it seems that adults react to these Down syndrome faces as they would to younger children. Fidler and Hodapp (1998) showed college undergraduates three sets of faces: one of children with Down syndrome, one of children with 5p- syndrome (who generally have longer, more angular, adult-like faces), and one of typically developing children. Each set consisted of one 8-year-old, one 10-year-old, and one 12-year-old, and respondents rated each face on the degree to which the face appeared physically baby-like, was likely to have baby-like traits (warmth, naiveté, kindness, honesty), and was likely to display baby-like behaviors (someone who would cuddle with mother, be compliant to others, or believe a far-fetched story).

Respondents rated the Down syndrome faces as younger looking, more dependent, and more likely to engage in immature behaviors. Combining across the faces of the 8-, 10-, and 12-year-olds, children with Down syndrome received a rating of 16.44 for having a "warm" face, whereas children with 5p- syndrome and typically developing age-mates received ratings of 13.05 and 12.84, respectively. There was also an interaction between age and group, such that the 10- and 12-year-old children with Down syndrome continued to receive high ratings on physical baby-faceness, traits, and behaviors. In contrast, the baby-faced physical, trait, and behavior ratings generally declined for older typically developing and 5p- syndrome children.

In a second portion of this study, we examined whether the "babyface overgeneralization" holds within the Down syndrome group. We asked respondents to rate pictures of twelve 10-year-old children with Down syndrome, but whose faces differed on their objectively measured degree of baby-faceness. Even though faces of 10-year-old children with Down syndrome did not show much within-group variance, adult judges still rated those faces that were more objectively immature as both more baby-like and as more dependent in both traits and behaviors. Thus, using both across- and within-group analyses, naive adult judges rated children with Down syndrome as having more baby-like faces and as possessing those attributes and behaviors that typically go along with such faces.

In understanding indirect effects of different genetic mental retardation disorders, then, both general and specific child characteristics seem to affect parents. Parents react to the child's under- or overreactivity, as well as to parents' own views and perceptions about their child's needs. At the same time, specific, etiologically related characteristics of children seem to affect parents. Using children with Down syndrome as an example, parents appear to react to children's pleasant and sociable personalities. Conversely, based on children with other genetic disorders, parents experience more stress when children show high levels of psychopathology. In addition to their reactions to the behavior of their children, parents and other adults may react to other characteristics, such as the child's more baby-like facial appearance.

IV. REMAINING ISSUES

Although some studies have begun to examine the ways in which persons with different genetic disorders affect adults, several important questions remain. These involve how one examines indirect effects, the underlying mechanisms by which such effects occur, and how one places single behaviors within ongoing child–adult relationships.

A. How Does One Study Interactional Effects?

Interactional research has always been considered difficult to do. Within mental retardation, one major issue concerns the question of general versus specific effects. Children with any genetic mental retardation disorder have both mental retardation and the genetic disorder. How can one tease apart the effects of each? One strategy is to compare adult reactions to children with one versus another type of mental retardation by resorting to pictures, stories, or videotapes and showing such stimuli to naive adults. This technique was used in the study of Down syndrome faces (Fidler & Hodapp, 1998). One can also compare parents, siblings, or peers of children with different etiologies, though it remains unclear whether children with different disabilities (or their families or peers) differ in ways other than in those child characteristics measured by the researchers.

So too do interactional researchers struggle with who affects whom, the heart of Bell's original critique of socialization studies. How does one tease apart the effects of the adult on the child as opposed to the effects of the child on the adult? Although such problems remain unresolved, statisticians examining typically developing children have recently come up with an array of helpful statistical techniques. Methods include path analysis, hierarchical linear modeling, and sequential analyses. Although each method has its limitations, each allows one to say with a specific degree of certainty that the child influences the adult or the adult influences the child.

Other methodological suggestions can be gleaned by returning to work studying typically developing child–adult dyads. Bell and Chapman (1986) propose four strategies for examining child effects on adults.

1. USING CONFEDERATE PARTICIPANTS

This strategy uses individuals trained to behave in a certain way to examine the effects of particular behaviors on adult interactors. The best example here might be the Brunk and Hengeller (1984) study that used two child confederates to act as conduct-disordered versus socially withdrawn children.

At first glance, this strategy might seem less useful for examining the effects on others of individuals with genetic disorders of mental retardation. Few studies have trained children or adults with mental retardation to act differently in order to examine the reactions of adult interactors. There may, however, be variations on this technique, as when one examines the reactions of naive interactors to children with mental retardation who generally differ in their behaviors. What, for example, is the reaction to off-task behavior of children with mental retardation syndromes that often feature ADHD (e.g., fragile X syndrome) compared to those in which attentional problems occur less frequently (Down syndrome)? As in Brunk and Henggeler (1984), the best evidence that the adults have been influenced by the child's general pattern of behaviors occurs in response to ambiguous behaviors, when the child with mental retardation does not answer, or misunderstands the request, or in other ways does not comply with the wishes of the adult interactor.

2. ALTERING BEHAVIOR OF THE CHILD

A good example of altered behavior occurred in Barkley and Cunningham's (1979) study of child effects on mothers. Using a double-blind placebo design, this study showed that mothers react differently to their children with ADHD once the child's behaviors were controlled by medications.

In many mental retardation syndromes as well, one can examine the effects on surrounding adults of child behavior that has been altered. As in ADHD, one can examine the effects on others when the child's behavior has been changed by psychotropic medication. In addition, however, one can examine how successful behavior-modification programs (which have changed the child's behavior) might influence the reactions of surrounding adults. For example, one might perform a pre–post study before and after the child's behavior has been changed by using behavioral modification, with different groups of naive adults as the pretest and posttest interactors or judges of videotaped interactions.

3. ALTERING PERCEPTION OF ADULT JUDGES

These studies involve such things as telling adults to describe the behaviors of children who they briefly interact with or see on videotape when the child is described as a boy versus a girl. The Rubin et al. (1974) study asking parents to describe their newborn infant based almost exclusively on their perceptions of gender roles and behaviors comes close to a study involving altered perception.

In mental retardation as well, one can alter the adult's perception and determine the effects of such altered perceptions on either descriptions or behavior. One might, for example, ask two groups of naive observers to describe the behaviors of a particular child when the child is described as having Down syndrome versus some other disorder (to determine the effects of the Down syndrome label). To determine the effects of the child's facial appearance on adult observers, one might ask naive adults to judge a videotape of parent–child interaction when examining the child from the front (full-face) versus from behind (not observing the face).

4. DISENTANGLING PARENT VERSUS ADULT REACTIONS (SAMPLE SELECTION)

These studies attempt to tease apart diagnostic versus relationship issues. A mother of a child with 5p- syndrome, for example, might be asked to interact with her own child, with another child with 5p- syndrome, and with a third, nonretarded child who functions at the same cognitive level. Or, conversely, different adult interactors might interact with a single child—for example, the child's mother, another mother of a child with the same condition, and a naive adult. One might even examine the behaviors of research assistants who are blind to the study's hypotheses to determine whether child behaviors differentially affect adult interactors in one versus another mental retardation syndrome.

Each of these research approaches has been successfully employed in earlier interactional work of adult–child interaction with typically developing children. Granted, many of these strategies may need to be adapted to children with different types of mental retardation, but it nevertheless appears that interactions between adults and children are open to study, and one can address the difficult question of who affects whom in interactions between adults and children with mental retardation.

B. How Does One Conceptualize the Mechanisms by Which Indirect Effects Operate?

Children do not influence adults by magic. Instead, such influences arise through a reasonably predictable set of behaviors and perceptions on the part of both. In mental retardation, we see that such behaviors and perceptions include some aspects that are general to all dyads in which the child has mental retardation, and other aspects that are specific to the child's particular type of mental retardation.

But even when considering child effects that are specific to a single type of mental retardation, one must consider particular child and adult characteristics. For the child, the main characteristic influencing others seems to be the child's degree of both social and maladaptive behavior. The most positive reactions from others appear when the child is socially oriented, has a pleasant personality, and is free from maladaptive behavior. Other behaviors, for instance the child's level of intellectual or adaptive functioning, seem less influential.

Table I presents a preliminary model of indirect effects of genetic disorders of mental retardation, but also hints at the many totally unexplored areas. Genetic disorder A predisposes individuals to a particular behavior or set of behaviors. These behaviors, in turn, elicit behavioral and emotional reactions from the child's surrounding interactors. But children with other genetic disorders do not generally show genetic disorder A's characteristic behaviors; the corresponding reactions from others also differ. Though this figure is overly static and does not highlight the back-and-forth interactions over time between children and adult interactors, it does provide a preliminary schematic of the workings of genetic disorders' indirect effects.

At the same time, Table I also implies the many aspects of indirect effects that remain unknown. For example, just how specific are the effects of such behaviors? Considering maladaptive behaviors, are parents and siblings reacting to the total amount of maladaptive behavior, or instead to specific behaviors such as hyperactivity or stubbornness? How does the feedback of parent reactions affect the child's future behaviors? How does the child's own cognitive, linguistic, and adaptive development complicate matters? How do parental reactions to child behaviors change when parents are older, divorced, or of lower SES, or when the family does or does not have additional children? All of these issues remain unresolved. At present, we can be reasonably certain only that child behaviors influence the

TABLE I
SIMPLIFIED MODEL OF INDIRECT EFFECTS OF GENETIC DISORDERS OF MENTAL RETARDATION

Etiology		Direct effects Child's behavior		Indirect effects Others' behavior
		Characteristic	➡	
A	➡	Presence of		Specific reaction(s)
		Specific behavior(s)	⬅	
B				
C				
D		Characteristic	➡	
E	➡	Absence of		Other reactions
F		Specific behavior(s)	⬅	
G				
H, etc.				

child's surrounding interpersonal environment, even if the conditions under which such behaviors operate remain unclear.

In addition, behavior is not the only salient child characteristic to adults. Parents and other adults are also influenced by the child's facial anomalies (Wasserman & Allen, 1987), by faces that are more baby-like (Fidler & Hodapp, 1998), and, possibly, by physical, medical, or other characteristics of the child. Indeed, social psychology has examined many variables that influence one person's perceptions of another; to date, few of these variables have been examined in mental retardation studies.

Parents, too, are affected by their perceptions of the child with disabilities, their goals for that child, and their sense of how the child's behaviors fit within parental goals and perceptions. To give but one example, parents of young children with Down syndrome report more concern about their child's cognitive and linguistic achievements than do parents of children with cerebral palsy, even though these children as well often show delays in cognitive-linguistic abilities (Hodapp, Dykens, Evans, & Merighi, 1992). As Bell (1979) noted 20 years ago, one cannot ignore the "thinking parent" within parent–child interactions.

C. How Do Adult Reactions to Child Behaviors Fit within Ongoing Relationships?

Finally, one must contrast behaviors and relationships. As Lollis and Kuczynski (1997) note, those studying parent–child interactions and those studying parent–child relationships have approached the issue of bidirectionality from very different perspectives. For the most part, interactional researchers have taken a more microanalytic perspective, whereas relationship researchers are more global.

And yet, behaviors occur within relationships. As in Brunk and Henggeler's (1984) short-term interactions between children acting as conduct disordered versus socially withdrawn, adults quickly realize what a child will do and how they should respond. Even more so in stable, longer-lasting relationships, both past experiences and future expectancies influence the behaviors of both the child and the adult interactors.

The behavior–relationship issue arises in other ways as well. Many parent–child researchers are realizing that interactions differ across different contexts, for example, when children are playing, being cared for, or being taught by their parents. So too are different interactors attuned to different behaviors. Consider, for instance, how preschoolers with Down syndrome often attempt to charm their way out of solving difficult intellectual problems by smiling or in other ways distracting adults (Pitcairn & Wishart, 1994). Are such behaviors, which parents consider as charming "party pieces," as charming to teachers? What about to children's siblings or peers? Certain behaviors might differentially affect diverse persons in the child's environment.

V. CONCLUSION

In considering the question of indirect effects, it is clear that we now have many more questions than answers. Thus, while indirect effects occur in adults' reactions both to children with mental retardation in general and to children with different genetic disorders, details remain sketchy as to how such reactions occur, in response to which stimuli, and how others' reactions operate within long-term, ongoing relationships. Just as in studies of typically developing child–adult dyads, mental retardation workers face a paradox (Dunn, 1997). On one hand, Bell's interactionism has been well known from the late 1960s on, and some studies have shown that specific behaviors of children with mental retardation—at this point, mainly the child's personality and maladaptive behavior—influence the coping of their parents. But on the other, the large majority of studies have yet to examine child effects in detail. Ultimately, if we are truly to understand the effects of both mental retardation and its different genetic syndromes, both direct and indirect effects must be examined.

ACKNOWLEDGMENTS

I would like to thank Elisabeth Dykens, Deborah Fidler, Len Abbeduto, and Laraine Glidden for their helpful comments on earlier drafts of this manuscript.

REFERENCES

Allanson, J. E., O'Hara, P., Farkas, L. G., & Nair, R. C. (1993). Anthropometric craniofacial pattern profiles in Down syndrome. *American Journal of Medical Genetics*, *47*, 748–752.

American Psychiatric Association (1994). *Diagnostic and statistical manual of mental disorders, 4th edition.* Washington, DC: Author.

Anderson, L. T., & Ernst, M. (1994). Self-injury in Lesch-Nyan disease. *Journal of Autism and Developmental Disorders*, *24*, 67–81.

Barkley, R., & Cunningham, E. (1979). The effects of methylphenidate on mother-child interaction in hyperactive children. *Archives of General Psychiatry*, *36*, 201–208.

Bell, R. Q. (1968). A reinterpretation of direction of effects in studies of socialization. *Psychological Review*, *75*, 81–95.

Bell, R. Q. (1979). Parent, child, and reciprocal influences. *American Psychologist*, *34*, 821–826.

Bell, R. Q., & Chapman, M. (1986). Child effects in studies using experimental or brief longitudinal approaches to socialization. *Developmental Psychology*, *22*, 595–603.

Bell, R. Q., & Harper, L. V. (1977). *Child effects on adults.* Hillsdale, NJ: Erlbaum.

Berry, D. S., & McArthur, L. Z. (1985). Some components and consequences of a babyface. *Journal of Personality and Social Psychology*, *48*, 312–323.

Brazelton, T. B., Koslowski, B., & Main, M. (1974). The origins of reciprocity: The early mother–infant attachment. In M. Lewis & L. A. Rosenblum (Eds.), *The effects of the infant on its caretaker.* New York: Wiley.

Brunk, W., & Henggeler, S. W. (1984). Child influences on adult controls: An experimental investigation. *Developmental Psychology*, *20*, 1074–1081.

Byrne, E. A., Cunningham, C. C., & Sloper, P. (1988). *Families and their children with Down's syndrome.* London: Routledge.

Cahill, B. M., & Glidden, L. M. (1996). Influence of child diagnosis on family and parent functioning: Down syndrome versus other disabilities. *American Journal on Mental Retardation, 101*, 149–160.

Carlin, M. E. (1990). The improved prognosis in Cri-du-Chat (5p-) syndrome. In W. I. Fraser (Ed.), *Proceedings of the 8th Congress of the International Association of the Scientific Study of Mental Deficiency* (pp. 64–73). Edinburgh: Blackwell.

Carr, J. (1995). *Down's syndrome: Children growing up.* Cambridge, UK: Cambridge University Press.

Dunn, J. (1997). Lessons from the study of bidirectional effects. *Journal of Social and Personal Relationships, 14*, 565–573.

Dunst, C. J. (1988). Stage transitioning in the sensorimotor development of Down's syndrome infants. *Journal of Mental Deficiency Research, 32*, 405–410.

Dunst, C. J. (1990). Sensorimotor development of infants with Down syndrome. In D. Cicchetti & M. Beeghly (Eds.), *Children with Down syndrome: A developmental perspective* (pp. 180–230). Cambridge, UK: Cambridge University Press.

Dykens, E. M. (1995). Measuring behavioral phenotypes: Provocations from the "New Genetics." *American Journal on Mental Retardation, 99*, 522–532.

Dykens, E. M. (1996). DNA meets DSM: The growing importance of genetic syndromes in dual diagnosis. *Mental Retardation, 34*, 125–127.

Dykens, E. M., & Cassidy, S. R. (1996). Prader-Willi Syndrome: Genetic, behavioral, and treatment issues. *Child and Adolescent Psychiatric Clinics of North America, 5*, 913–927.

Dykens, E. M., & Clarke, D. J. (1997). Correlates of maladaptive behavior in persons with 5p- (cri-du-chat) syndrome. *Developmental Medicine and Child Neurology, 39*, 752–756.

Dykens, E. M., Hodapp, R. M., & Leckman, J. F. (1994). *Behavior and development in fragile X syndrome.* Thousand Oaks, CA: Sage.

Dykens, E. M., & Kasari, C. (1997). Maladaptive behavior in children with Prader-Willi syndrome, Down syndrome, and non-specific mental retardation. *American Journal on Mental Retardation, 102*, 228–237.

Dykens, E. M., & Volkmar, F. R. (1997). Medical conditions associated with autism. In D. J. Cohen & F. R. Volkmar (Eds.), *Handbook of autism and developmental disorders* (2nd ed., pp. 388–407). New York: Wiley.

Erikson, M., & Upshure, C. C. (1989). Caretaking burden and social support: Comparison of mothers of infants with and without disabilities. *American Journal on Mental Retardation, 94*, 250–258.

Fidler, D. J., & Hodapp (1998). *Face perception and the Down syndrome difference.* Unpublished manuscript.

Gath, A., & Gumley, D. (1986). Behaviour problems in retarded children with special reference to Down's syndrome. *British Journal of Psychiatry, 149*, 156–161.

Glidden, L. M., & Cahill, B. M. (1998). Successful adoption of children with Down syndrome and other developmental disabilities. *Adoption Quarterly, 1*, 27–43.

Goldberg, S. (1977). Social competence in infancy: A model of parent-infant interactions. *Merrill-Palmer Quarterly, 23*, 163–177.

Hodapp, R. M. (1988). The role of maternal emotions and perceptions in interactions with young handicapped children. In K. Marfo (Ed.), *Parent-child interaction and developmental disabilities: Theory, research, and intervention* (pp. 32–46). New York: Praeger Publishers.

Hodapp, R. M. (1995). Parenting children with Down syndrome and other types of mental retardation. In M. Bornstein (Ed.), *Handbook of parenting.* Vol. 1. *How children influence parents* (pp. 233–253). Hillsdale, NJ: Erlbaum.

Hodapp, R. M. (1996). Down syndrome: Developmental, psychiatric, and management issues. *Child and Adolescent Psychiatric Clinics of North America, 5*, 881–894.

Hodapp, R. M. (1997). Direct and indirect behavioral effects of different genetic disorders of mental retardation. *American Journal on Mental Retardation, 102*, 67–79.

Hodapp, R. M., Dykens, E. M., Evans, D. W., & Merighi, J. R. (1992). Maternal emotional reactions to young children with different types of handicaps. *Journal of Developmental and Behavioral Pediatrics, 13*, 118–123.

Hodapp, R. M., Dykens, E. M., & Masino, L. L. (1997). Families of children with Prader-Willi Syndrome: Stress-support and relations to child characteristics. *Journal of Autism and Developmental Disorders, 27*, 11–24.

Hodapp, R. M., Fidler, D. J., & Smith, A. C. M. (1998). Stress and coping in families of children with Smith Magenis syndrome. *Journal of Intellectual Disability Research, 42*, 331–340.

Hodapp, R. M., & Mueller, E. (1982). Early social development. In B. Wolman (Ed.), *Handbook of developmental psychology* (pp. 284–300). Englewood Cliffs, NJ: Prentice-Hall.

Hodapp, R. M., Wijma, C. A., & Masino, L. L. (1997). Families of children with 5p- (cri du chat) syndrome: Familial stress and sibling reactions. *Developmental Medicine and Child Neurology, 39*, 757–761.

Holm, V. A., Cassidy, S. B., Butler, M. G., Hanchet, J. M., Greenswag, L. R., Whitman, B. Y., & Greenberg, F. (1993). Prader-Willi syndrome: Consensus diagnostic criteria. *Pediatrics, 91*, 398–402.

Holroyd, J., & MacArthur, D. (1976). Mental retardation and stress on parents: A contrast between Down's syndrome and childhood autism. *American Journal of Mental Deficiency, 80*, 431–436.

Hornby, G. (1995). Fathers' views of the effects on their families of children with Down syndrome. *Journal of Child and Family Studies, 4*, 103–117.

Kasari, C., & Sigman, M. (1997). Linking parental perceptions to interactions in young children with autism. *Journal of Autism and Developmental Disorders, 27*, 39–57.

Loeber, R., & Stouthamer-Loeber, M. (1986). Family factors as correlates and predictors of juvenile conduct problems and delinquency. In M. Tonry & N. Morris (Eds.), *Crime and justice: An annual review of research* (Vol. 7, pp. 29–149). Chicago: University of Chicago Press.

Loeber, R., Stouthamer-Loeber, M., & Green, S. M. (1991). Age of onset of problem behavior in boys, and later disruptive and delinquent behaviors. *Criminal Behaviour and Mental Health, 1*, 229–246.

Lollis, S., & Kuczynski, L. (1997). Beyond one hand clapping: Seeing bidirectionality in parent-child relations. *Journal of Social and Personal Relationships, 14*, 441–461.

Lytton, H. (1990). Child and parent effects in boys' conduct disorder: A reinterpretation. *Developmental Psychology, 26*, 683–697.

Marfo, K., Dedrick, C. F., & Barbour, N. (1998). Mother–child interactions and the development of children with mental retardation. In J. A. Burack, R. M. Hodapp, & E. Zigler (Eds.), *Handbook of mental retardation and development* (pp. 637–668). New York: Cambridge University Press.

Meyers, B. A., & Pueschel, S. M. (1991). Psychiatric disorders in persons with Down syndrome. *Journal of Nervous and Mental Disease, 179*, 609–613.

Mink, T., Nihira, K., & Meyers, C. E. (1983). Taxonomy of family life styles. I. Home with TMR children. *American Journal of Mental Deficiency, 87*, 484–497.

Noh, S., Dumas, J. E., Wolf, L. C., & Fisman, S. N. (1989). Delineating sources of stress in parents of exceptional children. *Family Relations, 38*, 456–461.

O'Brien, G. (1993). Behavioral phenotypes and their measurement. *Developmental Medicine and Child Neurology, 34*, 365–367.

O'Brien, G., & Yule, W. (Eds.) (1995). *Behavioural phenotypes.* London: MacKeith Press.

Olweus, D. (1980). Familial and temperamental determinants of aggressive behavior in adolescent boys: A causal analysis. *Developmental Psychology, 16*, 644–660.

Patterson, G. R. (1976). The aggressive child: Victim and architect of a coercive system. In E. J. Mash, L. Hamerlynck, & L. Handy (Eds.), *Behavior modification and families* (pp. 267–316). New York: Brunner/Mazel.

Pianta, R., Egeland, B., & Erickson, M. F. (1990). The antecedents of maltreatment: Results of the Mother-Child Interaction Research Project. In D. Cicchetti & V. Carlson (Eds.), *Child maltreatment: Theory and research on the causes and consequences of child abuse and neglect* (pp. 203–253). New York: Cambridge University Press.

Pitcairn, T. K., & Wishart, J. G. (1994). Reactions of young children with Down syndrome to an impossible task. *British Journal of Developmental Psychology, 12*, 485–489.

Pober, B. R., & Dykens, E. M. (1996). Williams syndrome: An overview of medical, cognitive and behavioral features. *Child and Adolescent Psychiatric Clinics of North America, 5*, 929–943.

Rodrigue, J. R., Morgan, S. B., & Geffken, G. R. (1990). Families of autistic children: Psychological functioning of mothers. *Journal of Clinical Child Psychology, 19*, 371–379.

Rubin, J. Z., Provenzano, F. J., & Luria, Z. (1974). The eye of the beholder: Parents' views on sex of newborns. *American Journal of Orthopsychiatry, 44*, 512–519.

Sanders, J. L., & Morgan, S. B. (1997). Family stress and adjustment as perceived by parents of children with autism or Down syndrome: Implications for intervention. *Child and Family Behavior Therapy, 19*, 15–32.

Scarr, S. (1993). Developmental theories for the 1990s: Development and individual differences. *Child Development, 63*, 1–19.

Seltzer, M. M., Krauss, M. W., & Tsunematsu, N. (1993). Adults with Down syndrome and their aging mothers: Diagnostic group differences. *American Journal on Mental Retardation, 97*, 496–508.

Stoneman, Z. (1998). Research on siblings of children with mental retardation: Contributions of developmental theory and etiology. In J. A. Burack, R. M. Hodapp, & E. Zigler (Eds.), *Handbook of mental retardation and development* (pp. 669–692). New York: Cambridge University Press.

Thomas, V., & Olsen, D. H. (1993). Problem families and the circumplex model: Observational assessment using the clinical rating scale (CRS). *Journal of Marital and Family Therapy, 19*, 159–175.

Walden, T. A. (1996). Social responsivity: Judging signals of young children with and without developmental delays. *Child Development, 67*, 2074–2085.

Wasserman, G. A., & Allen, R. (1987). Maternal withdrawal from handicapped toddlers. *Journal of Child Psychology and Psychiatry, 26*, 381–387.

Werner, E. (1993). Risk, resilience, and recovery: Perspectives from the Kauai Longitudinal Study. *Development and Psychopathology, 5*, 503–515.

West, D. J., & Farrington, D. P. (1973). *Who becomes delinquent?* London: Heinemann Education Books.

Wijma, C. A., & Hodapp, R. M. (1998). *Siblings of children with 5p- versus Down syndrome.* Unpublished manuscript.

Wishart, J. G. (1995). Cognitive abilities of children with Down syndrome: Developmental instability and motivational deficits. In C. J. Epstein (Ed.), *Etiology and pathogenesis of Down syndrome* (pp. 57–91). New York: Wiley-Liss.

Wishart, J. G., & Johnston, F. H. (1990). The effects of experience on attribution of a stereotyped personality to children with Down's syndrome. *Journal of Mental Deficiency Research, 34*, 409–420.

Zebrowitz, L. A. (1997). *Reading faces: Window to the soul?* Boulder, CO: Westview Press.

Zebrowitz, L. A., Kendall-Tackett, K. A., & Fafel, J. (1991). The influence of children's facial maturity on parental expectations and punishments. *Journal of Experimental Child Psychology, 52*, 221–238.

Zebrowitz, L. A., & Montepare, J. M. (1992). Impressions of babyfaced individuals across the life span. *Developmental Psychology, 28*, 1143–1152.

Zirpoli, T. J., & Bell, R. Q. (1987). Unresponsiveness of children with severe disabilities: Potential effects on parent-child interactions. *Exceptional Child, 34*, 31–40.

The Development of Basic Counting, Number, and Arithmetic Knowledge among Children Classified as Mentally Handicapped

ARTHUR J. BAROODY

COLLEGE OF EDUCATION
UNIVERSITY OF ILLINOIS AT URBANA-CHAMPAIGN
CHAMPAIGN, ILLINOIS

The National Council of Teachers of Mathematics (NCTM, 1989, 1991) has called for reforms so that instruction promotes the *mathematical power* of *all students*. Fostering mathematical power implies cultivating *adaptive expertise* (meaningful knowledge that can be applied to new tasks), which Hatano (1988) contrasts with *routine expertise* (rotely memorized knowledge that can be used effectively with familiar, but not unfamiliar, tasks). By *all students*, the NCTM (1991) includes "students who have not been successful in school" (p. 4)—including children with mental retardation (Thornton & Bley, 1994).[1] But is it realistic to expect such children to achieve adaptive expertise in mathematics and, thus, any real measure of mathematical power? Is there really reason to believe that we should change how and what mathematics is taught to children with mental retardation?

To answer these questions, it is important to understand the rationale for the current reform movement in mathematics education and the mathematical capabilities of children with mental retardation. So I begin this chapter with a brief discussion of the theoretical and empirical underpinnings of the NCTM's (1989, 1991) proposed reforms. Next, I describe my and other's research on the mathe-

[1]In this chapter, *children classified as mentally handicapped* (and referred to as *children with mental retardation*) include individuals up to 21 years old with an IQ less than 75. The term *people or individuals with mental retardation* includes adults. Most of the reported research studied children with moderate retardation (IQs 26–50) or those with mild retardation (IQs 51–75). A few reported studies included children with severe mental retardation (IQs 11–25).

INTERNATIONAL REVIEW OF RESEARCH IN
MENTAL RETARDATION, Vol. 22
0074-7750/99 $30.00

matical learning of children with mental retardation. I then end the chapter by tentatively answering the questions posed above and discussing what further research is needed.

I. RATIONALE FOR REFORMING MATHEMATICS INSTRUCTION

Business, governmental, and educational leaders now recognize that the way we teach mathematics in this country needs to change (e.g., Carnegie Forum on Education and the Economy, 1986; Davis, 1984; Lindquist, 1989; National Commission on Excellence in Education, 1983; NCTM, 1989, 1991). More specifically, the consensus among such leaders is that instruction should focus on fostering mathematical power (a positive disposition toward learning and using mathematics, an understanding of mathematical concepts and procedures, and inquiry skills such as problem solving and reasoning), rather than on memorizing definitions, facts, procedures, and formulas by rote. Reasons for this consensus include the following:

1. The advent of a rapidly changing technological- and information-based age makes mathematical thinking (e.g., problem solving and reasoning) and number sense (e.g., an ability to judge whether or not an answer makes sense) at least as important as arithmetic computational skills (e.g., Davis, 1984; Lindquist, 1989). Quantitative thinking and understanding is now needed in nearly all aspects of our personal and professional lives. Moreover, the availability of inexpensive electronic calculators and computers further puts a premium on thinking and understanding and reduces the importance of computational skills (e.g., Coburn, 1989; Fey, 1990).
2. Our economy faces increasingly stiff international competition, and our students must be on a par with those of other industrialized nations. However, cross-cultural research indicates that schoolchildren in this country score relatively low in mathematical achievement (e.g., McKnight et al., 1987; Stevenson, Lee, & Stigler, 1986).
3. Cognitive research has provided a better understanding of the nature of mathematical knowledge and learning. The "disaster studies" demonstrated that even high-achieving students did not understand the mathematics they were learning and, as a result, were unable to apply it to learning new material, solving mathematical problems, or dealing effectively with everyday situations (e.g., Davis, 1984).

In this section, I discuss further this third factor and its impact on the mathematics reform movement.

A. Changing Views

In the last 25 years, there has been a remarkable change in the way psychologists view the mathematical knowledge and learning of nonmentally handicapped (NMH) children. As cognitive theories became the predominant paradigm in psychology, a debate about how much young NMH children could learn and understand ensued. In this subsection, I describe the prevalent view held earlier, in the first three quarters of this century, and the prevalent view now.

1. EARLIER VIEW

Prior to 1975 or so, psychologists grossly underestimated NMH preschoolers' mathematical knowledge and capabilities. In particular, the following two assumptions were prevalent.

1. *Children just beginning school have little or no mathematical knowledge.* They were viewed as basically uninformed, blank slates, or empty vessels. Indeed, even the famous cognitive psychologist, Jean Piaget (1965), proposed that children before "the age of reason" (about 7 years of age) were capable of only "preoperational" (nonlogical) thinking, and hence, were incapable of constructing a true number concept. Moreover, Edward L. Thorndike (1922), the famous learning theorist, considered children so mathematically inept that he concluded: "It seems probable that little is gained by using any of the child's time for arithmetic before grade 2, though there are many arithmetic facts that can [be memorized by rote] in grade 1" (p. 198).
2. *Learning is essentially a passive process.* Because they have little or no useful mathematical knowledge, children are basically helpless when confronted with new learning tasks or new problems. Because they are uninformed and helpless, mathematical learning entails memorizing information provided by others with more expertise. In other words, it is essentially a process of absorbing knowledge from teachers, parents, older siblings, and so forth.

2. CURRENT VIEW

Research over the last 25 years paints a different picture of young children's mathematical knowledge (see, e.g., recent reviews by Baroody & Wilkins, 1999; Ginsburg, Klein, & Starkey, 1998; Sophian, 1998; Starkey, in press; Wynn, 1998).

1. *Children have a surprising amount of informal mathematical knowledge.* In contrast to formal knowledge, which is school taught and relatively abstract (largely symbolic, general, and impersonal in nature), informal mathematical knowledge is gleaned from everyday life and relatively concrete (largely the result of experience with real objects, often bound to a specific context, and almost always personally meaningful). The development of this knowledge begins well before

school (e.g., Court, 1920; Fuson, 1988, 1992; Gelman & Gallistel, 1978; Ginsburg, 1977). Children engage in all sorts of everyday activities that involve counting, numbers, and simple arithmetic and, as a result, develop a considerable body of informal knowledge about these domains (e.g., Carraher, Carraher, & Schliesmann, 1987; Ginsburg, Posner, & Russell, 1981; Hughes, 1986; Nunes, 1992; Resnick, 1992).

2. *Children actively construct meaningful mathematical knowledge* (e.g., Baroody, 1987a, 1998; Kamii, 1985; Koehler & Grouws, 1992). Substantive learning is an active problem-solving process—an effort to make sense of personally important tasks and to devise solutions for them (e.g., Cobb, Wood, & Yackel, 1991). It entails reorganizing our thinking—broadening our perspective—rather than merely accumulating information (e.g., Cobb et al., 1991). Even young children can draw on their everyday knowledge to informally construct new mathematical understandings and solve significant mathematical problems. For example, without instruction, they can deduce the concept of infinity. That is, from their counting experiences, children as early as kindergarten recognize that the counting numbers go on forever (Baroody, 1998; Gelman, 1982). Moreover, from their concrete experiences with adding and taking away items, they can comprehend simple addition and subtraction word problems and devise effective informal counting strategies to solve them, even before receiving formal arithmetic instruction (e.g., Baroody, 1987a; Carpenter & Moser, 1984; Ginsburg, 1977; Starkey & Gelman, 1982).

B. Educational Implications

In contrast to children's informal knowledge, which is characterized by adaptive expertise, their formal mathematical knowledge all too often consists merely of routine expertise. Whereas their informal knowledge is conceptually based, enabling them to actively and autonomously construct new mathematical understandings or devise their own solution to new mathematical problems, their school-learned mathematics is largely learned by rote, leaving them helpless and puzzled by even slightly new tasks. The contrast between children's powerful informal knowledge and their limited formal knowledge raised serious questions about the effectiveness of traditional instruction. In this subsection, I discuss the limitations of this instruction and summarize the instructional reforms recommended by the NCTM (1989, 1991).

1. THE TRADITIONAL SKILLS APPROACH: FOSTERING ROUTINE EXPERTISE

The nature of traditional instruction (a "skills approach") is summarized in the left-hand side of Table I. In a skills approach, children's informal knowledge is largely ignored, and instruction focuses on memorizing the definitions of symbols,

TABLE I
SKILLS VERSUS AN INVESTIGATIVE APPROACH

	Skills approach	Investigative approach
Aim	Foster routine expertise: the mastery (rote memorization) of basic skills (arithmetic and geometric facts, definitions, rules, formulas, and procedures)	Foster mathematical power including adaptive expertise (meaningful memorization of facts, definitions, rules, formulas, and procedures)
Focus	Procedural content (e.g., how to add multidigit numbers)	Conceptual content (e.g., why you carry when adding multidigit mathematical numbers) and the processes of mathmatical inquiry (problem solving, reasoning, and communicating)
Teacher's role	Teacher serves as an information dispenser.	Teacher serves as a guide.
Students' role	Because they are viewed as uninformed and helpless, students must be spoonfed knowledge (i.e., students are passive and dependent).	Because they have informal knowledge and an inherent need to understand, children are capable of inventing their own solutions and making (at least some) sense of mathematical situations themselves (i.e., students are active and somewhat independent).
Organizing principle	Bottom-up: Sequential instruction from most basic skills to most complex skills such as problem solving (like a phonetic/basal reader approach to reading)	Top-down: Posing a "worthwhile task" (one that is challenging and complex) as a way of exploring and practicing basic concepts and skills
Methods	• Teacher lectures and demonstrates.	• Students are encouraged to advance conjectures, ideas, and solutions.
	• Children work in isolation.	• Children work together in groups
	• Teacher provides feedback on correctness.	• Teacher responds to incorrect answers by posing a question, problems, or task that prompts student reflection
	• Practice with an emphasis on written, sterile worksheets	• Practice done purposefully by engaging students in interesting projects, problems, games, stories, and so forth
	• Little or no use of technology	• Use of technology is a key aim and central to many learning tasks

symbol facts, and procedures for manipulating symbols. Because children frequently cannot relate this formal instruction to what they understand, school mathematics typically makes little sense to them. In brief, the gap between the decontextualized and symbolic mathematics taught in school and children's informal knowledge promotes passive learning: It renders students helpless and requires them to resort to rote memorization that, in turn, makes them even more helpless and dependent later.

More specifically, fostering routine expertise means that children cannot apply (transfer) what they know to even moderately novel tasks or problems (e.g., Baroody, 1998; Wertheimer, 1945/1959). Consider, for example, learning the procedures for subtracting without renaming (e.g., Items A and C below do not require "borrowing") and subtracting with renaming (e.g., Items B, D, and E do require "borrowing"). Students who memorize by rote the procedures for subtracting two-digit numbers without renaming, two-digit numbers with renaming, and then three-digit numbers without renaming (e.g., for Items A, B, and C, respectively) often do not know what to do in situations that involve subtracting three-digit numbers with renaming (e.g., Item D). Indeed, even after memorizing the renaming procedure for subtracting three-digit numbers, they are often confused when expressions involving zero are introduced (e.g., Item E). In brief, when instruction focuses on fostering routine expertise, children must be spoonfed the whole mathematics curriculum.

A.	B.	C.	D.	E.
78	72	398	314	304
-35	-35	-126	-126	-126

In many cases, children fail to develop even routine expertise. Mystified by the math logic taught in school, many have difficulty memorizing assigned facts and procedures. Others do so, but quickly forget them. To foster rote memorization and counter the effects of forgetting, students are given huge amounts of often tedious practice. Moreover, with each successive grade, more and more time is spent reviewing previously taught (but unlearned or forgotten) material, until middle school where the entire mathematics curriculum consists of review. Incomprehensible and decontextualized instruction, massive and uninteresting practice, and constant review of meaningless and apparently pointless facts and procedures all too often create affective barriers to learning: a negative disposition towards mathematics or even math anxiety.

2. THE NATIONAL COUNCIL OF TEACHERS OF MATHEMATICS INVESTIGATIVE APPROACH: FOSTERING ADAPTIVE EXPERTISE

Fostering adaptive expertise makes sense pedagogically because, in the long run, it is more effective and efficient than promoting routine expertise. Children who understand mathematics are more likely to exhibit transfer and retain their mathematical knowledge, require less practice and review, autonomously invent and monitor strategies to new tasks or problems, and develop a positive disposition toward learning and using mathematics (e.g., confidence to tackle new learning tasks or problems and positive beliefs such as "everyone can achieve significant levels of mathematical competence") (e.g., Baroody, 1998). Moreover, students with mathematical adaptive expertise should be more successful in a technological work environment that is constantly changing.

To promote adaptive expertise, the NCTM (1989, 1991) has recommended a purposeful, meaningful, and inquiry-based approach to mathematics instruction. This "investigative approach" embodies the following key aspects of developmentally appropriate practices (Bredekamp, 1993): (a) carefully examining the developmental readiness of each student for a topic; (b) providing individualized remedial instruction of specific concepts and skills; (c) building on what students already understand, including their informal mathematical knowledge; (d) encouraging students to work in groups, share ideas, and arrive at their own solutions and conclusions; (e) refining solutions and conclusions through discussions and questioning by teachers and other students; (f) integrating instruction across mathematical topics and with other content areas; and (g) learning and practicing skills purposefully in the contexts of games, simple science experiments, projects, and solving developmentally appropriate problems. This approach is summarized in the right-hand side of Table I.

II. THE MATHEMATICAL LEARNING OF CHILDREN WITH MENTAL RETARDATION

Influenced by the cognitive research of NMH children, researchers in recent years have begun to explore the mathematical competencies and development of children with mental retardation. In this section, I describe how this research has helped to change our view of these special children and summarize some of the research on their basic informal and formal knowledge.

A. Changing Views

Paralleling the changed view of children's mathematical competence in general, there has been—in recent years—a remarkable change in the way psychologists view children with mental retardation. In this subsection, I contrast the traditional and an emerging view.

1. TRADITIONAL VIEW

Traditionally, children with mental retardation have been characterized as passive learners—capable of routine, but not adaptive, expertise. Indeed, a considerable amount of past research supported the following stereotypes: (a) children with mental retardation cannot devise an appropriate strategy for new learning or memory tasks (e.g., see reviews by Belmont & Butterfield, 1969; Bray, 1979; Brown, 1974; Cherkes-Julkowski et al., 1986); (b) such children can be trained to perform memory or learning tasks by rote, but such training will not transfer—that is, be adapted to meet the demands of even moderately new tasks (see, e.g., Bray & Turner, 1986; Brown, Bransford, Ferrara, & Campione, 1983; Butterfield & Belmont, 1977; Campione & Brown, 1974; Cherkes-Julkowski et al., 1986; Cherkes-Julkowski & Gertner, 1989). In brief, the inability of people with mental retardation to devise, transfer, or transform strategies has, in the past, been viewed as characteristic of low intelligence—of poor adaptive functioning (e.g., Binet & Simon, 1916; Grossman, 1983; Wechsler, 1958; all cited in Ferretti & Cavalier, 1991).

More specifically, various authorities have concluded that children with moderate mental retardation might learn to count and use small numbers in a limited way, such as recognizing sets of one, two, and three (Doll, 1931) but are incapable of acquiring functional academic skills (Burton, 1974; Goldberg & Rooke, 1967; Kirk, 1964; Louttit, 1957; McCarthy & Scheerenberger, 1966). Warren (1963) found that these children could memorize basic addition (and subtraction) facts by rote but that a concept of addition (and subtraction) and computational procedures for these operations appeared to be beyond their capacity. Using reinforcement procedures, children with moderate retardation have been trained to use concrete procedures for determining sums (Bellamy & Brown, 1972; Bellamy, Greiner, & Buttars, 1974), to count money (Bellamy & Buttars, 1975), and make change (Cuvo, Veitch, Trace, & Konki, 1978).

Research involving children with mild mental retardation has found that they were capable of basic addition and subtraction computation ability, but severely limited in terms of abstraction, concept formation, higher integrative abilities, and mathematical reasoning (Cornwall, 1974; Cruickshank, 1948a; Kirk, 1964; Noffsinger & Dobbs, 1970; Quay, 1963). For instance, Cruickshank (1948b) found their computational proficiency was impaired because of (a) a reliance on immature procedures such as finger counting and (b) a lack of understanding of subtraction procedures.

2. EMERGING VIEW

Recent research suggests that children with mental retardation can actively invent and transfer strategies for learning or memory tasks if presented clear-cut and simple tasks for which they are developmentally ready (e.g., see reviews by Bray & Turner, 1986; Cherkes-Julkowski & Gertner, 1989; Ferretti, 1989; Ferreti & Cavalier, 1991). Until recently, though, little was known about such children's conceptual understanding of school-related concepts or their strategic use of this knowledge (cf. Cherkes-Julkowski & Gertner, 1989; Mastropieri, Bakker, & Scuggs, 1991; Schied, 1990).

B. Evidence Supporting the Emerging View

This subsection will focus on three critical elements of basic mathematical knowledge: counting, numbers, and addition. Table II summarizes the focus and sample used in the principal studies ($n > 5$ subjects) discussed in this subsection.

1. COUNTING

Prior to 1975 or so, oral and object counting were basically considered to be skills that were learned by rote. Indeed, oral counting was often referred to as "rote counting" and considered by some to be a relatively unimportant development. For example, Piaget (1965) dismissed reciting the number-word sequence as a verbal and meaningless act. Moreover, evidence that object counting did not guarantee success on the number-conservation task led some psychologists to conclude that this skill did not guarantee an understanding of number (e.g., Piaget, 1965; Wohlwill & Lowe, 1962).

Gelman and Gallistel (1978), however, concluded that preschool children appear to understand, at least implicitly, fundamental counting principles (see Table III). Indeed, principle-first proponents have argued that basic counting principles develop first (as a result of an innate endowment) and guide the construction of counting skills (e.g., Gelman & Meck, 1992). Others (skills-first proponents) have countered that counting skills develop first and permit the discovery of counting principles (Briars & Siegler, 1984). In this view, children learn counting skills by means of imitation and reinforcement. Because skills are acquired in a piecemeal manner and are only gradually integrated, performance across even similar tasks is inconsistent. By applying their counting skills, children only slowly discover general counting principles and perform more coherently on counting tasks. Yet others have suggested that the development of counting concepts and skills is interwoven (see, e.g., Baroody, 1992a; Baroody & Ginsburg, 1986; Fuson, 1988). Although there is still an ongoing debate about the developmental relationship between counting concepts and counting skills, psychologists generally agree that rules or principles play an important role in the development of preschoolers' counting.

Evidence that NMH preschool children have a more conceptual understanding of counting than previously thought led some researchers to explore whether or not the same might be true for children with mental retardation. Below I discuss, in turn, the evidence that these children have any understanding of (a) general counting principles and (b) specific counting skills.

a. Evidence of Counting Principles. Research on the understanding of counting principles by children with mental retardation has yielded mixed, but encouraging, results.

i. EARLY EVIDENCE OF NONPRINCIPLED LEARNING. Cornwall (1974) concluded that his subjects with Down syndrome (DS) learned to count via rote associa-

TABLE II

SUMMARY OF THE FOCUS AND SAMLE OF THE PRINCIPAL STUDIES ON CHILDREN WITH MENTAL RETARDATION DISCUSSED IN THIS CHAPTER

Study	Focus	Sample			
		n	Classification[a]	IQ range	CA range (yrs.-mos.)[b]
Baroody (1986a)	Counting principles and skills	11	Moderate	33 to 49	6–10 to 12–10
		2	Mild	51 & 60	5–10 & 6–9
Baroody (1986b)	Counting principles and skills	13	K–5 moderate	33 to 50	6–0 to 10–10
		23	6–8 moderate	36 to 50	11–0 to 14–2
		37	K–5 mild	51 to 80	5–10 to 10–11
		27	6–8 mild	51 to 80	11–1 to 13–3
Baroody (1987b)	Commutative property of addition	34	Moderate	31 to 49	6–10 to 20–10
		17	Mild	52 to 75	10–2 to 20–11
Baroody (1988a)	Numeral writing	5	Moderate	30 to 45	10–3 to 12–8
		2	Mild	54 & 74	9–1 & 6–11
Baroody (1988b)	Mental addition	24	Moderate	31 to 49	6–10 to 20–10
		6	Mild	52 to 66	10–2 to 20–11
Baroody (1988c)	Number comparisons	22	Moderate and mild	36 to 74	6–6 to 16–4
Baroody (1995)	Informal addition	8	Moderate	<40 to 49	6–10 to 20–0
		3	Mild	56 to 66	10–2 to 20–6
Baroody (1996)	Informal addition	13	Experimental	33 to 57	6–10 to 20–6
		15	Control	31 to 66	10–2 to 20–10
Baroody & Snyder (1983)	Counting principles and skills	15	Moderate	30 to 47	17 to 20; $M = 19$
Caycho, Gunn, & Siegel (1991)	Counting principles and skills	15	DS NMH	40 to 60	(M 9–7; $SD = 1–2$)
		15	Preschool	(average)	($M = 4–6$; $SD = 0–8$)
Gelman & Cohen (1988)	Counting principles	10	DS group	43 to 73	10 to 13
		16	4-yr comparison	(average)	4–0 to 4–11
		16	5-yr comparison	(average)	5–0 to 5–11
Spradlin and others (1974)	Counting skills	49	Severe/moderate	12 to 50	8–10 to 15–1

[a]DS, Down syndrome; NMH, nonmentally handicapped.
[b]CA, chronological age.

TABLE III
COUNTING PRINCIPLES[a]

1. *Stable-order principle*: Numbers must be generated in the same sequence on every count.
2. *One-to-one principle*: Every item in a set has to be tagged once but only once.
3. *Abstraction principle*: Diverse items may be treated as elements of a set for counting purposes.
4. *Cardinality principle*: In counting a set, the last tag summarizes the count—i.e., represents the set.
5. *Order-irrelevance principle*: Elements of a set may be counted in any order, and this does not affect the outcome of counting (the cardinal designation of the set).

[a]From Gelman & Gallistel, 1978.

tive learning. Brown and DeLoache (1978), likewise, concluded that children with mental retardation learn to count by rote.

ii. EVIDENCE OF A CRITICAL MENTAL AGE? Gelman (1982) found some evidence that children with mental retardation used counting principles. However, she found no evidence of a stable-order or a cardinality principle in subjects with a mental age (MA) of less than 4 years. Gelman (1982) concluded that there may be a critical MA for applying or learning basic counting principles.

Baroody (1986a) studied 11 children with moderate retardation and 2 with mild retardation with MAs ranging from 3 to 4 years and drawn from classes that had a program that focused on basic counting skills. Although the performance of these children varied greatly, a few did exhibit evidence of counting principles. It appears that, with proper instruction, at least some children with mental retardation with an MA of less than 4 years are capable of using or learning counting principles.

iii. MORE RECENT EVIDENCE OF NONPRINCIPLED LEARNING? Gelman and Cohen (1988) compared the counting performance of children with DS with that of NMH children with similar MAs in order to demonstrate that development of counting is typically guided by innate principles.[2] They cited Cornwall (1974) and, interestingly, Gelman (1982) as evidence that children with DS learn to count by rote associative processes. Gelman and Cohen (1988) argued that if NMH children learned in the same way, their performance on novel counting tasks that required application of counting principles should be similar to that of children with DS. They further argued that, if NMH children had implicit knowledge of the counting principles, they should perform better on novel counting tasks or benefit more from explicit hints or repetitions of incorrect trials.

Gelman and Cohen's (1988) 4- and 5-year-old NMH children were more successful than eight of their 10 participants with DS on initial trials and even more

[2]Gelman and Cohen (1988) reported that they did not obtain MAs for their comparison group. Based on socioeconomic data, they estimated that these participants' MAs would be slightly higher than their CAs. Presumably, then, the MAs for the comparison group would have ranged from about 49 months to about 72 months. The range of MA for the DS sample was 48 months to 82 months.

so on repeated trials. These results were interpreted to mean that the NMH participants benefited from innate knowledge of basic counting principles. Gelman and Cohen (1988) further concluded that the eight participants with DS might have had the same innate endowment, but that such children have difficulty in mapping counting symbols to these underlying principles:

> It is . . . entirely possible that children with DS do have some early, implicit understanding of some counting principles but fail to develop them because of limits on their abilities to master mathematical meanings of count words and other mathematical symbols. (p. 93)

Gelman and Cohen's (1988) evidence and conclusions need to be considered cautiously because of difficulties with their methodology and analysis (see Baroody, 1992a, for a detailed critique). For example, their participants with DS were administered a somewhat different and, arguably, more difficult novel task than were their NMH participants (Baroody, 1992a; Caycho, Gunn, & Siegal, 1991).

What is particularly interesting about Gelman and Cohen's (1988) results is that two of their participants with DS *outperformed* the NMH preschoolers. Like the Baroody (1986a) study, then, this study found enormous individual differences in principled counting knowledge. Although the reasons for these individual differences are unclear, the performance of the two exceptional participants with DS raises the possibilities that such children can apply basic counting principles—whether innate or learned.

iv. More Recent Evidence of Principled Counting. Caycho et al. (1991) found that 15 children with DS (mean Peabody Picture Vocabulary Test—Revised [PPVT-R] = 4 years 7 months [4–7], mean IQ = 48) performed as well on counting-principle tasks as did NMH preschoolers with matching MAs and concluded that "counting by children with Down syndrome can be guided by counting principles" (p. 581). Again, though, significant individual differences were evident.

b. Development of Specific Counting Competencies. Discussed next is the evidence regarding the specific counting principles listed in Table III and the development of the following related counting skills: oral counting (generating the number-word sequence), object counting (counting a collection to determine its numerosity), cardinality (using the last number-word when counting a collection to represent the whole collection), and set production (counting out or creating a collection of a specified size).

i. Oral Counting. Although NMH children memorize the first twelve counting numbers by rote, they appear to master the rest of the number-word sequence by inducing a set of rules—that is, by discovering counting patterns and, at least, implicitly formulating prescriptions such as "two-digit numbers are formed by combining a decade term such as *twenty* with each of the first nine numbers (e.g., *twenty-one, twenty-two, twenty-three . . .*)."

Spradlin, Cotter, Stevens, and Friedman (1974) found that only 27% of their 48 participants with severe to moderate retardation (mean IQ = 35.2) could accurately count up to *five*. In other words, almost three-fourths of this sample appeared not to have even memorized most of the rote portion of the counting sequence. However, Fuson (1988) has cautioned that many children are not motivated to count orally when it has no purpose and recommended that oral counting be practiced and tested in the context of object counting. Interestingly, 45% of participants in the Spradlin et al. (1974) study accurately counted collections up to five—passed an object-counting task that required orally counting up to *five*. The moral here is that researchers should take care to test all children with engaging tasks.

Other research on children with mental retardation indicates that they are capable of rule-governed counting. Several studies suggest they can discover rules for counting to 30 or even 100 (Baroody, 1986b; Baroody & Snyder, 1983; Gelman, 1982). Baroody (1986b) found, for example, that—like NMH children—children with moderate or mild retardation made rule-governed errors, such as substituting "five-teen" for *fifteen*, "two-teen" for *twenty*, and "twenty-ten" for *thirty*. Ginsburg (1977) suggested that spontaneous systematic counting errors are a clear sign children are active learners. That is, given that it is highly unlikely that such errors were modeled or rewarded by teachers, parents, or others, they are almost surely the result of a relatively sensible overapplication of an induced counting rule.

Consider also the case of Katie, an elementary-level child with mild retardation (Baroody, 1998). Asked to count as high as she could, the girl counted up to 39 and then paused. She counted to herself, "One, two, three, four," and then announced, "40." Next, Katie quickly listed off 41 to 49 and paused again. She counted to herself, "One, two, three, four, five," announced, "Fifty," quickly listed off 51 to 59, and again determined the next decade by counting by ones. She repeated this process until she got to 100. In brief, this child recognized that the decade sequence parallels the one-to-nine sequence and is, in general, formed by adding the suffix *-ty* to these terms.

Ezawa (1996) extended previous findings. In case studies of two 18-year-olds with moderate retardation, she found that her participants exhibited some rule-governed counting to 1,000. For example, Anne counted, "498, 499, 400, 501, 502 . . ." (the substitution of the incorrect hundreds term *400* paralleled her incorrect substitutions of decade terms in counting to 100, e.g., ". . . 48, 49, *40*, 51, 52 . . .") or, later and more often, ". . . 508, 509, 600, 601, 602 . . .". Benno, who seemed to have better number sense for multidigit numbers, even recognized that there is no largest number; he deduced that the number-word sequence must go on indefinitely. He also once mentioned that neither the numbers from 1 to 100 and or 1 to 1000 had an exact middle value (e.g., the middle point of 1 to 100 is 50.5).

Baroody (1986a) attempted to assess whether or not children with mental retardation with MAs from 3 to 4.5 years know—at least implicitly—a stable-order principle (e.g., consistently use a conventional sequence or a combination of a conventional and nonconventional sequence, such as "one, two, three, seven, eight, nine, eleven, nineteen"). Most participants were not consistent over trials, and only four of 13 showed some consistency. Additional qualitative analyses suggested that only two children appeared to apply the stable-order principle. The data were consistent with that of young NMH children (see review by Fuson, 1988).

Caycho et al. (1991) obtained similar results with children with DS and a somewhat more advanced MA. Five of their 15 participants exhibited some knowledge of the stable-order principle, which was the same proportion of success of NMH preschools with matching MAs. None of the children, though, met the stringent criterion of a stable sequence—finished with a consistent nonconventional string of terms. This research, Baroody's (1986a) study, and research with NMH children (e.g., Fuson, 1988) suggest that a well-developed stable-order principle is a relatively sophisticated counting concept.

ii. Object Counting. To gauge a relatively explicit understanding of the one-to-one principle, Gelman and Cohen (1988) administered a novel object-counting task. This problem-solving task entailed, for example, pointing to the third item in a five-item array and asking children to count the whole collection starting with the third item (i.e., labeling it *one*). Gelman and Cohen (1988) found that two of their eight participants with DS were correct on about 90% of the trials and performed flawlessly when a tester provided help after an incorrect response. Indeed, these children outperformed both 4- and 5-year-old NMH children with similar mental ages. The remaining participants with DS, though, were less successful than those in the comparison group (about a 20% success rate) and benefited far less from the help provided by testers. Consistent with this latter finding, Caycho et al.'s (1991) 15 participants with DS had a mean success rate of only 0.7 trials on a five-trial novel object-counting task. Put differently, only five of their participants with mental retardation were correct on at least one trial. Four of the 15 NMH preschoolers in the comparison group had some success, and three were completely successful.

To gauge an implicit understanding of the one-to-one principle, Caycho et al. (1991) used an error-detection task. This task involves, for instance, showing a participant a hand puppet counting a collection of five small toys, correctly on some trials and incorrectly on others (e.g., not counting a middle item or counting an item twice). For each trial, a child is asked whether the puppet counted correctly or incorrectly. Even with a rigorous criterion (success = all six trials correct, $p = .016$, Sign test), these researchers found that 40% of their participants with moderate to mild retardation were successful on this task. To further gauge an implicit understanding of the one-to-one principle, Caycho et al. (1991) had their participants count collections of five and eight items. Two-thirds of their participants were successful on this task. Although Spradlin et al. (1974) found children with severe to moderate retardation had a lower success rate (45% successful with collections of 1 to 5), other researchers have found that children with moderate retardation had success rates with collections of about 5 to 8 items comparable to, or even higher than, that reported by Caycho et al. (1991) (e.g., Baroody, 1986b; Baroody & Snyder, 1983). Success rates for children with mild mental retardation of the same chronological age typically are even higher (Baroody, 1986b).[3] Although successfully counting collections does not guarantee that a child has an implicit understanding of the one-to-one principle because it is possible to learn this skill by rote, it does represent an important achievement.

To gauge an implicit understanding of the abstraction principle, Baroody and Snyder (1983) asked children with moderate retardation to count a collection of four different items (a domino, barrette, stamp, and paper clip). All 15 of their participants were willing to treat diverse items as a collection for the purpose of counting. Other studies have used counting tasks consisting of items that differed in size, color, or appearance and found that this did not prevent children with mental retardation from enumerating the collections (e.g., Baroody & Mason, 1984; Caycho et al., 1991). In brief, these children seemed to understand the abstraction principle, at least implicitly. Less clear is when and how this principle and the one-to-one principle develop and whether or not they could explain these principles.

iii. CARDINALITY. Various investigators (e.g., Fuson, 1988; Gelman & Gallistel, 1978; Schaeffer, Eggleston, & Scott, 1974) have found that young NMH children will use the last number word when counting a set to respond to "*How many*?" questions. Such behavior, sometimes taken as evidence for a cardinality principle, might more properly be taken as evidence for only a cardinality rule: The last number word has special significance because others accept it as the answer to *How many?* questions (Fuson & Hall, 1983; von Glasersfeld, 1982). More elaborate evidence is needed to demonstrate that children recognize the last number word represents the cardinal designation of the set.

Spradlin et al. (1974) found that only a minority (45%) of children with mental retardation could successfully count and state the number in a collection of up to five items. In contrast, Baroody and Snyder (1983) found all of their secondary-level participants with moderate retardation used the cardinality rule. Both Baroody (1986b) and Caycho et al. (1991) found that a majority of their participants with moderate or mild retardation were successful on collections of up to 10 items.

[3]Hoard, Geary, and Hamson (in press) found that 19 children (mean CA = 7-0) with low IQ (IQs of 65 to 84) recognized the standard left-to-right count of a collection as correct. Moreover, they also accepted right-to-left counting as correct and were able to identify object-counting errors at least for smaller collections. They did poorly on a pseudotrial that involved starting with a middle chip, counting the chips of one color, and then returning to the left end to count the chips of a different color. However, their performance on this last task was not significantly different from children with average IQ (IQs 85 to 115) or children with high IQ (IQs > 115).

Furthermore, there is at least some evidence that children with mental retardation can be successful on tasks that suggest a deeper understanding of cardinality: order-irrelevance, finger-correspondence, and set-production tasks.

1. The order-irrelevance task serves to evaluate whether or not a child recognizes that a collection will have the same number of item (cardinality) regardless of the order in which items are counted. Baroody and Snyder (1983) found that 80% of their participants with moderate retardation were successful on such a task involving four items. In contrast, Baroody (1986b) found that only 38% and 31% of his participants with moderate retardation were successful on at least three of four order-irrelevance trials involving sets of 2 to 5 and 6 to 10, respectively. A majority (59%) of children with mild retardation had similar success on the smaller sets, but only a minority (49%) were largely successful on the larger sets.
2. The finger-correspondence task entails asking children to display a specified number of fingers (create a model of a cardinal value). Baroody (1986b) found that a majority of his participants with moderate retardation and nearly all of his participants with mild retardation could automatically display up to five fingers, and many could quickly display up to 10 fingers.
3. The set-production task requires what Fuson (e.g., 1988) calls the *cardinal-count concept*, an appreciation that, for example, the cardinal term "five" predicts the outcome of counting a set of five objects. In a sense, this concept is the reverse of the cardinality (count-cardinal) rule. Whereas the former involves starting with a cardinal label or the total for a collection and recognizing that it is equivalent to counting the collection (e.g., *Five* = "one, two, three, four, five"), the latter begins with counting the collection and recognizing that the last tag designates its cardinal value or the total (e.g., "One, two, three, four, five" = *five*). Spradlin et al. (1974), Baroody and Snyder (1983), and Baroody (1986b) all found that only a minority of children with moderate retardation could produce sets of up to five items (31%, 20%, and 38%, respectively). Caycho et al. (1991) found that 8 of their 15 children with moderate to mild retardation could produce a set of five items, and 7 could produce a set of eight items—a performance identical to NMH children with a similar MA. Baroody (1986b) found that 81% of his participants with mild retardation successfully produced sets of 2 to 5 items, and most could do so with 6 to 10 items.

Gelman (1982), however, found no evidence of the cardinality rule in children with mental retardation with mental ages of less than 4.5 years. Contrary to Gelman's (1982) finding, though, Baroody (1986a) found that 9 of his 13 participants with mental retardation with a MA of 3 to 4.5 consistently used the last number word counted to answer *How many?* questions. Indeed, it appears that some understood or could apply more sophisticated aspects of cardinality. Five children appeared to understand that changing the order of a count would not affect the cardinal designation of a set (the order-irrelevance principle). Over half were capable of creating cardinal models of the numbers one to five with their fingers, and most could do so automatically (finger correspondence). Finally, three children counted out two to five items correctly on at least half of the trials (set production).

iv. SET PRODUCTION. Counting out a specified number of items is a relatively difficult counting task because of the multiple demands put on working memory: (a) register the target (the cardinal term requested); (b) label each object taken with a tag from the number-word sequence; and (c) compare the tags against the target in order to stop the counting process. A common error among young NMH children and children with mental retardation is a failure to stop the counting process after reaching the target (Baroody & Snyder, 1983; Spradlin et al., 1974; Wang, Resnick, & Boozer, 1971). For example, Matt, a child with mental retardation, was shown eight pencils and asked to take five. The child simply counted all eight pencils (Baroody, 1987a).

"No-stop" errors have been attributed to two types of memory failures (e.g., Resnick & Ford, 1981). According to the "register-deficit" hypothesis, children may fail to register the specified amount or become so involved in the counting process, they forget the target value. In short, children do not have a basis for stopping the production process, because they do not have or hold the target in working memory. According to the "matching-failure" hypothesis, a work overload prevents working memory from simultaneously processing required information. That is, even though children register (and may later recall) the target, the counting process so taxes working memory they fail to match the target to the number words of the counting process. Thus, according to the register-deficit and matching-failure hypotheses, no-stop errors are due to either not having or not keeping the goal of the task in mind.

However, some NMH toddlers (Wagner & Walters, 1982) and children with mental retardation (Baroody, 1986b) have set-production difficulties even when they remember the target. For example, Fred, a child with moderate retardation, made what can be called an *end-with-the target* error: Asked to count out three objects from a pile of five items, he responded, "1, 3, 4, 6, 11" and then *retagged* the last item "*3*." Asked to produce five items from a pile of nine things, the child responded: "1, 2, 3, 4, 5, 6, 8, 9, *5*." In brief, he typically exhibited a no-stop error but frequently *ended* his count with the target number. Although the child failed to stop when the target was first produced, he frequently appeared to remember it and so made sure that the last item was given this number. Brian, another boy with moderate retardation, regularly made this "end-with-the-target error," but usually after abbreviating his count. For example, in response to a request to count out four items, he responded, "1, 2, *4*." Asked for 12 items, Brian counted, "1, 2, *12*." Again, it appeared this child kept the goal in mind.

Note that end-with-the-target errors cannot be reconciled with a register-deficit hypothesis. Such errors, however, are not inconsistent with a matching-failure hypothesis. Fred, for example, may have failed to make the match because he could not simultaneously count objects and match the resulting tags to the target. At the end of the counting process—freed of executing two processes simultaneously—the child focused on the goal of the task and so labeled or relabeled the last item with the target number. Furthermore, Brian may have dealt with the overload on working memory posed by counting objects and matching by abbreviating the counting process (rather than losing track of the goal).

Another possibility is that some end-with-the-target errors are due to a conceptual deficit: the absence of a cardinal-count concept. That is, some children may not realize that they are supposed to match the target to their count. To evaluate the viability of the conceptual-deficit hypothesis, Baroody and Mason (1984) conducted a follow-up case study with Brian, who was 10 years old and had an IQ of 45.

Consistent with his previous test results discussed above, Brian—at least for the first two sessions—regularly abbreviated his counting and made the end-with-the-target error. His responses to the last two trials in session 1 are especially interesting. In each case, Brian paused at a critical point in the count and looked at the tester as though he were seeking guidance. In one case, he proceeded to produce the correct amount but, in the second, the lad proceeded to make a no-stop error. In this latter case, it was clear Brian remembered the target: He paused after counting out five objects but then continued counting out items. In response to the check question, Brian correctly indicated that he was supposed to have gotten *five* items. Moreover, he appeared to make some effort at matching the target value to his count but appeared unsure whether this was what he was supposed to do. That is, he apparently made an effort to simultaneously count and match, but was uncertain whether or not the *five* tag in his count represented the same quantity as the cardinal designation “five.”

During the course of the case study, Brian's production ability improved somewhat. During session 3, he correctly produced sets involving numbers he had never previously been successful with: five and, on second efforts, three and four. Because of the repeated testing, it may be that Brian was attempting to come to terms with the production task conceptually. This interpretation and a conceptual-deficit hypothesis are supported by his performance on cardinal-count tasks. It appeared that Brian's grasp of the cardinal-count concept was not secure or automatic. For example, given the cardinal designation “two” and asked to predict what the outcome of counting the set would be, he responded by counting “one, two.” For trials involving “three” and “five,” however, he could not predict the outcome of a count. In brief, it appeared that Brian did not know he had to match a number *in his count* to the target (rather than forgetting to make this match). Another possibility is that until applying the cardinal-count concept becomes automatic, it presents an extra processing burden and, thus, may help overload working memory.

By logical extension, no-stop errors may also be due to a conceptual deficit as well as memory failures. Indeed, a conceptual deficit may help to explain why some children fail to register the target or make a match. If children do not appreciate the cardinal-count concept, they have no reason to register the target or attempt a match. If the cardinal-count concept is less than automatic, the extra load on working memory may cause them to forget the target or overlook the matching process. Clearly, though, further research is needed to investigate what role conceptual factors play in production deficiencies.

2. NUMBER CONCEPTS

Counting experiences with a single collection of real things provide a key foundation for a concept of number. In time, children use their counting knowledge to construct more advanced number concepts and skills, such as precisely comparing the relative size of two (or more) collections of real things and, later, two (or more) cardinal numbers (representations of concrete collections). Moreover, concrete counting experiences provide a conceptual basis for understanding written number symbols (numerals). In this section, I discuss research on the basis of the following basic number skills: comparing numbers, connecting counting knowledge with written representations of numbers, and reading and writing numerals.

a. Comparing Numbers. An ability to gauge the relative magnitude of two numbers is a basic mathematical skill that has countless applications. For example, if a child has \$4 and an item costs \$5, the child must realize that five is greater than four to conclude that more money is needed to buy the item.

Research (e.g., Schaeffer et al., 1974; Siegler & Robinson, 1982; Wagner & Walters, 1982) indicates that, without formal training, young NMH children learn to use their mental representation of the number-word sequence to make magnitude comparisons (Resnick, 1983). Typically, they discover quite early that *the later a number comes in the sequence, the greater the quantity it represents.* This knowledge enables the typical 4-year-old to accurately compare numbers that are relatively far apart—to make *gross* comparisons between, say, 1 and 8, or 10 and 2. Children further discover the $N + 1 > N$ rule (The "number neighbor" coming later in the number-word sequence represents the larger quantity), a rule that allows them to compare familiar *adjacent* numbers, such as four and five or nine and eight (Ginsburg & Baroody, 1983; Schaeffer et al., 1974).

Knowledge of number-after relationships facilitates making number-neighbor comparisons (Resnick, 1983). Typically, 4- and 5-year-olds can automatically cite the next number for familiar portions of the number-word sequence (e.g., "after four comes five") (Fuson, 1988, 1992; Fuson, Richards, & Briars, 1982).

Baroody and Snyder (1983) found that secondary-level children with moderate retardation were correct on only 20% and 13% of the number-neighbor comparisons with numbers up to 5 and with numbers from 6 to 10, respectively (cf. Hoard et al., in press). These researchers also found that their participants generally lacked the prerequisite for mentally and efficiently comparing number neighbors.

Specifically, their sample was correct only 13% of the time when given 1 to 10 in random order and asked to specify the number after it.

Interestingly, Baroody and Snyder's (1983) participants had a much higher (73%) success rate on the written number-after task than on the verbal version. The most likely explanation for this discrepancy is that the former—unlike the latter—effectively provided the students a "running start" (i.e., encouraged them to count from *one* to the last listed number and then state the next number). For example, the written task involved presenting participants with the sequence 1, 2, 3, 4, __ and asked them to fill in the blank, instead of simply asking what number comes after *four*? as was done with the verbal task. Research with NMH children indicates that determining the number after another is easier with a running start than without one (e.g., Fuson, 1988, 1992).

If children with mental retardation can learn to specify the number after another with a running start, then they might be able to learn how to do so without a running start. If such children could become proficient in this latter skill, then they might be able to use it in the service of determining which of two number neighbors is larger (implementing the $N + 1 > N$ rule). To evaluate this hypothesis, Baroody (1988c) undertook a training experiment involving 22 children with mental retardation (mean IQ = 52). Half were randomly assigned to an experimental group, and the other half, to a control group. The experimental training focused on helping children master, in turn, number-after, gross number comparisons, and number-neighbor comparisons up to *five* (using the $N + 1 > N$ rule). On both immediate and delayed posttests, the experimental participants outperformed control participants on the trained number pairs (number-neighbor comparisons to *five*). The experimental participants also outperformed the control participants on three of the four transfer tasks on either the immediate or delayed posttest. On the immediate posttests, the difference was significant for the age comparison task (e.g., "Who is older—a 5-year-old or a 4-year-old?"), a near-transfer task. On the delayed posttest, the difference reached a significant level on two far-transfer tasks: number-neighbor comparisons of (a) 6 to 10 and (b) hundreds (e.g., 100 vs. 200 or 400 vs. 300). On both posttests, the scores of the two groups were essentially identical on the third far-transfer tasks, comparisons of 20s to 25 (e.g., 22 vs. 21 or 24 vs. 25).[4] Regression analyses indicated that IQ was not a significant factor in who was or was not successful on the trained number pairs or the transfer tasks.

[4]Although preliminary screening established that participants could count to *ten*, some may not have been familiar with the twenties number-word sequence, and, thus, the number-after another in this range. Participants could have solved the problem by focusing on the second or units place of the twenty terms (e.g., twenty-*two* vs. twenty-*one*, [twenty-]; the number with the *two* is larger), but did not. The experimental participants may have been more successful on the hundreds task because some focused on the first portion of the hundreds term (e.g., *two* hundred vs. *one* hundred). Clearly, though, this conjecture needs to be tested.

The results of Baroody (1988c) are consistent with more recent evidence that individuals with mental retardation can learn and apply a symbolic ordered sequence (see, e.g., Mackay, Kotlarchyk, & Stromer, 1997; Maydak, Stromer, Mackay, & Stoddard, 1995; Stromer, Mackay, Cohen, & Stoddard, 1993). Maydak et al. (1995), for example, studied a 30-year-old with a MA of about 7–9 and a 49-year-old with a MA of about 3–6. Pretesting or training established that these participants could correctly match collections of one to five items to a number word or a numeral (e.g., associated ••• with *three* or 3), recognize which of two collections or numerals was larger (e.g., identified ••• as larger than •• or 3 as larger than 2), and could correctly order collections or numerals (e.g., put in order the unordered set of numerals 1 to 5). Participants then were trained to equate each collection or numeral to a geometric form (e.g., 2 = ◇). Without further training, the participants correctly ordered the geometric forms (e.g., apparently viewed ◇ as the "second" geometric form). In other words, they appeared to transfer the ordinal relationships inherent in their knowledge of numbers.

Ezawa's (1996) work explored the ability of children with moderate retardation to compare multidigit numbers as well as one-digit numbers. Both of her participants could compare single-digit numbers, and Benno could compare two- or three-digit numbers (e.g., he recognized that 75 is greater than 57). Over a period of several years, Anne learned a rule for judging which of two three-digit numbers is larger: compare the left-most digit first (e.g., 345 is greater than 289 because three [hundred] is greater than two [hundred]).

b. Connecting Counting Knowledge to Written Representations of Numbers. Written representations of numbers include tallies (e.g., | | |), numerals (e.g., 3), and written number words (e.g., three). The connection between verbal number words and latter two (e.g., "three" → three) is discussed below.

i. Connection between Verbal Number Words and Numerals. Wang et al. (1971) found that, among NMH children, object-counting skills developed prior to numeral skills such as reading and writing numerals and matching numerals to sets. They concluded that, although numeral skills could be acquired by rote memorization "in a paired-associated-like fashion" prior to counting, functional counting typically serves as a basis for the meaningful learning of numeral skills and, thus, facilitates such learning.

Spradlin et al. (1974) found that children with moderate retardation were far more proficient on numeral skills than object-counting skills. They concluded that such children, unlike NMH children, entered school without a repertoire of informal counting skills. Because many curriculum designers and teachers assume that all children have functional counting skills, little or no time was spent on these foundational competencies. Instead, instruction focused on mastering numeral skills. Without the conceptual basis provided by counting experience, children with mental retardation simply learned numeral skills by rote. However, given the evidence that many of these children can learn functional counting skills (e.g., Baroody, 1986a, 1986b; Baroody & Snyder, 1983), there is no reason to believe that this outcome is inevitable.

Indeed, consider the case of Jay, a 10-year-old boy with severe retardation (Mackay et al., 1997). Pretesting established that the child had functional counting skills (e.g., he could count out a collection of three items upon request) and had some numeral skills (i.e., verbally given a number such as "three," he could correctly identify its corresponding numeral or, given a numeral, he could correctly create a corresponding collection). However, although Jay could orally state the numbers "one" to "nine" in the correct order, he could not correctly order the numerals 0 to 9. After training ordering the numerals 0 to 3, posttesting indicated he could correctly order the numerals 0 to 10. This transfer was probably aided by his knowledge of the oral counting sequence.

ii. CONNECTION BETWEEN VERBAL NUMBER WORDS AND WRITTEN NUMBER WORDS. Gast, VanBiervlient, and Spradlin (1979) found evidence that children with mental retardation can also spontaneously transfer counting knowledge to written number words. Pretesting established that three children with IQs of 50, 53, and 67 could, given a verbal number, identify the corresponding numeral (e.g., "three" → choose the numeral 3) or count out an appropriate number of items (e.g., "three" → produce three items). Moreover, given a numeral, they could identify a corresponding collection (e.g., 3 → choose the set •˙•) or verbally identify it (e.g., 3 → state "three"). Training focused on equating the written number words one to six to the corresponding verbal number word (e.g., "three" → choose the written number word *three*). Posttesting showed that, given a written number name, the participants could successfully complete the following unpracticed tasks: (a) count out a corresponding collection (e.g., three → produce three items), (b) identify the corresponding numeral (e.g., three → choose the numeral 3), and (c) identify a corresponding collection (e.g., three → choose the set •˙•). Maydak et al. (1997) obtained similar results with a child with severe retardation.

c. Numeral Literacy. Most children learn to read and write numerals with relatively little difficulty. However, some—particularly children with mental retardation—have considerable difficulty mastering these basic skills and, for a few, the difficulties continue well after the primary grades. In the past, difficulties such as reading a 6 as "nine" or writing a numeral in reverse were blamed on "associative confusions" or insufficient practice to establish an association or motor habit. Special educators have also commonly attributed numeral-reading and -writing difficulties to perceptual-motor deficiencies (e.g., Frostig, LeFever, & Whittlesey, 1964; Mann & Suiter, 1974; Sears, 1986). Cognitive theory and research suggests a different cause for these difficulties.

i. NUMERAL READING. In order to read numerals, children must be able to distinguish among these symbols. This requires constructing a mental image of each numeral: knowing its component parts and how the parts fit together to form the whole (Baroody, 1987a, 1998). For example, the numeral 6 consists of two parts (a curved line and a loop), which distinguishes it from all other numerals except 9. The relationship between these parts (the loop of a 6 joins the lower right-hand side of the curved line) distinguishes it from a 9 (in which the loop joins the *upper left-hand* side of the curved line).[5]

Children typically have little difficulty constructing a mental image of the numerals 1 to 9. Not surprisingly though, some may confuse numerals that share similar characteristics (2 and 5 or 6 and 9). A 6 and a 9, for example, are difficult to distinguish, because these numerals have the same parts and differ only in how the parts fit together: where the curve joins the loop.

Spradlin et al. (1974) found that 52% of their participants with moderate retardation could read the numerals 1 to 5. Baroody (1988b, 1988c, 1996) used reading the numerals 1 to 10 as a screening test item and consistently found that large numbers of children with mental retardation have mastered this basic skill (see also the case of Steven described below and in Baroody, 1988a).

Hoard et al. (1998) found that their young children with low IQs had difficulty reading numerals. These researchers suggested that this difficulty might be attributed to deficits in the system that transcodes (translates) numerals into number words (see McCloskey, Carmazza, & Basili, 1985, for a detailed discussion of such cognitive deficits). They also concluded that a more mundane explanation is that the children had not yet learned what number-word name corresponded to each numeral (i.e., had not yet constructed a mental image of each numeral). Although it is possible that some children with mental retardation have organic cognitive deficiencies that prevent translating from one symbol system to another, the fact that so many do learn to read numerals suggest the more prevalent source of difficulty is in constructing a mental image of each numeral. To distinguish between these causes of reading difficulties, researchers and educators need to assess learning potential (i.e., whether or not a particular child can benefit from instruction that focuses on helping him/her construct a mental image).

ii. NUMERAL WRITING. In order to write numerals, children must have an accurate mental image and a motor plan (a preplanned course of action for translating a mental image into motor actions). A motor plan specifies where to start (e.g., at the top of a line or just below it), in what direction to head (left, right, up, down, diagonally), what needs to be drawn (e.g., a straight line, an arc), when to stop a given step, how to change directions, how to begin the next step, and where to stop (Goodnow & Levine, 1973).

Unless children have an accurate step-by-step plan of execution in mind *before* they start writing a numeral, they may begin in the wrong place or head off in the

[5]In fact, a completely accurate mental image is not necessary to distinguish among, identify, or read numerals. Children could, for example, distinguish between a 6 and a 9 without left–right orientation. If a child recognized that the loop of the 6 is at the bottom, not the top, there is no need to know also that the loop is on the right-hand side of the line. A completely accurate mental image is, however, necessary in order to write numerals correctly.

wrong direction. The result may be writing a numeral backwards (Ɣ) or some other error (⌐). Without an accurate motor plan, children may make a mistake repeatedly, despite efforts to get them to look carefully at a model numeral.

Consider the case of Steven, an 11-year-old student with moderate retardation (Baroody, 1988a). Diagnostic testing indicated that he could read the numerals 1 to 10. However, except for 1, 2, and 4, he was unable to write the single-digit numerals. Asked to draw a seven, he drew † and commented, "Oh, this is a 't,' this isn't right." For "three," he drew s and said, "This is a 's.' How do you make a three?" Steven could *see* that his seven and three were drawn incorrectly. Although he apparently realized that the written forms did not match his mental image of the numerals, Steven did not have a preplanned method for translating the mental image into appropriate motor actions. Aware of his problem at some level, the lad, in effect, requested guidance in constructing a motor plan for the numeral 3.

Baroody (1988a) undertook a demonstration project to check the feasibility of using a cognitive-based instructional approach with children with mental retardation. The training focused on helping participants with moderate or mild retardation learn motor plans for each numeral 1 to 10. To aid in giving step-by-step instructions for writing each numeral, writing paper from the *Recipe for Reading Program* (Traub, 1977) was used. Figures on the paper aided in giving left–right and up–down directions. Instructors described motor plans as they modeled writing a numeral, physically guided a child's writing, or while a child practiced numeral writing. Participants were also encouraged to rehearse motor plans themselves.

Posttesting after 12 weeks of training indicated that six of the seven participants had made substantial progress. More specifically, the children were, on average, able to write 3.9 numerals correctly before training and 8.1 numerals after the training. The results are particularly impressive because the participants were tested using a blank sheet of paper, not the paper with directional cues used in the training. In brief, the demonstration project indicated that children with mental retardation could successfully internalize a motor plan.

3. ADDITION

Research indicates that informal addition knowledge of NMH children is surprisingly rich (e.g., Ginsburg, 1977; Starkey, in press). For example, without instruction, they first construct concrete counting strategies for determining sums, then verbal (abstract) counting strategies, and finally more advanced reasoning and retrieval strategies (e.g., Steinberg, 1985). Furthermore, they informally discover important mathematical regularities such as additive commutativity: the order in which addends are added does not affect the sum (e.g., $5 + 3 = 3 + 5 = 8$). Mentally retarded children's development of addition strategies, with an emphasis on the concrete and abstract counting strategies, is discussed first. Their mental-arithmetic ability, which includes the more advanced strategies of reasoning and retrieval, is treated second. Their knowledge of additive commutativity is then addressed.

a. Strategy Development. Recent research suggests that NMH children spontaneously invent increasingly efficient counting procedures to compute sums (see, e.g., literature reviews by Baroody & Ginsburg, 1986; Carpenter, 1986; Fuson, 1992; Resnick & Ford, 1981; Siegler & Jenkins, 1989). Table IV lists the main achievements in strategy development, including the milestone of counting-on, and illustrative strategies.

A lack of self-initiated learning, including the inability to transform existing strategies into more sophisticated strategies, is often considered a key distinguishing characteristic of children with mental retardation (see, e.g., reviews by Cherkes-Julkowski & Gertner, 1989; Ferretti & Cavalier, 1991). Perhaps because of this assumption, earlier research efforts focused on teaching these children addition strategies by rote. For example, Bellamy et al. (1974) taught children with moderate retardation to count-on by rote. Until recently, there is almost no evidence that such children can spontaneously invent more sophisticated addition strategies.

i. Evidence of Spontaneous Inventions and Progress. Baroody (1987a) reported a case study of a 19.5-year-old male with moderate retardation who seemed to adjust his computational strategy when he encountered more difficult addition combinations. With small items such as 3 + 5, Mike concretely represented each addend with a finger pattern and counted all the fingers (a shortcut for direct modeling; Achievement 2 in Table IV). Apparently aware that this strategy would not work well with larger items such as 2 + 8 and 6 + 3, he represented only the smaller added, verbally counted up to the cardinal value of the larger addend, and then continued the count while pointing to each of the previously extended figures (i.e., switched to a strategy that involved disregarding addend order and indirectly modeling the starting amount; Achievements 5 and 3 in Table IV, respectively). It is unlikely that anyone taught Mike this computational shortcut. Unfortunately, he was not provided further computational opportunities, and follow-up testing 5 months later found no evidence of this adaptation. Mike had reverted to using direct modeling or inappropriate strategies.

Baroody (1996) undertook a training experiment that included 30 children with moderate or mild retardation to see if they could spontaneously invent more efficient addition strategies for determining simple sums (e.g., 5 + 3); apply these strategies to larger, unpracticed combinations (e.g., 8 + 3); and retain these strategies after 5 months. A pretest provided baseline data for strategy use. Less than a fourth of the children used an appropriate strategy, typically a direct-modeling strategy (concrete counting-all or a shortcut for this procedure; Achievement 1 or 2 in Table IV). The remaining children had no organized strategy for adding and had to be taught the concrete counting-all procedure.

Interestingly, the vast majority of the children showed high learning potential,

TABLE IV
MAJOR ACHIEVEMENTS IN THE DEVELOPMENT OF ADDITION STRATEGIES AND ILLUSTATIVE STRATEGIES USING 3 + 5 AS AN EXAMPLE

Achievement	Strategy
1. *Direct modeling.* Children's first appropriate addition strategy typically involves using objects concretely to represent and to answer problems.	*Concrete counting-all strategy*—a counting strategy that involves (a) directly modeling *both* addends and (b) a separate sum count. For 3 + 5, for example, a child might count out three blocks to concretely represent the starting amount 3, count out five blocks to concretely represent the added-on amount 5, and then count all eight blocks to determine the sum.
2. *Shortcutting the direct model.* Children take a small, but useful, step by using patterns to shortcut one or more steps in the concrete counting-all procedure.	*Concrete counting-all shortcut strategies* include using finger patterns to represent each addend. For 3 + 5, for example, a child could automatically raise three fingers on one hand and five on the other hand to represent the addends, instead of counting and successively raising three fingers on one hand and five fingers on the other hand.
3. *Indirect modeling.* Children take an important step forward when they no longer have to concretely represent an addend.	*Concrete counting of added-on amount strategies*—counting strategies that involve indirectly modeling the starting amount and directly modeling the added-on amount with objects either sequentially or simultaneously *before* the sum count. For 3 + 5, for example, a child might first count and successively extend five fingers to represent the added-on amount. Next, the child would *verbally* count up to the cardinal value of the starting amount (*one, two, three*) and then continue this count as she pointed, in turn, to each of the previously extended fingers (*four, five, six, seven, eight*). Such strategies are particularly useful when at least one addend is larger than five, making it difficult or impossible to represent both addends on the fingers of two hands.
4. *Keeping track.* This watershed development enables children to continue a verbal count from a number for a specified interval and, thus, permits	*Abstract counting strategies*—counting strategies that involve indirectly modeling both the starting amount and the added-on amount and, thus, require a sequential

continues

TABLE IV. *(continued)*

Achievement	Strategy
the development of relatively abstract counting strategies	keeping-track process done in tandem with a sum count. For 3 + 5, for instance, a child might "count-all beginning with the first addends." Verbally count out the starting amount ("One, two, three") and then count "four [is one more], five [is two more], six [is three more], seven [is four more], eight [is five more]." Note that the portion in brackets is the keeping-track process.
5. *Disregarding addend order*. Simultaneously executing a sum count and a keeping-track count puts a heavy burden on working memory. With small-addend-first combinations such as 3 + 5, disregarding the order of the addends can minimize the keeping-track count and, thus, greatly reduce the load on working memory.	*Abstract counting strategies that disregard addend order* such as "counting-all beginning with the larger addend." For 3 + 5, this could take the form of starting with one, counting up to the cardinal value of the larger addend ("one two, three, four, five . . ."), and then continuing the count for three more terms: "six [is one more], seven [is two more], eight [is three more]."
6. *Counting-on*. Counting-on (starting with the cardinal value of the starting amount) —instead of counting all (counting up to the value of the cardinal value of the starting amount)—is a significant advance.	*Abstract counting strategies that involve counting-on* such as "counting-on from the larger addend." For 3 + 5, for instance, this might take the form of stating the larger addend ("five") and counting on three more times: "six [is one more], seven [is two more], eight [is three more]."
7. *Reasoning and recall*. Using known combinations to reason out the sums of unknown combinations (e.g., Because 3 + 3 is 6 and 4 is one more than 3, then 4 + 3 must be 7) and recalling sums from memory represent momentous achievements.	*Reasoning strategy*—an advanced strategy that involves deriving a sum by reasoning from a known fact (e.g., if 3 + 1 is four, then 3 + 2 must be five because 2 is one more than 1). *Fact recall*—an advanced strategy that involves generating a sum in 2 seconds or less without any apparent computing or reasoning.

as they required only one or two demonstrations of the strategy in order to learn it. Moreover, one-third of the children began to use shortcuts soon after they were shown a basic addition procedure. That is, they spontaneously began to use patterns to short-cut the direct modeling procedure (Achievement 2 in Table IV). The most common shortcut involved representing each addend with a finger pattern. Although incorporating finger patterns into a counting strategy for computing sums does not represent a major advance in addition sophistication, it nevertheless is an adaptation.

Over a 6-month period, the experimental group was given regular opportunities to practice computing sums. On both the immediate and the delayed posttest, these participants used significantly more sophisticated strategies than did the control participants on practiced items and were significantly more likely to use an appropriate strategy on larger unpracticed items. More specifically, without explicit instruction, most experimental children invented shortcuts for the concrete counting-all procedure they were taught or already knew (Achievement 2 in Table IV), and some participants adopted a variety of strategies. Many apparently recognized that their existing knowledge of finger patterns was useful for short-cutting the representation of an addend or the sum count. Moreover, a number of experimental participants appeared to make major advances. Two invented abstract counting strategies that involved a keeping-track process and disregarding addend order (Achievements 4 and 5, respectively, in Table IV). Indeed, one of these children invented and retained a strategy that also involved counting-on (Achievement 6 in Table IV). Furthermore, several experimental participants began using recall during the course of the study (Achievement 7).

The evidence pointed to spontaneous strategy development and transfer. Although trainers provided feedback about the correctness of answers, they neither modeled nor described more advanced procedures. Training records indicated that on several occasions, telling experimental participants their answer was incorrect apparently had the effect of prompting them to reflect on their strategy and to make adjustments. In many other cases, though, strategy adjustments appeared to be a way of short-cutting an *already accurate and rewarded strategy*. (Correct responses were rewarded in the sense that a child did not have to recompute an answer. Note that such a reward is risked by trying a new and unproven strategy.) For example, given 4 + 5 on the immediate posttest, Chris initially tried to use, but abandoned, an abstract counting strategy that honored addend order. In an apparent effort to minimize the keeping-track process, he then switched to an abstract counting strategy that disregarded addend order.

In a case study of an 8-year-old whose intellectual performance was two to three years below age level, Bråten (1996), likewise, found evidence of self-initiated strategy development, differentiation, and flexibility. Initially, the child used a concrete counting-all (a direct-modeling) strategy. Over the course of several months, she invented the abstract strategy of counting-on from the larger addend (Achievements 3, 4, 5, and 6 in Table IV).

ii. Counting-on. How children invent a counting-on strategy has long remained a mystery. Using a microgenetic methodology, Siegler and Jenkins (1989), for example, found that children had relatively long solution times both on the trial before inventing a counting-on procedure and on the trial itself. They concluded that invention of this important strategy was accompanied by heightened cognitive activity but did not specify the cause or nature of this activity. Speculation about the basis for inventing counting-on has run the gamut from nonconceptual factors (e.g., Neches, 1987) to conceptual learning (e.g., Fuson, 1982, 1992; Secada, Fuson, & Hall, 1983). For instance, Resnick and Neches (1984), attributed this invention to the nonconceptual factor of saving mental labor, namely eliminating redundancy and minimizing the load on working memory. At the other extreme, Cobb (1986) concluded that both counting-on and mastering $n + 1$ combinations such as 5 + 1 or 8 + 1 are due to the construction of an elaborated cardinality concept, namely the cardinal-count concept.

The case study of Steven (IQ = 46; chronological age [CA] = 11–9) led Baroody (1995) to propose a plausible developmental mechanism for counting-on. The child's mastery of a few $n + 1$ combinations suddenly extended to include all such combinations, suggesting he had discovered the number-after-*n* rule: The sum of $n + 1$ is the number after *n* in the number-word sequence. Shortly after Steven began responding to $n + 1$ combinations automatically, he spontaneously invented a counting-on strategy. Follow-up analyses of nine other children with mental retardation and five NMH kindergartners were consistent with this finding.

Apparently, the number-after-*n* rule for $n + 1$ combinations serves as a scaffold for constructing a counting-on strategy (Baroody, 1995). That is, children appear to realize, for example, that if the sum of 7 + 1 is eight (the number after *seven*), then 7 + 2 must be two numbers after *seven* in the number-word sequence.

b. Mental Arithmetic. How children memorize the single-digit (basic) addition combinations such as 8 + 3 = 11 and why they make such mental-addition errors as 8 + 3 = 10 has long been debated (see, e.g., reviews by Ashcraft, 1992; Baroody, 1994a). Thorndike (1922), for instance, argued that children master a combination by making and strengthening an association with the correct answer. In his associative-learning view, the key to mastery was repetitive practice of each basic combination. In this view, mental-arithmetic errors are basically the by-product of associative confusion (e.g., responding to 8 + 3 with 10, because a child had previously practiced and learned the closely related fact 8 + 2 = 10). Brownell (1935), on the other hand, argued that mastery was facilitated by taking into account regularities among combinations. In his meaningful-learning view, a key to mastery was discovering patterns or relationships and devising reasoning strategies, such as "If 8 + 2 = 10 and 3 is one more than 2, then 8 + 3 must equal 11" (Brownell & Carper, 1943). In this view, mental-arithmetic errors can reflect inaccurate or incomplete reasoning processes.

Siegler's (e.g., Siegler & Shipley, 1995; Siegler & Shrager, 1984) influential distribution-of-associations model is based squarely on Thorndike's (1922) associative-learning view. According to this model, the representation of a basic multiplication combination consists of a set of possible answers of varying associative strength. Three factors are presumed to influence the development of the associative network and, hence, the probability of correct and incorrect answers: (a) related knowledge, (b) the difficulty of executing computational or other backup strategies, and (c) the frequency of combination exposure. The first factor affects the initial formation of the representation and, thus, the frequency of early mental-arithmetic errors. The second and third factors affect the relative frequency of incorrect and correct answers, and this, in turn, shapes the evolution of mental-arithmetic errors and the development of an efficient retrieval strategy.

As children with mental retardation are often characterized as rote learners, Siegler's (e.g., Siegler & Shipley, 1995; Siegler & Shrager, 1984) distribution-of-association model should be particularly descriptive of their mental-addition development. Baroody's (1988b) training experiment with 30 children with moderate or mild mental retardation provided an opportunity to test key assumptions of this model.

i. INITIAL STATE: FLAT DISTRIBUTION OF ASSOCIATIONS AND INTERFERENCE ERRORS. Siegler and Shrager (1984) argued that, with little or no computational experience, children would have a relatively flat distribution of associations because associative strength is, with one exception, dispersed evenly among all known numbers. The exception arises because prior learning of the number-word sequence interferes with the associative network for addition. More specifically, with a combination such as 2 + 5 or 3 + 5, there is a somewhat greater probability that a child will state *six* than other answers, because six is the "counting-string associate" (i.e., *six* follows *five* in the number-word sequence and, hence, is somewhat more strongly associated with *five* than with other numbers). The end result is that, initially, children should respond to an addition combination with a broad set of answers with more or less the same frequency—except for the counting-string associate, which should generally be the most common answer.

In his sample, Baroody (1988b) identified five participants with no prior addition training. After a familiarization phase, these children (and the other 25 participants) were administered a mental-addition task consisting of four combinations involving zero (e.g., 0 + 5 and 6 + 0), four combinations involving one (e.g., 1 + 4 and 8 + 1), and eight other combinations (e.g., 5 + 8 and 9 + 3). To gauge the distribution of associations, the set of combinations was administered 20 times over 7 or 8 sessions over the course of 4 weeks.

Contrary to what would be predicted from the distribution-of-associations model, the five novices almost always responded to a combination with an extremely narrow set of answers. Four almost always responded to all combinations with one of the addends (e.g., for 5 + 8, answered *five* or *eight*). The fifth novice, typically responded to combinations involving 0 with an answer of *ten* and, over 85% of the time, responded to the remaining combinations with an answer one more than an addend (e.g., for 5 + 8, answering *six* or *nine*). Thus, except for the one child, the counting-string associate was *never* stated.

Baroody (1988b) concluded that, as with NMH novices (Baroody, 1989b), the highly regular error patterns were due to the inflexible application of a prescription. In other words, because novices have little prior knowledge to draw on, they adopt mechanical estimation strategies to produce some answer.

These results also have two clear methodological implications.

1. Siegler (e.g., Siegler & Shrager, 1984) assumed that a response without overt computing was—regardless of reaction time—typically a retrieved answer. The results of Baroody's (e.g., 1988b) studies indicate that many or, even most, mental-arithmetic responses of children may stem from covert nonretrieval processes.

2. Siegler (e.g., Siegler & Shrager, 1984) analyzed data collapsed over subjects. Baroody's (e.g., 1988b) results indicate that analyses of individual data should be done before, or instead of, pooling data. Siegler and Shrager's (1984) finding that counting-string associates are relatively common among novices, for example, may be due to pooling the data of many children who never state a counting-string associate with a few who almost always use the mechanical estimation strategy of adding one to an addend.

ii. The Transition State: The Error-Learning Hypothesis. According to Siegler's (e.g., Siegler & Shipley, 1995; Siegler & Shrager, 1984) model, the initial distribution of associations for a combination is transformed by practice. Every time an answer is calculated or stated, whether correct or incorrect, a trace is laid down in long-term memory. Because children's computational errors are most often off by only one or two, responses that are ± 1 or 2 from the correct sum gain in relative associative strength, while other incorrect responses decrease in relative strength. According to this error-learning hypothesis, then, the relative mental-addition error rates by older children, and even adults reflects the relative frequency of computational errors made during the transition state.

The Baroody (1988b) study is currently the only effort to test Siegler's (e.g., Siegler & Shipley, 1995; Siegler & Shrager, 1984) error-learning hypothesis directly. After pretesting, half of the 30 participants were given computational training and practice on a subset of addition combinations for a total of 51 20-minute sessions over a period of 20 weeks. Trainers kept a record of all items practiced and all responses given or computed during the training phase. Posttesting immediately after the training included both practiced and nonpracticed combinations.

One notable finding was that the most common errors made by the experimental participants on the posttest were different than those on the pretest—even for nonpracticed combinations. Another notable finding was that the most common posttest errors on the practiced combinations were stated or computed a negligible number of times during the training phase. In brief, the error-learning hypothesis is not necessary to explain changes in error frequency. Baroody (1988b) concluded that, as with NMH children (e.g., Baroody, 1989b), the computational experience enabled his participants to construct more sensible and accurate estimation strategies that could be applied to even novel, unpracticed items. In other words, these children with mental retardation appeared to have developed a better "operation sense" for addition.

iii. EXPERT STATE: MASTERY OF BASIC NUMBER COMBINATIONS. According to the distribution-of-associations model (e.g., Siegler & Shipley, 1995; Siegler & Shrager, 1984), as children's calculational efficiency increases, the correct answer to a combination is given more and more often and, thus, its relative associative strength increases. With practice, the distribution of associations for a combination becomes more and more peaked until the correct answer is stated almost exclusively.

Baroody (1988b) found that experimental participants mastered significantly more practiced and unpracticed combinations involving 0 to 1 than did control participants. Some of the former apparently discovered a $n + 0/0 + n = n$ rule and $n + 1/1 + n =$ the number-after-n rule, rules that they could apply to novel, unpracticed combinations. In brief, because of rule-based learning, practicing *all* $n + 0$ and $n + 1$ combinations thousands of times, as suggested by Siegler and Shrager's (1984) model, was not necessary.

These results are consistent with those found in more recent studies. In a training experiment involving children with moderate or mild retardation, Baroody (1995) found that 8 of 13 participants in his experimental (computation-practice) group appeared to discover the number-after-n rule for $n + 1/1 + n$ combinations. Moreover, he (Baroody, 1996) later reported that although there was no clear-cut evidence of other thinking strategies on the posttests, several experimental participants appeared to use reasoning strategies to figure out the sums of unknown combinations during the training.

Ezawa (1996) reported that, in addition to using $n + 0$ and $n + 1$ rules, her two participants with moderate retardation had at least some ability to use knowledge of basic addition combinations to determine the differences of subtraction combinations (e.g., $5 - 3 = ?$ can be thought of as $3 + ? = 5$, and because $3 + 2 = 5$, it follows that $5 - 3 = 2$). Moreover, one child (Benno) used a $n + 10 = n +$ teen rule (e.g., $7 + 10 =$ seven + teen) and a $n + 9$ reasoning strategy (e.g., $7 + 9 = [7 - 1] + [9 + 1] = 6 + 10 = 16$). Clearly, though, we need further and clear-cut evidence that most, or at least many, children with mental retardation can—under the right conditions—spontaneously discover rules or invent reasoning strategies for determining basic sums and differences.

c. Additive Commutativity. Research with NMH children indicates that the principle of additive commutativity is frequently discovered before formal instruction on the topic (e.g., Baroody & Gannon, 1984; Baroody, Ginsburg, & Waxman, 1983; but see Baroody, Berent, & Packman, 1982). Moreover, despite claims to the contrary (e.g., Cowan & Renton, 1996; Ganetsou & Cowan, 1995; Sophian, Harley, & Martin, 1995), the empirical evidence indicates that commutativity performance is related to informal computational experience (Baroody, Wilkins, & Tiilikainen, in press).

Resnick (1992) proposed that in any given mathematical domain, children begin with concrete thinking and successively add three levels of increasingly abstract thinking. Only with the achievement of the last level do children supposedly develop the capacity for general arithmetic principles. For example, Resnick (1992) suggests that children first understand additive commutativity only as it applies to familiar situations and numbers. Only when they achieve the last phase do children recognize additive commutativity as a general principle. Put differently, children should first exhibit a size effect—understand the principle with small, relatively familiar numbers but not with large relatively unfamiliar numbers.

Baroody (1987b) examined 34 children with moderate retardation and 17 with mild retardation in order to gauge the salience of the commutative relationship to this population and to determine if they would exhibit a size effect. Participants were tested by presenting them an equation such as $5 + 2 = 7$ and then asking them if a second expression such as $2 + 5 =$ __ (a commuted expression) or $4 + 2$ (a different expression) had the same answer or not. (The latter trials served to discourage or check for a response bias.) Small-number trials had sums less than 10, and large-number trials had sums in the teens.

In contrast to Baroody and Snyder (1983), who found that only one-fifth of their sample of children with moderate retardation understood the principle, Baroody (1987b) found that about three-fifths of his sample was successful on the additive-commutativity task. Similar to results with NMH children (Baroody et al., in press), there were no significant size effects. That is, the children appeared to understand additive commutativity as a general principle. Although IQ or category of retardation was not related to performance, the extent of computational experience was. That is, children who had or were receiving substantial computational practice were significantly more likely to be successful on the additive commutativity task.

Note that using the commutativity principle to short-cut computational effort can be considered a simple form of intelligent problem solving. That is, recognizing that both $9 + 7$ and $7 + 9$ have the same sum means a student need make only one computational or retrieval effort.

III. IMPLICATIONS

In this section, I discuss the theoretical and empirical implications of the research reviewed above and then the educational implications. I end with some general conclusions about the need for additional research on the mathematical learning and teaching of children with mental retardation.

A. Theoretical and Empirical Issues

In this subsection, general and then specific implications are addressed.

1. GENERAL IMPLICATIONS

In psychology, the behavioristic paradigm reached its zenith as a general theory of learning in the 1950s. As it became evident that this paradigm was adequate to explain simple instances of learning, but not more complex learning such as that required by language acquisition and meaningful school learning, cognitive theorizing emerged as the predominant paradigm. In the field of special education, this paradigm shift has been much slower, partly perhaps, because of the widely held assumption that special children are capable of only simple forms of learning (routine expertise). Below I discuss the contributions of the emerging cognitive paradigm to the field of special education and how research with special education enriches the cognitive paradigm.

a. Contributions of Cognitive Theory and Research. One general implication of this review is that cognitive theorizing and research on NMH handicapped children's mathematical learning have been indispensable tools in guiding research and constructing a better understanding about children with mental retardation (Baroody, 1986b; see Bråten, 1996, for a similar conclusion). For example, 15 years ago, there was little or no discussion of such children's *understanding* or *transfer* of counting, number, and arithmetic rules and concepts. What little research that was done by behaviorists on these topics focused on routine expertise. As evidence of NMH children's adaptive expertise grew, researchers began to explore the possibility that children with mental retardation too might be capable of greater mathematical competence than previously believed possible. As evidence of mathematical adaptive expertise in both of these populations has slowly accumulated, neobehaviorists have incorporated such phenomena as rule learning and transfer into their theories of learning (see, e.g., Brown, Bellamy, & Gadberry, 1971; Holcomb, Stromer, & Mackay, 1997; Mackay et al., 1997; Maydak et al., 1995; Stromer et al., 1993).

b. Contributions to Cognitive Theory. Another general implication of this review is that the relationship between cognitive psychology and research on children with mental retardation is not a one-way street. The latter also informs and enriches the former. For example, the studies by Baroody (1995) and Baroody and Mason (1984) underscore a possible advantage in studying children with mental retardation when exploring general developmental issues. With NMH children, progress can occur quickly in spurts, making it difficult for researchers to witness important transition phases or developmental changes. Studying analogous developments with children with mental retardation, whose progress may be slower, may enable researchers to better examine transition phases or catch developmental changes.

2. SPECIFIC IMPLICATIONS

Discussed below are the implications of the reviewed research regarding the adaptive expertise of children with mental retardation and related issues.

a. Adaptive Expertise. As with children in general, there has been a trend in the last 15 years to focus on what children with mental retardation can do mathematically, rather than what they can't do. In contrast to the vast amount of earlier research that fostered the pessimistic stereotype that these children are capable of only routine expertise (see, e.g., reviews by Cherkes-Julkowski & Gertner, 1989; Ferretti & Cavalier, 1991; Scheid, 1990), more recent research (e.g., Baroody, 1988c; Ezawa, 1996; Mackay et al., 1997; Maydak et al., 1995) suggests more optimistically that they—under the right conditions—are capable of at least some adaptive intelligence. Discussed below are two critical aspects of developing adaptive expertise: informal knowledge and active construction of knowledge.

i. INFORMAL KNOWLEDGE. The bad news suggested by this review of the research is that preschoolers with mental retardation typically do not construct the powerful informal mathematical knowledge that NMH preschoolers do. The good news is that many children with mental retardation appear capable of learning the counting, number, and arithmetic concepts and skills that provide the foundation for the meaningful learning of school (formal) mathematics.

ii. ACTIVE CONSTRUCTION OF KNOWLEDGE. If the research in the last 15 years does not completely counter the argument that children with mental retardation are passive learners (e.g., Burton, 1974; Noffsinger & Dobbs, 1970; Quay, 1963; Warren, 1963), then it certainly dilutes the claim. Although only further research will determine whether or not most of these children are capable of active learning, recent results (e.g., Baroody, 1988a, 1988b, 1988c, 1996; Bråten, 1996; Ezawa, 1996; Mackay et al., 1997; Maydak et al., 1995) demonstrate that at least some can engage in such self-initiated behavior as discovering patterns or relationships, adapting or devising strategies, and applying extant knowledge to simple, but novel, mathematical tasks (see also the Editor's Note to Foti, 1959). This surely means that children with mental retardation must be treated as individuals rather than automatically categorized as passive learners.

b. Related Issues. A fundamental assumption of cognitive psychology is that meaningful learning depends on developmental readiness. This assumption has important implications for conducting training studies with children with mental retardation, the value of labels, and the relative importance of metacognitive training.

i. GENERALIZABILITY VERSUS READINESS. Although screening may limit sample size and, thus, generalizability, it is necessary for training studies in which the goal is fostering adaptive expertise. Screening for prerequisite knowledge is consistent with a cognitive perspective that constructing an understanding of a new concept or procedure must build on what a child already understands. If the conceptual underpinnings are not there or cannot be fostered within the time frame of a study, the best that can be hoped for is routine expertise.

ii. LABELS VERSUS READINESS. Time and time again, studies have found that labels, such as *DS*, *moderate retardation*, and *mild retardation* are not particularly helpful in predicting successful performance on mathematical tasks or in mathematical training studies (Baroody, 1986a, 1987b, 1988c, 1994b, 1996; Caycho et al., 1991). For example, Caycho et al. (1991) found that developmental level, rather than syndrome, determines counting behavior. Baroody (1996) found that children who actively invented more sophisticated addition strategy did not have higher IQs than did more passive learners. Specifically, regression analyses indicated that IQ was not predictive of posttest performance (see Baroody, 1994b, for details). Indeed, the only two experimental subjects who invented relatively sophisticated abstract counting strategies had IQs of less than 50. If IQ has validity as a measure of adaptiveness, the results of these two children raise the hope that under the right circumstances, other children with mental retardation—including those who are moderately handicapped—can likewise exhibit active learning.

iii. Metacognitive Training versus Meaningful Instruction. Although there is relatively little research on the topic, metacognitive skills (e.g., knowledge about the relative usefulness of strategies and self-monitoring of procedures) are presumed to make an important contribution to primary-level children's mathematical development (see review by Bråten, 1996). Not surprisingly, a popular explanation for why children with mental retardation are so often passive learners (e.g., for why they are able to learn, but not invent or transfer strategies) has been that they lack the self-management processes necessary to control and monitor strategy use (e.g., Brown, 1978; Scheid, 1990; but see Cherkes-Julkowski & Gertner, 1989; Ferretti & Cavalier, 1991). It follows from this view that such children need training on general metacognitive skills in order to develop the self-management proficiencies necessary to become active learners.

An alternative explanation for the passivity of individuals with mental retardation is that they lack well-connected knowledge that is the bedrock of conceptual understanding (Cherkes-Julkowski & Gertner, 1989). Extant knowledge, particularly conceptual knowledge, affects what is noticed about novel situations (Rosch, 1977) and how one processes information about it (e.g., Chi, 1978).

Indeed, this author's informal observations of spontaneous self-corrections of object counting and addition errors by children with mental retardation suggests that self-monitoring may be a natural outcome of adaptive expertise. That is, if children conceptually understand what they are doing, they will be prone to watch for, recognize, and correct errors or dubious answers. For example, Baroody (1996) found that the experimental subjects in his study spontaneously modified their strategy for adding without self-management training. These results, then, are consistent with other data demonstrating that specific-strategy training can be as effective as specific-strategy training coupled with self-management training (e.g., Burger, Blackman, & Clark, 1981).

iv. Metacognitive or Conceptual Deficits versus Processing Deficits. Yet another explanation for the passivity of individuals with mental retardation is cognitive-processing deficiencies. Two processes, in particular, have been identified as contributing to individual differences in counting, number, and arithmetic skills: working memory and processing speed (Geary, 1993; Jensen, 1998).[6]

Working memory enables an individual to remember information for a very short period of time and is crucial for mental tasks that require using several processes or bits of information simultaneously. It has been hypothesized that because individuals with mental retardation have a limited working-memory capacity, they can process only a limited amount of information (see, e.g., Ferretti & Cavalier, 1991). This would explain why they can respond effectively to simple and clear (cognitively undemanding) tasks, but not more complex tasks. More specifically, Hoard et al. (1998) offered that many of the difficulties their participants with low IQ had in detecting correct and incorrect examples of object counting with larger collections, comparing numbers, reading numerals, and informally calculating sums might be the result of working-memory difficulties. For example, their overreliance on less sophisticated or less efficient strategies for determining sums might be due to difficulties with or an inability to keep track of the amount added on, while simultaneously counting to determine the sum (Achievement 4 in Table IV) (see, e.g., Baroody, 1987a, or Baroody & Ginsburg, 1986, for a more complete explanation).

Processing speed includes the ability to accurately store and retrieve numerical information and affects how quickly and to what extent skills become automatized (Hoard et al., 1998). A lack of automatized basic skills can delay, disrupt, or prevent the development of more advanced skills. For example, as suggested earlier, automatic knowledge of the number after another is important for efficiently judging which of two number neighbors is larger and for efficiently using the number-after-n rule for $n + 1$ combinations. Specifically, Baroody (1988c) hypothesized that transfer of learned comparisons to larger nontrained numbers may have been hampered, in part, because participants were probably unfamiliar with the number-after relationships for the larger numbers. Furthermore, if number-after knowledge is not automatic, it seems less likely that children of any ability level will notice the relationship between this knowledge and adding one (i.e., discover the number-after-n rule for $n + 1$ combinations).

Although deficiencies in general cognitive processes undoubtedly play an important role in the learning difficulties of children with mental retardation, research is needed to address a number of questions: To what extent are such difficulties characteristic of the whole population? Do children with moderate retardation have greater cognitive-processing deficiencies than those with mild retardation? Might such deficiencies vary significantly even within a broad classification such

[6]Yet another often identified source of difficulty is an attention-deficit disorder. For example, Ezawa (1996) reported that while Benno knew the conventional order of spoken and written to 100 and even 1000, his ability to generate these sequences was often disturbed by uncontrollable impulsiveness.

as *mild retardation*? To what extent are deficiencies in cognitive processing organic or due to other factors, such as the lack of conceptual knowledge or purposeful practice? For instance, are difficulties inventing advanced informal addition strategies due to deficiencies in working memory, in conceptual prerequisites, or both? To what extent can measurable deficiencies in cognitive processes be modified or circumvented?

Needed are long-term training/learning studies that explore the learning potential of children with mental retardation and their ability to automaticized meaningfully learned skills. Methodologies that separate processing deficiencies from other causes of learning difficulties such as a lack of conceptual understanding need to be developed.

B. Educational Implications

Cognitive theory and research has important general and specific implications for special education. In this subsection, I discuss each in turn.

1. GENERAL ISSUES

Cognitive theory and research has provided a crucial underpinning of the mathematics education reform movement in this country. Its growing application to the field of special education suggests that changing how and what mathematics is taught to children with mental retardation may be helpful also.

a. Adaptive Expertise. A growing amount of research by cognitive psychologists (e.g., Baroody, 1986b, 1996) and now neobehaviorists (e.g., Mackay et al., 1997; Maydak, 1995; Stromer et al., 1993) indicate that the mathematical instruction of children with mental retardation should not be limited to rote memorization—merely fostering routine expertise (cf. Burton, 1974; Noffsinger & Dobbs, 1970; Quay, 1963; Warren, 1963). There is now good reason to believe that with patience and effective instruction, these children can achieve adaptive expertise of basic mathematical knowledge: counting, number, and simple arithmetic.

Achieving adaptive expertise in primary-level mathematics is essential for the meaningful learning and successful use of subsequent school mathematics, such as multidigit addition, percents, and decimals and their applications to everyday life. In effect, it provides the cognitive building blocks necessary to develop the adaptive expertise needed for functioning independently in our complex society. Fostering the mathematical adaptive expertise of students with mental retardation at all levels of school is particularly important now, given the increasing emphasis on deinstitutionalization. Only with adaptive expertise will they develop the necessary self-reliance to manage their personal affairs, particularly their finances. As Brown et al. (1971) noted over 25 years ago:

> Obviously, the abilities and concepts necessary for functioning in a community setting greatly exceed those required for institutional living. . . . It is no longer acceptable for special educators

> to assume that [students with mental retardation] cannot learn to count, work, travel, shop, tell time, etc. The students are now in the community. We must find ways to teach them the necessary skills and concepts. (pp. 178–179)

More recently, Massey, Noll, and Stephenson (1994) noted that

> parents and professionals agree that the most appropriate and desired educational outcome for students with moderate and severe retardation is the ability to participate meaningfully in the activities of daily living. Ultimately, this means living in the community and working in integrated competitive-employment settings. (p. 353)

i. INFORMAL KNOWLEDGE. Informal knowledge is a critical basis for the meaningful learning of formal knowledge—for expanding their adaptive expertise to school-taught and largely symbolic mathematics (Ginsburg & Baroody, 1983). Thus, it is essential that special educators assess the entry knowledge of children classified as mentally handicapped. Study after study indicates that special education teachers cannot take for granted that children with mental retardation just beginning school will have the same level of informal mathematical knowledge that NMH children bring to school (e.g., Baroody, 1986a, 1996; Caycho et al., 1991; Spradlin et al., 1974). For example, Baroody (1986b) found that a majority of elementary- and secondary-level children with moderate retardation were successful on only 4 of 10 counting skills commonly demonstrated by NMH kindergarten children (namely, counting collections 1 to 5, displaying up to five fingers on request, and applying the cardinality rule to collections 1 to 5 and 6 to 10; but not orally counting to 29, producing sets of up to five items, recognizing number patterns up to 5, recognizing the order-irrelevance principle with collections of 2 to 5 and 6 to 10, and gauging the equivalence of collections with three to five items). Thus, with children with mental retardation, it is important to examine their basic counting skills and concepts, understanding of numerical relationships, ability to identify and read numerals, and understanding of addition.

ii. ACTIVE LEARNING. Like teachers of NMH children, special education teachers need to support and encourage mentally retarded children's efforts to actively construct knowledge and to do as much thinking for themselves as possible. In effect, they need to consider being more of "a guide on the side" instead of always serving as "a sage on the stage." There is ample evidence that instruction of children with mental retardation can and should include, for example, searching for patterns and relationships (inductive reasoning), formulating and applying general rules (inductive and deductive reasoning), and devising computational strategies (e.g., Baroody, 1987a, 1987b, 1988b, 1996). Projects and games are two ways of actively involving students in their own learning (e.g., Beattie & Algozzine, 1982; Foti, 1959; Taylor & Watkins, 1974). For example, Ross (1970) found that children with mild retardation who received game-playing instruction exhibited considerable incidental learning of basic number concepts. More specifically, they significantly outperformed children in the control group that received direct instruction on the nine tested concepts and skills, including oral counting to 10, object counting, and recognizing the numerical value of small quantities.

b. Related Issues. To foster adaptive expertise among children with mental retardation, it is essential that special education teachers consider the issues of readiness, individual differences, and conceptual understanding.

i. READINESS. It follows from Piaget's (1964) principle of assimilation that "the most important single factor influencing learning is what the learner already knows" (Ausubel, 1968, p. vi). Meaningful instruction involves building on what children already know. As Foti (1959) suggested 40 years ago: "The teacher would do well to determine what [mathematical] knowledge [a child with mental retardation] already has and seize every possible social situation and opportunity from which she can provide meaningful concepts of terms relating to time, quantity, space, measurement, and [commerce]" (p. 156).

Two common mistakes made by special education teachers are overlooking informal strengths and weaknesses and proceeding through a curriculum before a child understands basic concepts and skills. If children lack basic informal concepts and skills, they will have to be spoonfed and memorize by rote basic formal knowledge. Likewise, if they don't understand basic formal concepts, more advanced concepts such as multidigit addition, fractions, decimals, and percents will make little or no sense and be unduly difficult to learn, if learned at all.

ii. INDIVIDUAL DIFFERENCES. Differences in background knowledge (e.g., informal mathematical experiences) and cognitive-processing capabilities may mean that not every child will be ready to understand and to learn the same material at the same time and in the same way. Even within what are often presumed to be "homeogeneous" groups of children (e.g., "children with moderate retardation"), there can be huge individual differences in readiness and capacity to learn a particular mathematical concept or skill. Recent research has repeatedly underscored the need to consider individual strengths and weaknesses.

iii. CONCEPTUAL UNDERSTANDING. In order to foster adaptive expertise of formal mathematics, it is crucial that mathematics instruction of all children—including children with mental retardation—focus on fostering meaningful learning (understanding). Although training on general metacognitive strategies may well be helpful, it cannot be a substitute for helping children with mental retardation conceptually understand skills or procedures. Without conceptual understanding, children—including those with mental retardation—will not be able to use what they have learned flexibly or adaptively.

Meaningful instruction may be particularly important for children classified as mentally handicapped. These children may be less able to shed the ill effects of poor (meaningless and decontextualized) instruction, and more prone to learned helplessness (passivity). Moreover, meaningful learning can eliminate the need for "overlearning"—the dubious practice of assigning huge amounts of often tedious practice (Moyer & Moyer, 1985). With understanding, children with mental retardation may be able to master and retain skills with a moderate amount of practice.

iv. PURPOSEFUL PRACTICE. It is essential that basic counting, number, and arithmetic skills become automatic so that their processing in working memory requires minimal effort and attention. This will allow these skills to be used as the components of more advanced mathematical skills. It will also free up attention to focus on finding mathematical patterns, relationships, and shortcuts—essential elements in advancing mathematical knowledge. Teachers need to keep in mind that practice should follow meaningful learning and be purposeful or, at least, interesting in order to motivate students and to be as effective as possible.

2. SPECIFIC ISSUES

Briefly outlined below are instructional recommendations for teaching counting, number, and addition to children with mental retardation. For more detailed advice, see, for example, Baratta-Lorton (1976), Baroody (1987a, 1989a, 1992b, 1998), Kamii (1985), and Wynroth (1986).

a. Counting.

i. ORAL COUNTING. For children who have not yet learned the rote portion of number-word sequence to *twelve*, there are numerous examples of children's literature and rhymes that can provide entertaining exposure to it (see, e.g., Burns, 1992; Whitin & Wilde, 1992). For children who have learned the number-word sequence to *twelve*, instruction should focus on finding patterns—that is, inducing counting rules.

ii. OBJECT COUNTING. Instruction should be purposeful. Find or create situations where there is a real need to enumerate a collection (e.g., as part of an art lesson on drawing people, counting how many fingers a person has). Many games, particularly those involving dice, involve counting. Start with small, easily counted collections (e.g., two or three items in a row). Help a child learn keeping-track strategies (e.g., separating counted items from uncounted items).

iii. CARDINALITY. By regularly being involved in counting collections, children should discover, for instance, the cardinality rule and the order-irrelevance principle. If children have difficulty discovering the cardinality rule themselves, this shortcut can be modeled and practiced by playing the "Hidden-Stars" Game: Have the child count a card on which several stars have been pasted, then cover the stars, and ask the child, "How many stars am I hiding?" To deepen a child's understanding, encourage them to model numbers with their fingers. To encourage the discovery of the order-irrelevance principle, ask a child, for instance, to count a small set of steps on the way up and again on the way down.

b. Number.

i. COMPARING NUMBERS. Again, find or create a real need to compare numbers, such as determining who is older (e.g., "Is a 5-year-old or a 4-year-old older?"), playing a game (e.g., "Would you rather move your race car three spaces or four spaces?"), or choosing a treat (e.g., "Would you rather have three candies or two candies?"). Start with comparing small collections that children can easily count and then introduce somewhat larger collections. Help children to recognize that the further one counts, the larger the number. Once children understand this and have mastered number-after relationships, help them discover and master the $N + 1 > N$ rule.

ii. COUNTING–NUMERAL CONNECTION. Help children master oral- and object-counting first. Then a numerical symbol such as 3 can be related to various arrangements of three items (e.g., ooo, o°o, 8, o°o) and the number-word "three."

iii. NUMERAL READING AND WRITING. Help children to construct a mental image of each numeral 0 to 9 by having them consider its parts and how the parts fit together. Easily confused numerals such as 2 and 5 or 6 and 9 should be introduced together in order to highlight the differences between them. If need be, explicitly point out how numerals differ in their parts and how the parts fit together (e.g., "See, the loop of the six is on the bottom, and the loop of the nine is at the top"). Analogies can be particularly helpful in forming and remembering mental images of numerals (e.g., a *six* is like a nose 6 and a nine is like a balloon on a stick or a zero with a tail hanging down 9).

Once children have a complete and accurate mental image of a numeral, including the proper left-right orientation, they are ready to learn how to write it. If a child encounters difficulty or asks for help (e.g., "How do you write a three?"), provide an explicit motor plan and encourage the child to rehearse and internalize it.

c. Addition

i. STRATEGY DEVELOPMENT. Pose simple problems (real or otherwise) and encourage children to devise an appropriate strategy. If a child has difficulty with this, try modeling concrete counting-all. Once children can use this direct-modeling strategy, encourage the invention of shortcuts by providing purposeful practice and having children share their invented shortcuts. Counting-on can be fostered by encouraging children to induce the number-after rule for adding one.

ii. ARITHMETIC RELATIONSHIPS. Prompt children to discover arithmetic relationships. For example, the discovery of additive commutativity can be promoted by posing, for instance, $3 + 5$ and $5 + 3$ one after the other, and encouraging children to record the answer to each.

iii. MENTAL ARITHMETIC. Foster a number sense by encouraging children to estimate sums and to reflect on and discuss the effects of adding zero (nothing), one, two, or more. Encourage the students to look for patterns and relationships—to discover, for example, $n + 0 = n$ and $n + 1 =$ number-after-n rules.

C. Conclusions

Although we should guard against being overly optimistic or unrealistic, recent research suggests that—like NMH children—children with mental retardation are capable of more mathematics competence than previously thought possible. There are also some signs that they can benefit from a more purposeful, meaningful and inquiry-based approach than traditional instruction provides. Nevertheless, much remains to be learned about the mathematical learning and teaching of these special children. Below I summarize some of the issues that need to be addressed.

1. LEARNING

Although mathematical literacy is becoming ever more important in our technology- and information-based society, and although mathematical disabilities may be more widespread than reading disabilities, we know significantly less about the former than the latter (Jordan, Blanteno, & Uberti, in press). In particular, although recent research suggests that at least some children with mental retardation can develop adaptive expertise in the areas of counting, number, and simple addition, many questions remain. Under the right conditions, can practically all, or at least most, children with mild retardation develop adaptive expertise in these basic mathematical domains? Might not the same be true even for children with moderate retardation? Can children with mental retardation build on these foundational competencies to learn in a meaningful fashion more advanced concepts and skills such as place-value, multidigit addition, fractions, decimals, or percent? Put differently, can such children use elementary mathematical concepts to achieve adaptive expertise of more advanced topics on school mathematics—to devise their own strategies, to learn new material without direct intervention, or to solve unfamiliar problems?

2. TEACHING

Analogous to the argument over how NMH children should be taught mathematics, there is currently heated debate over how to best teach mathematics to children with special needs, including those with mental retardation. On the one hand, some proponents of reform argue that the traditional direct-instruction approach should be entirely replaced by a child-centered approach that embodies developmentally appropriate practices (e.g., Gestwicki, 1995). On the other hand, others have countered that developmentally appropriate practices may not be effective with children with special needs and that special educators should rely on direct instruction (e.g., the teacher modeling correct procedures and providing special feedback) (see, e.g., Atwater, Carta, Schwartz, & McConnell, 1994; Carta, 1995; Carta, Schwartz, Atwater, & McConnell, 1991).

Yet others who basically support the philosophy of developmentally appropriate practices—including the NCTM (1989, 1991)—take a more moderate view. Rowen and Cetorelli (1990), for example, noted that there is no one correct way to teach mathematics. According to the National Research Council (1987), effective teachers use a variety of methods to enhance the mathematical power of their students. In other words, effective teachers may implement the investigative approach in various ways: from teacher-guided inquiry or discovery learning to open-ended projects (Baroody, 1998). Indeed, although instruction should, for the most part, be meaningful, purposeful, and inquiry-based, there may be times another approach is needed (Baroody, 1998).

In the past, there have been sporadic reports that children with mental retardation can benefit from a purposeful, meaningful, and inquiry-based approach to mathematics instruction (see, e.g., Beattie & Algozzine, 1982; Ross, 1970). For instance, the editor's note to Foti (1959) pointed out:

> Some twenty years ago, the editor experimented with a combination of shop work and mathematics with some retarded boys ages ten to thirteen. Our outgrowth of the experiment was the "discovery" by pupils of non-conventional methods of obtaining answers to simple computational exercises. The carpenters' steel square became a most useful device. (p. 158)

Recent research (Ezawa, 1996; personal communication, August 27, 1997) further raises the hope that children with mental retardation can profit from an investigative approach that focuses on *patiently* helping them construct basic counting, number, and arithmetic concepts and skills. For example, teachers can foster the development of informal addition strategies by taking advantage of everyday situations and introducing projects, games, or simple word problems. As children invent more sophisticated strategies, they can encourage them to share their inventions with others. Moreover, teachers can prompt their classes to discuss these new procedures. While it may take several years before children with mental retardation invent advanced strategies such as counting-on, they may learn, for instance, the value of sharing or discussing ideas or strategies and that there are different ways to doing things (Ezawa, personal communication, August 27, 1997). These "lessons" and the construction of meaningful knowledge may help to promote greater flexibility—a hallmark of adaptive expertise.

Even so, to date there is little hard evidence that the investigative approach recommended by the NCTM (1989)—and proponents of "developmentally appropriate practices" (Bredekamp, 1993)—is effective with most, or even many, children with mental retardation. Still unanswered, then, are the following questions: What instructional approach can best foster the adaptive expertise of school mathematics among the majority of children with mental retardation? For example, will a purposeful, meaningful, inquiry-based approach that integrates mathematics with children's literature, science, and other subjects be more effective than a traditional skills approach in helping most of these children learn basic skills such as mastering the basic number facts, constructing key concepts such as place value and functions, inventing procedures such as counting-on or carrying, and applying problem-solving heuristics? What form of the investigative approach might best be suited for fostering adaptive expertise with different topics? For example, might guided discovery learning be helpful or not in inventing informal addition strategies, devising reasoning strategies to determine simple sums and differences, understanding key place-value concepts, or constructing multidigit arithmetic, none of the above, or all of the above?

There are significant, but not insurmountable, barriers to implementing and evaluating an investigative approach with children with mental retardation. One is that inadequate attention has been given to developing effective instructional methods for implementing the NCTM reforms with children having learning difficulties (Giordano, 1993; Hofmeister, 1993; Mallory, 1994; Rivera, 1993). Clearly, much more thought and effort must go into developing mathematics programs that are engaging, understandable, and thought provoking for all children, but especially for children with mental retardation. Another barrier is a widespread pessimism about children with mental retardation, a disposition that has been fueled, in part, by their lack of progress when taught in a developmentally inappropriate manner. For example, because many special education teachers do not believe that children with learning difficulties are capable of adaptive expertise, they incorporate the NCTM's (1989, 1991) recommendations into their traditional instructional approach in such a way as to distort or defeat the intent of the reforms (Grobecker, 1999). Clearly, educational programs are needed to help special education teachers, administrators, parents, curriculum developers, and others overcome the stereotypes associated with mental retardation—the stereotypes that result all too often in a self-fulfilling prophecy.

Although there is no guarantee that the investigative approach will be effective in promoting even a modest level of adaptive expertise among children with mental retardation, how will we know if we do not give it a genuine try? Until it is empirically established to be invalid, the mathematical instruction of these children, whatever its form, should be evaluated by the criterion proposed by Trafton and Claus (1994): "Are we teaching mathematics so that all students will be empowered to use it flexibly, insightfully, and productively?" (p. 19)

ACKNOWLEDGMENTS

Preparation of this chapter was supported, in part, by a grant from the University of Illinois Research Board ("Early Arithmetic Development").

REFERENCES

Ashcraft, M. H. (1992). Cognitive arithmetic: A review of data and theory. *Cognition*, *44*, 74–106.

Atwater, J. B., Carta, J. J., Schwartz, I. S., & McConnell, S. R. (1994). Blending developmentally appropriate practice and early childhood special education: Redefining best practice to meet the needs of all children. In B. L. Mallory & R. S. New (Eds.), *Diversity and developmentally appropriate practices* (pp. 1–14). New York: Teachers' College, Columbia University.

Ausubel, D. P. (1968). *Educational psychology: A cognitive view*. New York: Holt, Rinehart, & Winston.

Baratta-Lorton, M. (1976). *Mathematics their way*. Menlo Park, CA: Addison-Wesley.

Baroody, A. J. (1986a). Basic counting principles used by mentally retarded children. *Journal for Research in Mathematics Education, 17*(5), 382–389.

Baroody, A. J. (1986b). Counting ability of moderately and mildly mentally handicapped children. *Education and Training of the Mentally Retarded, 21*, 289–300.

Baroody, A. J. (1987a). *Children's mathematical thinking: A developmental framework for preschool, primary, and special education teachers*. New York: Teachers College Press.

Baroody, A. J. (1987b). Problem size and mentally retarded children's judgment of commutativity. *American Journal of Mental Deficiency, 91*, 439–442.

Baroody, A. J. (1988a). A cognitive approach to writing instruction for children classified as mentally handicapped. *Arithmetic Teacher, 36*, 7–11.

Baroody, A. J. (1988b). Mental-addition development of children classified as mentally handicapped. *Educational Studies in Mathematics, 19*, 369–388.

Baroody, A. J. (1988c). Number comparison learning by children classified as mentally handicapped. *American Journal of Mental Deficiency, 92*, 461–471.

Baroody, A. J. (1989a). *A guide to teaching mathematics in the primary grades*. Boston: Allyn and Bacon.

Baroody, A. J. (1989b). Kindergartners' mental addition with single-digit combinations. *Journal for Research in Mathematics Education, 20*(2), 159–172.

Baroody, A. J. (1992a). The development of preschoolers' counting skills and principles. In J. Bideaud, C. Meljac, & J. P. Fischer (Eds.), *Pathways to number* (pp. 99–126). Hillsdale, NJ: Erlbaum.

Baroody, A. J. (1992b). Remedying common counting difficulties. In J. Bideaud, C. Meljac, & J. P. Fischer (Eds.), *Pathways to number* (pp. 307–323). Hillsdale, NJ: Erlbaum.

Baroody, A. J. (1994a). An evaluation of evidence supporting fact-retrieval models. *Learning and Individual Differences, 6*, 1–36.

Baroody, A. J. (1994b, April). *Individual differences in self-invented addition strategies by children classified as mentally handicapped.* Paper presented at the annual meeting of the American Educational Research Association, New Orleans.

Baroody, A. J. (1995). The role of the number-after rule in the invention of computational short cuts. *Cognition and Instruction, 13*, 189–219.

Baroody, A. J. (1996). Self-invented addition strategies by children classified as mentally handicapped. *American Journal on Mental Retardation, 101*, 72–89.

Baroody, A. J. (1998). *Fostering children's mathematical power: An investigative approach to K-8 mathematics instruction*. Mahwah, NJ: Erlbaum.

Baroody, A. J., Berent, R., & Packman, D. (1982). The use of mathematical structure by inner city children. *Focus on Learning Problems in Mathematics, 4*(2), 5–13.

Baroody, A. J., & Gannon, D. E. (1984). The development of the commutativity principle and economical addition strategies. *Cognition and instruction, 1*, 321–329.

Baroody, A. J., & Ginsburg, H. P. (1986). The relationship between initial meaningful and mechanical knowledge of arithmetic. In J. Hiebert (Ed.), *Conceptual and procedural knowledge: The case of mathematics* (pp. 75–112). Hillsdale, NJ: Erlbaum.

Baroody, A. J., Ginsburg, H. P., & Waxman, B. (1983). Children's use of mathematical structure. *Journal for Research in Mathematics Education, 14*, 156–168.

Baroody, A. J., & Mason, C. A. (1984). The case of Brian: An additional explanation for production deficiencies. In J. Moser (Ed.), *Proceedings of the Sixth Annual Meeting of the North American Chapter of the International Group for the Psychology of Mathematics Education* (pp. 2–8). Madison, WI: Wisconsin Center for Educational Research.

Baroody, A. J., & Snyder, P. M. (1983). A cognitive analysis of basic arithmetic abilities of TMR children. *Education and Training of the Mentally Retarded, 18*, 253–259.

Baroody, A. J., & Wilkins, J. L. M. (1999). The development of informal counting, number, and arithmetic skills and concepts. In J. Copeley (Ed.), *Mathematics in the early years, birth to five*. Reston, VA: National Council of Teachers of Mathematics.

Baroody, A. J., Wilkins, J. L. M., & Tiilikainen, S. (in press). The development of children's understanding of additive commutativity: From protoquantitive concept to general concept? In A. J. Baroody & A. Dowker (Eds.), *The development of arithmetic concepts and skills: The construction of adaptive expertise*. Mahwah, NJ: Erlbaum.

Beattie, J., & Algozzine, B. (1982). Improving basic academic skills of educable mentally retarded adolescents. *Education and Training of the Mentally Retarded, 17*, 255–258.

Bellamy, T., & Brown, L. (1972). A sequential procedure for teaching addition to trainable mentally retarded students. *The Training School Bulletin, 69*, 31–44.

Bellamy, T., & Buttars, K. L. (1975). Teaching trainable level retarded students to count money: Toward personal independence through academic instruction. *Education and Training of the Mentally Retarded, 10*, 18–26.

Bellamy, T., Greiner, C., & Buttars, K. L. (1974). Arithmetic computation for trainable retarded students: Continuing a sequential instructional program. *The Training School Bulletin, 70*, 230–240.

Belmont, J. M., & Butterfield, E. C. (1969). The relations of short-term memory to development and intelligence. In L. Lipsitt & H. Reese (Eds.), *Advances in child development and behavior* (Vol. 4, pp. 29–84). New York: Academic Press.

Bråten, I. (1996). *Cognitive strategies in mathematics*. Report No. 10, 1996. Oslo, Norway: Institute for Educational Research, University of Oslo.

Bray, N. W. (1979). Strategy production in the retarded. In N. R. Ellis (Ed.), *Handbook of mental deficiency: Psychological theory and research* (2nd ed., pp. 699–726). Hillsdale, NJ: Erlbaum.

Bray, N. W., & Turner, L. A. (1986). The rehearsal deficit hypothesis. In N. R. Ellis & N. W. Bray (Eds.), *International review of research in mental retardation* (Vol. 14, pp. 47–71). Orlando, FL: Academic Press.

Bredekamp, S. (1993). The relationship between early childhood education and early childhood special education: Healthy marriage or family feud? *Topics in early childhood special education, 13*(3), 258–273.

Briars, D. J., & Siegler, R. S. (1984). A featural analysis of preschoolers' counting knowledge. *Developmental Psychology, 20*, 607–618.

Brown, A. L. (1974). The role of strategic behavior in retardate memory. In N. R. Ellis (Ed.), *International review of research in mental retardation* (Vol. 7, pp. 55–111). New York: Academic Press.

Brown, A. L. (1978). Knowing when, where, and how to remember: A problem of metacognition. In R. Glaser (Ed.), *Advances in instructional psychology* (Vol. 1, pp. 77–165). New York: Wiley.

Brown, A. L., Bransford, J. D., Ferrara, R. A., & Campione, J. C. (1983). Learning, remembering, and understanding. In J. H. Flavell & E. M. Markman (Eds.), *Handbook of child psychology* (4th ed., pp. 77–166). New York: Wiley.

Brown, A. L., & DeLoache, J. S. (1978). Skills, plans, and self-regulation. In R. S. Siegler (Ed.), *Children's thinking: What develops?* (pp. 3–55). Hillsdale, NJ: Erlbaum.

Brown, L., Bellamy, T., & Gadberry, E. (1971). A procedure for the development and measurement of rudimentary quantitative concepts in low functioning trainable students. *The Training School Bulletin, 68*, 178–185.

Brownell, W. A. (1935). Psychological considerations in the learning and the teaching of arithmetic. In D. W. Reeve (Ed.), *The teaching of arithmetic* (Tenth yearbook, National Council of Teachers of Mathematics) (pp. 1–50). New York: Bureau of Publications, Teachers College, Columbia University.

Brownell, W. A., & Carper, D. V. (1943). *Learning multiplication combinations*. Durham, NC: Duke University Press.

Burger, A. L., Blackman, L. S., & Clark, H. T. (1981). Generalization of verbal abstraction strategies by EMR children and adolescents. *American Journal of Mental Deficiency, 85*, 611–618.

Burns, M. (1992). *Math and literature (K-3)*. Sausalito, CA: Math Solutions Publication.

Burton, T. A. (1974). Education for trainables: An impossible dream? *Mental Retardation, 12*, 46.

Butterfield, E. C., & Belmont, J. M. (1977). Assessing and improving the cognition of mentally retarded people. In I. Bialer & M. Sternlicht (Eds.), *Psychology of mental retardation: Issues and approaches* (pp. 277–318). New York: Psychological Dimensions.

Campione, J. C., & Brown, A. L. (1974). The effects of contextual changes and degree of component mastery on transfer of training. In H. W. Reese (Ed.), *Advances in child development and behavior* (Vol. 9). New York: Academic Press.

Carnegie Forum on Education and the Economy. (1986). *A nation prepared: Teachers for the 21st century*. New York: Carnegie Corporation.

Carpenter, T. P. (1986). Conceptual knowledge as a foundation for procedural knowledge: Implications from research on the initial learning of arithmetic. In J. Hiebert (Ed.), *Conceptual and procedural knowledge: The case of mathematics* (pp. 113–132). Hillsdale, NJ: Erlbaum.

Carpenter, T. P., & Moser, J. M. (1984). The acquisition of addition and subtraction concepts in grades one through three. *Journal for Research in Mathematics Education, 15*, 179–202.

Carraher, T. N., Carraher, D. W., & Schliemann, A. D. (1987). Written and oral mathematics. *Journal for Research in Mathematics Education, 18*, 83–97.

Carta, J. J. (1995). Developmentally appropriate practice: A critical analysis applied to young children with disabilities. *Focus on exceptional children, 27*(8), 1–14.

Carta, J. J., Schwartz, I. S., Atwater, J. B., & McConnell, S. R. (1991). Developmentally appropriate practice: Appraising its usefulness for young children with disabilities. *Topics in early childhood special education, 11*(1), 1–20.

Caycho, L., Gunn, P., & Siegal, M. (1991). Counting by children with Down syndrome. *American Journal on Mental Retardation, 95*, 575–583.

Cherkes-Julkowski, M., Davis, L., Fimian, M., Gertner, N., McGuire, J., Norlander, K., Okolo, C., & Zoback, M. (1986). Encouraging flexible strategy usage in handicapped learners. In J. M. Berg (Ed.), *Science and service in mental retardation* (pp. 189–196). London: Methuen.

Cherkes-Julkowski, M., & Gertner, N. (1989). *Spontaneous cognitive processes in handicapped children*. New York: Springer-Verlag.

Chi, M. T. H. (1978). Knowledge structure and memory development. In R. S. Siegler (Ed.), *Children's thinking: What develops*? (pp. 73–96). Hillsdale, NJ: Erlbaum.

Cobb, P. (1986). An investigation into the sensory-motor and conceptual origins of the basic addition facts. *Proceedings of the 10th International Conference of the International Group for the Psychology of Mathematics Education* (pp. 141–146). London: University of London Institute of Education.

Cobb, P., Wood, T., & Yackel, E. (1991). A constructivist approach to second grade mathematics. In E. von Glasersfeld (Ed.), *Constructivism in mathematics education* (pp. 157–176). Boston: Kluwer.

Coburn, T. G. (1989). The role of computation in the changing mathematics curriculum. In P. R. Trafton & A. P. Shulte (Eds.), *New directions for elementary school mathematics* (pp. 43–58). Reston, VA: National Council of Teachers of Mathematics.

Cornwall, A. C. (1974). Development of language, abstraction and numerical concept formation in Down's syndrome children. *American Journal on Mental Retardation, 79*, 179–190.

Cowan, R., & Renton, M. (1996). Do they know what they are doing? Children's use of economical addition strategies and knowledge of commutativity. *Educational Psychology, 16*, 407–420.

Court, S. R. A. (1920). Numbers, time, and space in the first five years of a child's life. *Pedagogical Seminary, 27*, 71–89.

Cruickshank, W. M. (1948a). Arithmetic ability of mentally retarded children: Ability to differentiate extraneous materials from needed arithmetical facts. *Journal of Educational Research, XLII*(3), 161–170.

Cruickshank, W. M. (1948b). Arithmetic work habits of mentally retarded boys. *American Journal of Mental Deficiency, 52*, 318–330.

Cuvo, A. J., Veitch, V. D., Trace, M. W., & Konke, J. L. (1978). Teaching change computation to the M. R. *Behavior Modification, 2*, 531–548.

Davis, R. B. (1984). *Learning mathematics: The cognitive science approach to mathematics education*. Norwood, NJ: Ablex.

Doll, E. A. (1931). *A survey and program for special types of education in Trenton, NJ*. White House Conference on Child Health and Protection, Section III, Washington, D.C.

Ezawa, B. (1996). *Zählen und rechnen bei geistig behinderten schülern: Leistungen, konzepte und strategien junger erwachsener mit hirnfunktionsstörungen* [Counting and calculating of students with mental retardation: Capabilities, concepts and strategies of young adults with brain dysfunction]. Frankfurt, Germany: Peter Lang.

Ferretti, R. P. (1989). Problem solving and strategy production in mentally retarded persons. *Research in Developmental Disabilities, 10*, 19–31.

Ferretti, R. P., & Cavalier, A. R. (1991). Constraints on the problem solving of persons with mental retardation. In N. W. Bray (Ed.), *International review of research in mental retardation* (Vol. 17, pp. 153–192). San Diego, Academic Press.

Fey, J. T. (1990). Quantity. In L. A. Steen (Ed.), *On the shoulders of giants* (pp. 61–94). Washington, DC: National Research Council.

Foti, F. T. (1959). Teaching the mentally handicapped. *Arithmetic Teacher*, April, 156–157.

Frostig, M., LeFever, D. W., & Whittlesey, J. R. (1964). *The Marianne Frostig developmental test of visual perception*. Palo Alto, CA: Consulting Psychologists Press.

Fuson, K. C. (1982). An analysis of the counting-on solution procedure in addition. In T. P. Carpenter, J. M. Moser, & T. A. Romberg (Eds.), *Addition and subtraction: A cognitive perspective* (pp. 67–82). Hillsdale, NJ: Erlbaum.

Fuson, K. C. (1988). *Children's counting and concepts of number*. New York: Springer-Verlag.

Fuson, K. C. (1992). Research on whole number addition and subtraction. In D. Grouws (Ed.), *Handbook of research on mathematics teaching and learning* (pp. 243–275). New York: Macmillan.

Fuson, K. C., & Hall, J. W. (1983). The acquisition of early number word meanings: A conceptual analysis and review. In H. P. Ginsburg (Ed.), *The development of mathematical thinking* (pp. 49–107). New York: Academic Press.

Fuson, K. C., Richards, J., & Briars, D. J. (1982). The acquisition and elaboration of the number word sequence. In C. Brainerd (Ed.), *Progress in cognitive development: Children's logical and mathematical cognition* (Vol. 1, pp. 33–92). New York: Springer-Verlag.

Ganetsou, E., & Cowan, R. (1995, September). *The development of commutativity*. Paper presented at the conference on Language and Mathematical Thinking, London, England.

Gast, D. L., VanBiervliet, A., & Spradlin, J. E. (1979). Teaching number-word equivalences: A study of transfer. *American Journal of Mental Deficiency, 83*, 524–527.

Geary, D. C. (1993). Mathematical disabilities: Cognitive, neuropsychological, and genetic components. *Psychological Bulletin, 114*, 345–362.

Gelman, R. (1982). Basic numerical abilities. In R. J. Sternberg (Ed.), *Advances in the psychology of intelligence* (Vol. 1, pp. 181–205). Hillsdale, NJ: Erlbaum.

Gelman, R., & Cohen, M. (1988). Qualitative differences in the way Down's syndrome and normal children solve a novel counting problem. In L. Nadel (Ed.), *The psychobiology of Down's syndrome* (pp. 51–99). Cambridge, MA: M.I.T./Bradford Press.

Gelman, R., & Gallistel, C. (1978). *Young children's understanding of number*. Cambridge: Harvard University Press.

Gelman, R., & Meck, E. (1992). Early principles and concepts of number. In J. Bideaud, C. Meljac, & J. P. Fischer (Eds.), *Pathways to number* (pp. 171–189). Hillsdale, NJ: Erlbaum.

Gestwicki, C. (1995). *Developmentally appropriate practice: Curriculum and development in early childhood education*. Delmar, NY: Delmar Publishers.

Ginsburg, H. P. (1977). *Children's arithmetic*. New York: D. Van Nostrand.

Ginsburg, H. P., & Baroody, A. J. (1983). *The Test of Early Mathematics Ability* (TEMA). Austin, TX: Pro-Ed.

Ginsburg, H. P., Klein, A., & Starkey, P. (1998). The development of children's mathematical knowledge: Connecting research with practice. In I. E. Sigel & K. A. Renninger (Eds.), *Handbook of child psychology: Vol. 4. Child psychology in practice* (5th ed., pp. 401–476). New York: Wiley & Sons.

Ginsburg, H. P., Posner, J. K., & Russell, R. L. (1981). The development of mental addition as a function of schooling. *Journal of Cross-Cultural Psychology*, *12*, 163–178.

Giordano, G. (1993). Fourth invited response: The NCTM Standards: A consideration of the benefits. *Remedial and Special Education*, *14*, 28–32.

Goldberg, I. I., & Rooke, M. L. (1967). Research and educational practices with mentally deficient children. In N. G. Haring & R. L. Schiefelbusch (Eds.), *Methods in special education*. New York: McGraw-Hill.

Goodnow, J., & Levine, R. A. (1973). "The grammar of action": Sequence and syntax in children's copying. *Cognitive Psychology*, *4*, 82–98.

Grobecker, B. (1999). *Mathematics reform and learning differences. Learning Disability Quarterly*, *22*, 43–58.

Hatano, G. (1988). Social and motivational bases for mathematical understanding. In G. B. Saxe & M. Gearhart (Eds.), *Children's mathematics* (pp. 55–70). San Francisco: Jossey-Bass.

Hoard, M. K., Geary, D. C., & Hamson, C. O. (in press). *Numerical and arithmetical cognition: Performance of low- and average-IQ children. Mathematical Cognition*.

Hofmeister, A. M. (1993). Elitism and reform in school mathematics. *Remedial and Special Education*, *14*, 8–13.

Holcomb, W. L., Stromer, R., & Mackay, H. A. (1997). Transitivity and emergent sequence performances in young children. *Journal of Experimental Child Psychology*, *65*, 96–124.

Hughes, M. (1986). *Children and number: Difficulties in learning mathematics*. New York: Basil Blackwell.

Jensen, A. R. (1998). *The g factor: The science of mental ability*. Westport, CT: Praeger.

Jordan, N., Blanteno, L. M., Uberti, H. Z. (in press). Development of calculation and problem-solving skills in children with mathematics difficulties. In A. J. Baroody & A. Dowker (Eds.), *The development of arithmetic concepts and skills: The construction of adaptive expertise*. Mahwah, NJ: Erlbaum.

Kamii, C. (1985). *Young children reinvent arithmetic: Implication of Piaget's theory*. New York: Teachers College Press.

Kirk, S. A. (1964). Research in education. In H. A. Stevens & R. Heber (Eds.), *Mental Retardation: A review of research*. Chicago: University of Chicago.

Koehler, M. S., & Grouws, D. (1992). Mathematics teaching practices and their effects. In D. A. Grouws (Ed.), *Handbook of research on mathematics teaching and learning* (pp. 115–126). New York: Macmillan.

Lindquist, M. M. (1989). It's time for change. In P. R. Trafton & A. P. Shulte (Eds.), *New directions for elementary school mathematics* (pp. 1–13). Reston, VA: National Council of Teachers of Mathematics.

Louttit, C. M. (1957). *Clinical psychology of exceptional children* (3rd ed.). New York: Harper & Bros.

Mackay, H. A., Kotlarchyk, B. J., & Stromer, R. (1997). Stimulus classes, stimulus sequences, and generative behavior. In D. M. Baer & E. M. Pinkston (Eds.), *Environment and behavior* (pp. 124–137). Boulder, CO: West View.

Mallory, B. L. (1994). Inclusive policy, practice and theory for young children with developmental differences. In B. L. Mallory & R. S. New (Eds.), *Diversity and developmentally appropriate practices* (pp. 44–62). New York: Teachers' College, Columbia University.

Mann, P. H., & Suiter, P. (1974). *Handbook in diagnostic teaching: A learning disabilities approach.* Boston: Allyn & Bacon.

Massey, A., Noll, M. B., & Stephenson, J. (1994). Spatial sense and competitive-employment options for students with mental retardation. In C. A. Thornton & N. S. Bley (Eds.), *Windows of opportunity: Mathematics for students with special needs.* Reston, VA: National Council of Teachers of Mathematics.

Mastropieri, M. A., Bakken, J. P., & Scruggs, T. E. (1991). Mathematics instruction for individuals with mental retardation: A perspective and research synthesis. *Education and Training of the Mentally Retarded,* June, 115–129.

Maydak, M., Stromer, R., Mackay, H. A., & Stoddard, L. T. (1995). Stimulus classes in matching to sample and sequence production: The emergence of numeric relations. *Research in Developmental Disabilities, 16,* 179–204.

McCarthy, J. J., & Scheerenberg, R. C. (1966). A decade of research on the education of the mentally retarded. *Mental Retardation Abstracts, 3,* 481–501.

McCloskey, M., Caramazza, A., & Basili, A. (1985). Cognitive mechanisms in number processing and calculation: Evidence from dyscalculia. *Brain and Cognition, 4,* 171–196.

McKnight, C. C., Crosswhite, F. J., Dossey, J. A., Kifer, E., Swafford, J. O., Travers, K. J., & Cooney, T. J. (1987). *The underachieving curriculum: Assessing U.S. school mathematics from an international perspective.* Champaign, IL: Stipes.

Moyer, M. B., & Moyer, J. C. (1985). Ensuring that practice makes perfect: Implications for children with learning difficulties. *Arithmetic Teacher, 33*(1), 40–42.

National Commission on Excellence in Education. (1983). *A nation at risk.* Washington, DC: U.S. Government Printing Office.

National Council of Teachers of Mathematics. (1989). *Curriculum and evaluation standards for school mathematics.* Reston, VA: Author.

National Council of Teachers of Mathematics. (1991). *Professional standards for teaching mathematics.* Reston, VA: Author.

National Research Council. (1987). *The teacher of mathematics: Issues for today and tomorrow.* Washington, DC: National Academy Press.

Neches, R. (1987). Learning through incremental refinement procedures. In D. Klahr, P. Langley, & R. Neches (Eds.), *Production system models of learning and development* (pp. 163–219). Cambridge, MA: MIT Press.

Noffsinger, T., & Dobbs, V. (1970). Teaching arithmetic to educable mentally retarded children. *Journal of Educational Research, 64*(4), 177–184.

Nunes, T. (1992). Ethnomathematics and everyday cognition. In D. A. Grouws (Ed.), *Handbook of research on mathematics teaching and learning* (pp. 557–574). New York: Macmillan.

Piaget, J. (1964). Development and learning. In R. E. Ripple & V. N. Rockcastle (Eds.), *Piaget rediscovered* (pp. 7–20). Ithaca, NY: Cornell University.

Piaget, J. (1965). *The child's conception of number.* New York: Norton.

Quay, L. C. (1963). Academic skills. In N. R. Ellis (Ed.), *Handbook of mental deficiency.* New York: McGraw-Hill.

Resnick, L. B. (1983). A developmental theory of number understanding. In H. P. Ginsburg (Ed.), *The development of mathematical thinking* (pp. 109–151). New York: Academic.

Resnick, L. B. (1992). From protoquantities to operators: Building mathematical competence on a foundation of everyday knowledge. In G. Leinhardt, R. Putnam, & R. A. Hattrup (Eds.), *Analysis of arithmetic for mathematics teaching* (pp. 373–425). Hillsdale, NJ: Erlbaum.

Resnick, L. B., & Ford, W. W. (1981). *The psychology of mathematics for instruction.* Hillsdale, NJ: Erlbaum.

Resnick, L. B., & Neches, R. (1984). Factors affecting individual differences in learning ability. In R. J. Sternberg (Ed.), *Advances in the psychology of human intelligence* (Vol. 2, pp. 275–323). Hillsdale, NJ: Erlbaum.

Rivera, D. M. (1993). Third invited response: Examining mathematics reform and the implications for students with mathematics disabilities. *Remedial and Special Education, 14*, 24–27.

Rosch, E. (1977). Classification of real-worlds objects: Origins and representations in cognition. In P. N. Johnson-Laird & P. C. Wason (Eds.), *Thinking* (pp. 264–273). New York: Cambridge University Press.

Ross, D. (1970). Incidental learning of number concepts in small group games. *American Journal of Mental Deficiency, 74*, 718–725.

Rowen, T. E., & Cetorelli, N. D. (1990). A model for teaching elementary school mathematics. In T. J. Cooney & C. R. Hirsch (Eds.), *Teaching and learning mathematics in the 1990s* (1990 Yearbook, pp. 62–68). Reston, VA: National Council of Teachers of Mathematics.

Schaeffer, B., Eggleston, V., & Scott, J. (1974). Number development in young children. *Cognitive Psychology, 6*, 357–379.

Scheid, K. (1990). *Cognitive-based methods for teaching mathematics to students with learning problems*. Columbus, OH: LINC Resources, Inc.

Sears, C. J. (1986). Mathematics for the learning disabled child in the regular classroom. *Arithmetic Teacher, 33*(5), 5–11.

Secada, W. G., Fuson, K. C., & Hall, J. (1983). The transition from counting-all to counting-on in addition. *Journal for Research in Mathematics Education, 14*, 47–57.

Siegler, R. S., & Jenkins, E. (1989). *How children discover new strategies*. Hillsdale, NJ: Erlbaum.

Siegler, R. S., & Robinson, M. (1982). The development of numerical understanding. In H. W. Reese & L. P. Lipsitt (Eds.), *Advances in child development and behavior* (Vol. I, pp. 241–312). New York: Academic Press.

Siegler, R. S., & Shipley, C. (1995). Variation, selection, and cognitive change. In G. Halford & T. Simon (Eds.), *Developing cognitive competence: New approaches to process modeling* (pp. 31–76). Hillsdale, NJ: Erlbaum.

Siegler, R. S., & Shrager, J. (1984). Strategy choices in addition: How do children know what to do? In C. Sophian (Ed.), *Origins of cognitive skills* (pp. 229–293). Hillsdale, NJ: Erlbaum.

Sophian, C. (1998). A developmental perspective on children's counting. In C. Donlan (Ed.), *The development of mathematical skills* (pp. 27–46). Hove, East Sussex: Psychology Press.

Sophian, C., Harley, H., & Martin, C. S. M. (1995). Relational and representational aspects of early number development. *Cognition and Instruction, 13*, 253–268.

Spradlin, J. E., Cotter, V. W., Stevens, C., & Friedman, M. (1974). Performance of mentally retarded children on pre-arithmetic tasks. *American Journal of Mental Deficiency, 78*, 397–403.

Starkey (in press). Informal addition. In A. J. Baroody & A. Dowker (Eds.), *The development of arithmetic concepts and skills: The construction of adaptive expertise*. Mahwah, NJ: Erlbaum.

Starkey, P., & Gelman, R. (1982). The development of addition and subtraction abilities prior to formal schooling in arithmetic. In T. P. Carpenter, J. M. Moser, & T. A. Romberg (Eds.), *Addition and subtraction: A cognitive perspective*. Hillsdale, NJ: Erlbaum.

Steinberg, R. M. (1985). Instruction on derived fact strategies in addition and subtraction. *Journal for Research in Mathematics Education, 16*, 337–355.

Stevenson, H. W., Lee, S. Y., & Stigler, J. W. (1986). Mathematics achievement of Chinese, Japanese, and American children. *Science, 231*, 693–699.

Stromer, R., Mackay, H. A., Cohen, M., & Stoddard, L. T. (1993). Sequence learning in individuals with behavioral limitations. *Journal of Intellectual Disability Research, 37*, 243–261.

Taylor, G. R., & Watkins, S. T. (1974). Active games: An approach to teaching mathematical skills to the educable mentally retarded. *Arithmetic Teacher*, December, 674–678.

Thorndike (1922). *The psychology of arithmetic*. New York: Macmillan.

Thornton, C. A., & Bley, N. S. (Eds.). (1994). *Windows of opportunity: Mathematics for students with special needs*. Reston, VA: National Council of Teachers of Mathematics.

Trafton, P. R., & Claus, A. S. (1994). A changing curriculum for a changing age. In C. A. Thornton & N. S. Bley (Eds.), *Windows of opportunity: Mathematics for students with special needs* (pp. 19–39). Reston, VA: National Council of Teachers of Mathematics.

Traub, N. (1977). *Recipe for reading*. New York: Walker.

von Glasersfeld, E. (1982). Subitizing: The role of figural patterns in the development of numerical concepts. *Archives de Psychologie*, *50*, 191–218.

Wagner, S., & Walters, J. (1982). A longitudinal analysis of early number concepts: From numbers to number. In G. Forman (Ed.), *Action and thought* (pp. 137–161). New York: Academic Press.

Wang, M. C., Resnick, L. B., & Boozer, R. F. (1971). The sequence of development of some early mathematics behaviors. *Child Development*, *42*, 1767–1778.

Warren, S. A. (1963). Academic achievement of trainable pupils with five or more years of schooling. *The Training School Bulletin*, *60*, 75–86.

Wertheimer, M. (1959). *Productive thinking*. New York: Harper & Row. (Original work published 1945).

Whitin, D. J., & Wilde, S. (1992). *Read any good math lately: Children's books for mathematical learning. K-6.* Portsmouth, NH: Heinemann.

Wohlwill, J., & Lowe, R. (1962). Experimental analysis of the development of the conservation of number. *Child Development*, *33*, 153–167.

Wynn, K. (1998). Numerical competence in infants. In C. Donlan (Ed.), *The development of mathematical skills* (pp. 3–25). Hove, East Sussex: Psychology Press.

Wynroth, L. (1986). *Wynroth math program: The natural numbers sequence*. Ithaca, NY: Wynroth Math Program.

The Nature and Long-Term Implications of Early Developmental Delays: A Summary of Evidence from Two Longitudinal Studies

RONALD GALLIMORE, BARBARA K. KEOGH,
AND LUCINDA P. BERNHEIMER

DEPARTMENT OF PSYCHIATRY
UNIVERSITY OF CALIFORNIA, LOS ANGELES
LOS ANGELES, CALIFORNIA

I. HISTORY AND CURRENT STATUS OF THE CATEGORY AND CONCEPT OF DEVELOPMENTAL DELAY

Developmental delay is generally defined as the failure of a child to reach developmental milestones at the expected age (First & Palfrey, 1994). Delay rather than disability is commonly used to describe young children who perform poorly on developmental tests or who otherwise display a slower-than-expected rate of development when a more specific diagnosis is absent (Bernheimer & Keogh 1982, 1986). Drillien, Pickering, and Drummond (1988) reported a 10% prevalence rate for developmental delay. A survey of 65 Early Education Programs for Children with Disabilities (EEPCD) indicated that 36% of the children being served were labeled delayed with no specific diagnosis, 21% were considered at risk for developmental delays, and only 3% of the children were labeled with mental retardation (Stayton & Karnes, 1994). As states are now permitted to serve children using relatively broad criteria for defining developmental delay, it is probable that increasing numbers of young children with problems will receive this nonspecific label.

Like developmental disabilities, the term *developmental delay* came into use over the past two decades as an umbrella category signifying a continuum of problems. In reference to younger children, developmental disabilities and develop-

INTERNATIONAL REVIEW OF RESEARCH IN
MENTAL RETARDATION, Vol. 22
0074-7750/99 $30.00

mental delays are often treated as synonymous and as substitutes for more specific diagnoses. Bernheimer and Keogh (1986) suggest that despite the nonspecific diagnosis, the referential breadth and lack of diagnostic specificity of the term *delay* signals the need for early interventions with children and families. It also offers clinicians a relatively benign way to describe problem development to parents with less ominous overtones for the future. Because of the substantial variation in children's development, describing a child as "delayed" offers the possibility of a "catch-up" to age norms and the hope "the child will grow out of it" (First & Palfrey, 1994, p. 478). The long-term implications of early delay are discussed in subsequent sections of this chapter.

One of the puzzling aspects of children exhibiting nonspecific developmental delays is that the etiology is often uncertain or unknown. The delays cannot be attributed with certainty to either biological or environmental factors such as initial biologic insult, chromosomal abnormalities, genetic conditions, to maternal prenatal drug or alcohol usage, or to postnatal neglect or abuse. The number of children with developmental delays of unknown or uncertain etiology has been estimated to be from 50 to 80% of the overall population of persons with retardation (Batshaw & Perret, 1981; Hayden & Beck, 1982). Many of these children display varying delays in language, behavior, social, and cognitive development. In contrast to known diagnostic conditions (e.g., Down syndrome) relatively little information is available to describe long-term outcomes or likely developmental paths. Early identification remains problematic (First & Palfrey, 1994), as before age 3 or 4 it is often difficult to diagnose a wide range of problems including language/speech, behavioral/emotional, learning disabilities, and mild to moderate retardation (Palfrey, Singer, Walker, & Butler, 1987). It is likely that some children identified as developmentally delayed would meet criteria for Pervasive Developmental Disorders (PDD), a medical/psychiatric diagnostic category defining "a group of neuropsychiatric disorders characterized by specific delays and deviance in social, communicative, and cognitive development" (Volkmar, 1991, p. 489). Like developmental delay, the term *PDD* describes a heterogeneous set of problems (including autism) that are apparent early in a child's life but that may not receive specific early diagnoses. The ambiguity of these conditions presents troubling problems for families and professionals alike, some children remaining low profile until age 4 or older, with questions being raised only after entrance into preschool or kindergarten.

To address the lack of information about outcomes for children with early developmental delays, in 1977 a research team at UCLA's Graduate School of Education organized a longitudinal study of a cohort of 44 3- and 4-year-olds with ambiguous, uncertain delays (Project REACH, Keogh & Kopp, 1982). Research in REACH focused on questions of child characteristics, issues of measurement, and features of the broader environment. Not quite 10 years later, a second UCLA longitudinal study (Project CHILD, Gallimore, Weisner, Kaufman, & Bernheimer,

1989; Keogh, Bernheimer, & Guthrie, 1997) replicated the REACH sampling procedure and expanded the scope of investigation to include family adaptations. Drawing on the results of both projects, in this chapter we summarize the results of 15 years of longitudinal study of children exhibiting delayed development in preschool. Our review includes a summary of the characteristics of the two longitudinal samples of children with developmental delays, Projects REACH and CHILD. For both two samples, we summarize the changes over time in the children's cognitive and developmental status and their social/behavioral competence and problems. For Project CHILD, we summarize the results of our longitudinal analyses of family responses and adaptations to developmental delay. Finally, we offer some observations on our experiences in the conduct of two longitudinal studies.

II. REACH AND CHILD CHILDREN IN THE PRESCHOOL YEARS

Before summarizing the cognitive/developmental characteristics of the children, we note briefly some issues in sample selection. Uncertainties in diagnosing young children with developmental delays pose formidable sampling problems for researchers. Because the term, *developmental delay*, is a nonspecific diagnosis, we found a range of problems in both REACH and CHILD samples. Delays were often expressed across developmental and behavioral domains or in some cases the delay was focused primarily in one. Furthermore, although all developmental and cognitive testing was done by trained and experienced assessors in the children's homes, we sometimes questioned the appropriateness of standardized tests and assessment procedures for evaluating the status of young children with problems. We also had occasional concerns about the accuracy of retrospective reports of parents when describing their child's developmental and health histories. In both the REACH and CHILD projects we used multiple measures and multiple probes over time in our efforts to gather reliable and interpretable data about the children's development. In this section we describe sampling procedures and provide summary information about the developmental status of our sample children in the initial stages of our studies. These findings provide a picture of the developmental characteristics and early histories of children with delays.

A. Project REACH

In the initial research 69 children between the ages of 18 and 42 months were studied over a 3-year period. The children had been recruited from pediatricians, early intervention programs, regional centers, and preschools. All children evidenced suspect or known delays in major developmental domains. Although the concept of developmental delay is represented across the continuum of infancy through preschool, it was apparent that the patterns of abilities and disabilities and the expression of problems varied relative to age such that the infant/toddlers and preschoolers comprised discrete groups, the infants demonstrating more serious problems. Reports of the infant studies may be found in Krakow and Kopp (1982) and in Kopp, Krakow, and Johnson (1983). The findings reported here are based on study of the preschool children. The mean chronological age (CA) of the 44 preschool children (29 boys and 15 girls) was 33.8 month, SD = 3.7, range 25 to 42 months. Mean developmental quotient (DQ) was 74.9, SD = 16.8, range 50–85. Twenty-two children were firstborns, 16 second borns, and 15 were only children. Age of parents when the study child was born was 26 (4.4) years for mothers, and 29 (4.7) years for fathers. All children were Caucasian and in English-speaking families. Mean maternal and paternal education levels were 13.4 years and 14.5 years, respectively. Occupations of parents ranged from unskilled to professional, with 83% of the fathers holding skilled, managerial, or professional positions. All but five children were enrolled in intervention programs, and many were receiving additional speech, physical, or occupational therapy. Health histories of the children suggested a high number of complications. The mean birthweight was 6.4 (SD = 2.0) pounds, range = 1.4–11.7 pounds. Twenty-three percent of the sample were preterm, and 59% were reported to have health problems in the first month of life. Forty-five percent did not leave the hospital with their mothers, 32% were hospitalized, and 27% had some kind of surgery prior to entering the REACH study.

At the time of entry into the study the children were assessed with standard developmental and language tests (the Gesell, Sequenced Inventory of Communication Development, Bayley, and the McCarthy where appropriate); all testing was done by trained and experienced assessors in the children's homes. The Caldwell Preschool Home Inventory was administered at the same time, and parents were asked to complete the short form (Keogh, Pullis, & Cadwell, 1979) of the Thomas and Chess Parent Temperament Questionnaire. Children were reassessed five times at 6-month intervals based on time of entry, and parents were asked to update information at the same time points. REACH children were assessed twice in the elementary school years and again as adolescents. These findings are reported in a subsequent section.

B. Project CHILD

Project CHILD used similar sampling procedures to those in REACH, thus providing reasonable comparability of samples. Children had been identified by pediatricians, teachers, early interventionists, and/or regional center professionals as having mild to moderate nonspecific developmental delays. A total of 313 children were reviewed for possible entry into the CHILD cohort and 103 were entered into the sample with parental consent. About 5% of the 313 children met our sampling criteria but were not studied, primarily because parents declined to participate. The final CHILD sample consisted of 103 children in 102 families. In all cases, the etiology and prognosis were unknown or uncertain. Children were excluded from the sample if they were known to have chromosomal abnormalities and/or genetic conditions associated with mental retardation, or if the delays were associated with either known prenatal drug or alcohol usage, or with postnatal neglect or abuse. The children were all Euro-American from English-speaking, primarily middle class families. Sixty-two percent of the mothers and 49.5% of the fathers had some college education; 80.4% of the fathers held skilled, managerial, or professional positions. Only two children received no formal services at entry and over one-third of the children were receiving three or more services or therapies. As with the REACH sample, many children had health problems in the first 3 years of life: 28% of the sample were preterm, 39% had some kind of surgery, and 47% were hospitalized at least once prior to entering the study. At entry, the mean CA was 41.8 months (*SD* = 6.2; range = 32 to 55). The mean Gesell DQ was 72.3 (*SD* = 16.0; range 38 to 117). All but 18 of the children had DQs below 90, and all 103 had significant delays in one or more areas (motor, speech, or cognition). Fifty-eight percent of the children were boys.

The initial data collection at age 3 included the Gesell, the short form of the Stanford-Binet, the Communication and Daily Living Subscales of the Vineland, the Caldwell HOME, and the short form of the Parent Temperament Questionnaire (Keogh et al., 1979). Teachers also completed a teacher version of the Temperament Questionnaire (Keogh, Pullis, & Cadwell, 1982) as well as a project-developed questionnaire about the child's problems and competencies in the program setting. Concurrent with the child testing, parents were interviewed at length about the daily lives of their family when raising a child with delays. Fieldworkers gathered parents' reports of behavior, medical, and communication "hassle," with hassles defined as the extent of the child's impact on the daily routine of family life. Based on the interviews fieldworkers also made ratings of family accommodations or adaptations made in response to the child with delays. Accommodations were defined as the family's functional responses or adjustments (Gallimore et al., 1989; Bernheimer & Keogh, 1995) and included actions taken, avoided, or delayed in order to create and sustain an everyday routine of life.

C. Cognitive and Developmental Status in the Preschool Years: Summary Findings

For the REACH sample, results of the developmental testing over time (5 time points) confirmed the reality of the delays recognized early on. Means and standard deviations for the Gesell DQ from time points 1 to 5 were 74 (16.9), 73 (16.90), 72 (17.7), 69 (15.5), and 67 (17). Examination of the correlations between test scores across time points, regardless of specific test, also confirmed the stability of developmental rate for the REACH preschool sample as a whole. Correlation between the Bayley mental age (MA) from time 1 to time 4 was .93; the r for the Gesell DQ from time 1 to 4 was .94. Relationships among scores from the different tests within time periods were also strong and consistently significant. At assessment time 2 for REACH, the Gesell language scores correlated .81 and .76 with the SICD expressive and receptive subscales; at time 5 both the SICD scales were significantly associated with the Gesell language and personal-social scales, values of r .60 and .93. Also to be noted were the significant correlations among subtests within any assessment measure. At time 1 the strength of association among the five subtests of the Gesell ranged from .67 to .81. Finally, there were moderate and generally significant relationships between the REACH children's CAs and their performance on the developmental tests. At time 1 the correlations between CA and Bayley MA was .38; the comparable value of r for CA and the Gesell developmental age (DA) was .56.

Turning to the CHILD sample, at entry, the mean Gesell DQ was 72.3 (SD = 16.0); the mean Binet IQ was 70.6 (SD = 13.8); means for the Vineland Daily Living and Communication Subscales were 71.8 (SD = 11.2) and 72.5 (SD = 10.5), respectively. Over 50% of the CHILD parents reported problems in speech, language, learning, physical, and behavioral areas. The mean number of problems reported by parents was 4.4, with a range from 0–8; number of problems was moderately associated with the developmental test scores (range of $r = -.24$ to $-.48$). As with the REACH sample, CHILD parents struggled to make sense of the ambiguity of their children's diagnoses and prognoses. It was not uncommon for children to have more than one diagnosis or label, and at entry 90% of the parents reported multiple, sometimes conflicting diagnoses. The most common diagnoses at age 3, reported by 50% of parents or more, were developmental delays and language/communication problems. Other labels/diagnoses, in descending order of frequency, included cerebral palsy, mental retardation, normal development, visual impairment, hearing impairment, and attention deficit disorder (ADD)/hyperactivity. CHILD parents' expectations regarding the future reflected their confusion: 53.4% predicted that their children would catch up and participate in regular education programs when they entered school, whereas 46.6% felt it was likely their child would retain a marginal status and require continuing special education services.

In addition to being strikingly similar in terms of their developmental status at entry, the REACH and CHILD cohorts shared other characteristics when the children were 3, in spite of being recruited 10 years apart. Examples included the mean age of parents' first concern that there was a problem (9.1 months for both samples); and mean age of diagnosis by a professional (12.7 months for REACH, 13.7 months for CHILD). The CHILD sample entered intervention earlier than did the REACH sample (20.3 months vs. 25.3 months), a predictable difference given the passage of PL 99-457 in 1986.

D. Generalizations from REACH and CHILD Preschool Studies

A number of generalizations emerged from the findings during the preschool years. Not surprisingly, children who are delayed at age 2–3 had a high probability of being delayed at age 4–5. The cognitive/developmental scores underscored the stability of the delays, even when CA was taken into account. The magnitude of the correlations among the various tests lent support to their reliability in assessing young children with delays. In addition to strong agreement between different tests, there were significant relationships among the various subscales within tests suggesting that the scales may in fact tap one broad ability factor (Bernheimer & Keogh, 1982, 1986). Although they have labels that have meaning on a construct level (e.g., fine motor, adaptive, personal/social), the tests may measure a global aptitude. This may be especially so for children with developmental delays, as the various ability domains may not be well differentiated early on, as shown in the significant correlations among subtest scores. When patterns of change scores for individual children were examined it was clear that the children who made the most overall gain during the 3 years of the REACH study had change scores on the language subscales which exceeded the corresponding change in CA (e.g., 31-months gain in a 24-month period).

Although it was clear that there was real stability of cognitive/developmental level over time based on group data, our findings also showed that predictions about individual children must be made with caution, especially on the basis of findings from a single test session. Within our samples a few children made rapid progress while others maintained a stable pace and still others declined in developmental level. The reasons for these differences in patterns were unclear, but provided direction to many of the follow-up efforts that were the focus in Project CHILD. For detailed information regarding the range and distribution in developmental patterns, see Bernheimer and Keogh (1988).

E. Stability of Cognitive Development over Time

The stability of cognitive status of children with developmental disabilities has been confirmed by a number of different investigators (Shonkoff, Hauser-Cram, Krauss, & Upshur, 1992). REACH correlation coefficients between DQ and IQ at different time points ranging from .74 to .81 were reported by Bernheimer and Keogh (1988). These findings are consistent with those reported by Goodman (1977); Stavrou (1990); Truscott, Narrett, and Smith (1994); and Vanderveer and Schweid (1974) in studies focused on children with identified diagnoses such as Down syndrome or other genetic conditions. The questions of stability of cognitive development over time may be less certain when the etiology of the delay is unknown or uncertain, as was the case with the children in our studies. In this section we focus primarily on the results of the CHILD studies in which children's cognitive status was assessed when the children were ages 3, 7, and 11 years chronologically.

Results of the cognitive tests by age are shown in Table I for the CHILD sample and for boys and girls separately. These analyses were based on children (N = 82) for whom we had complete data over time. Correlations between cognitive scores over time are also shown in Table I for the total group and for boys and girls separately. The magnitude of the associations suggest that early signs of delay signal the probability of continuing delays.

Scores for the CHILD group as a whole decreased over time, but examination of individual growth curves suggested that there were differences in the amount and direction of change. Between ages 3 and 11 years the majority of children (61%) had cognitive scores with ± 1 *SD*, some (33%) decreased by more than 1 *SD*, and only five children (6%) increased by 1 *SD* or more. Use of a random coefficient technique identified differences in rates of decline (Keogh et al., 1997). Variations in scores documented stable declines in DQ/IQ (estimated means slope $= -1.52$ IQ points per year, $Z = -4.03$, $p = .001$) for boys and for girls. Tests of possible child and family covariates of change (e.g., number of child problems, DQ, temperament, family socioeconomic status and family accommodation) confirmed that only the children's entering DQ and their temperaments were significantly associated with rate of decline. The relationship between temperament and

TABLE I

MEANS AND STANDARD DEVIATIONS OF DEVELOPMENTAL/COGNITIVE SCORES AT THREE TIME POINTS FOR TOTAL GROUP, BOYS AND GIRLS

	Child age					
	Age 3		Age 7		Age 11	
	M	*SD*	*M*	*SD*	*M*	*SD*
DQ/IQ						
Total = 82	72.22	(15.34)	69.60	(16.89)	66.13	(20.37)
Boys = 45	72.85	(14.06)	68.46	(14.90)	66.00	(20.19)
Girls = 37	71.46	(16.94)	70.99	(19.16)	66.30	(20.87)

Stability coefficients for developmental/cognitive scores over three time points

	r ages 3–6	*r* ages 3–11	*r* ages 6–11
Total = 82	.76***	.74***	.85***
Boys = 45	.75***	.67***	.83***
Girls = 37	.77***	.81***	.88***

***$p < .001$; **$p < .01$

DQ was nonsignificant. Of particular interest was the counterintuitive finding that it was difficult temperament rather than easy temperament that was associated with a slower decline in cognitive scores. We speculate that difficult children with delays may elicit more interaction and attention from other family members than do delayed children with easy temperaments, thus providing the difficult children with more opportunities for stimulation. Consistent with this interpretation were the findings of significant relationships between parents' views of behavioral hassle and children's temperaments at age 3. Values of r were $-.35$ and .29 for hassle scores and easy and difficult temperaments, respectively. This interpretation is also consistent with the findings of Maziade, Cote, Boutin, Bernier, and Thivierge (1987) in Canada, and with morbidity studies in Africa by DeVries (1984). The findings raise interesting questions about the possible influence of experience on the cognitive development of children with delays.

Cognitive/developmental scores were also examined relative to possible etiologic conditions of the children (Keogh & Bernheimer, 1995). Review of records of 102 CHILD children identified 28 who had signs of perinatal or immediate postnatal stress (e.g., low birthweight, anoxia, or other medical conditions); 41 had no histories of pre- or perinatal trauma or stress. There were no differences in mean values for DQ or IQ between the groups at ages 3 and 7, but the patterns of associations between early developmental scores and outcomes varied by subgroup. The most robust correlations between early measures and subsequent outcomes ($r = .80$) were in the group composed of the children with unknown etiologies; the comparable value of r was .47 for the group with known perinatal stress. The relationships between early measures and outcome was particularly strong for girls with disabilities of unknown etiology. For this subgroup of girls significant relationships were found between developmental measures at both ages 3 and 7 and behavioral characteristics at 9 or 10. For example, correlations between the Gesell DQ at age 3 and subsequent Vineland communication and daily living skills were $-.58$ and $-.64$, respectively. The correlation between the age 3 DQ and number of problems reported by parents at age 9 were .55. Similarly, the early DQ was also significantly associated with teachers' views of competencies and problems. In contrast to the findings for the girls whose disabilities were of unknown etiology, there were few significant associations for girls with identified pre- or perinatal stress, findings similar to those for boys. We have no powerful explanation for the gender-by-etiology findings. However, a reasonable inference about etiology without regard to gender is Kopp's theory (Keogh & Kopp, 1982) that the children of unknown etiology experienced trauma in the early gestational months, leading to pervasive delays in many domains, whereas perinatal stress occurred when the infants were more mature and thus more resilient.

Results of the REACH and CHILD studies of delayed children were strikingly similar, despite the 10 years between the projects, a period which has seen changes in policies, services, and attitudes. Findings from both REACH and CHILD were consistent in documenting the stability of cognitive development across ages 3–11 years. Stability was related to etiology (unknown vs. suspect) and gender; the strongest associations between early delays and subsequent problems were for girls with delays of unknown etiology. Declines in cognitive scores were associated with early developmental status and children's temperament. For both samples, the findings document long-term and continuing cognitive limitations when delays are evident in the preschool years. They also underscore the need to consider different areas of outcomes—cognitive/academic, personal/social, and behavioral. A consistent finding from work to date is that personal/social competencies and the number and expression of problem behaviors of children and youth with developmental delays are related to, but not highly correlated, with cognitive status. That is, the problem behaviors cannot be "explained" on the basis of IQ. Rather they are associated with other characteristics of the children and families and are, in part at least, age related. These findings led us to broaden our study of the children with delays to take into account a range of personal/social and behavioral and educational outcomes.

III. COMPETENCE AND PROBLEMS OF CHILDREN WITH DELAYS

Our studies of competence and problems of children with delays was guided in part by the model proposed by Masten, Garmezy, and their colleagues at the University of Minnesota (Masten, Best, & Garmezy, 1990) and by the work of Werner and Smith (1982, 1992) in their research in Hawaii. We also were influenced by the literature defining the major developmental tasks of the middle years of childhood and adolescence (Erikson, 1959; Havighurst, 1972). There is considerable evidence suggesting gender and age differences in normal developmental patterns through these time periods, but less is known about the developmental paths of children with nonspecific delays. Having documented the stability of cognitive development over time, we focused on progress and outcomes in two related areas: education/schooling; personal/social and behavioral competence and problems. In the following sections we summarize findings from both REACH and CHILD projects.

A. Schooling and Educational Achievement

We consider first the school placements of children in both REACH and CHILD cohorts as they entered and proceeded through elementary school. The majority of the children moved directly into special education placements, a finding consistent with the earlier work of Edgar, McNulty, Gaetz, and Maddox (1984), Edgar, Hegglund, and Fischer (1988), and Walker et al. (1988). We note that much of the earlier work on placement was done before the movement toward inclusion was well established, and when separate classes were the placement of choice. Consistent with earlier REACH findings, however, examination of the placements of 87 CHILD children at ages 9–10 in elementary school indicated that 78% were in separate special education classes full- or part-time, and only 22% were placed in regular education (Keogh, Coots, & Bernheimer, 1995). CHILD children in special education programs were served in categories of learning handicaps (25%); severe handicaps (30%); visual, physical, or communication handicaps (23%); or other. For most children, integration was limited to recesses, lunch periods, and assemblies; only one child at age 9–10 was integrated academically for more than half a day. Follow-up of the CHILD children when they were age 11 documented that 50% remained in separate full-day special education classes, and 21% were based in separate classes but also spent time in regular or mainstreamed classes. Similarly, 50% of the REACH sample were in separate special education programs in middle and high school, and another 30% continued to receive special help on a part-time basis (Bernheimer & Keogh, 1996).

There were significant differences across CHILD elementary school placement groups in cognitive scores. IQ means and *SD*s for the regular education, learning handicapped, severely handicapped, and other groups were 87 (15.86), 75.90 (12.79), 52.94 (14.43), and 66.06 (13.32), respectively. Similar differences were found for communication test scores and daily living competence scores, and on teachers' ratings of children's educational problems, suggesting that placements reflected individual differences in children's cognitive status. Examination of the placement groups in terms of the children's characteristics in preschool or at entrance to elementary school showed clearly that the severity of problems predicted the need for subsequent special services.

B. Personal and Social Competence and Problems

In contrast to direct testing of cognitive level, children's competencies and behavior problems are defined and assessed primarily through the reports of others, usually parents and teachers. Thus, both competencies and problems reflect the observers' perceptions as well as possible situational or setting effects (Keogh & Bernheimer, 1998). In an effort to take into account both observer and situational effects, where possible we assessed our children's competencies and problems drawing on the views of both parents and of teachers.

In an early study as part of Project REACH when the children were age 6 (Keogh, Bernheimer, Haney, & Daley, 1989), parents were asked to complete a measure of personal care competencies (Alpern & Boll, 1972) and of behavior problems (Achenbach, 1981). Results confirmed that as a group the children exhibited lower personal competency scores and higher behavior problem scores than expected from either mental or CA norms. There were no statistically significant differences in behavior problem scores by gender, although the number of problems reported was greater for boys than girls. Importantly, the correlations between the behavior problem scores and the children's IQ or mental ages (MA) were not statistically significant. Further study of the REACH children at ages 7, 8, and 9 years of age (Keogh, Ratekin, & Bernheimer, 1992), using ratings from both parents and teachers, confirmed the higher than normal rates of behavior problems at home and at school. The relationships between scores for rater groups became stronger as the children grew older (r for intensity at CA 7 = .38, r at CA 9 = .55). Salient problems for both parents and teachers focused on immaturity, clumsiness, impulsivity, and inattention, characteristics which appeared to represent the "hard-core" problems evident at home and at school. Not surprisingly, teachers also emphasized problems related to learning and classroom behavior, while parents were more concerned with personal and social interactions.

In a survey of the REACH sample at adolescence (CA mean = 18.2 years), parents were asked to describe their child's living arrangements, employment, education, health, social life, and problems. The majority of the adolescents were living at home, were autonomous in self-help skills, and were still in special education programs. Few were employed, even on a part-time basis. Of particular interest was the finding that almost half of the high-frequency behavior problems identified by parents when the children were age 6 were still considered problems by parents when their children were age 17–18. Specific problems included acts too young (73%), speech problems (57%), stubborn (67%), likes to be alone (53%), and can't concentrate (43%).

Detailed examination of the personal and social and behavioral compentencies of the children with delays was carried out with the CHILD sample when the children were 11 years of age (Keogh & Bernheimer, 1998). Data were collected from both teachers and mothers using the Teacher–Child Rating Scale (T-CARS; Hightower, Spinell, & Lotyczewski, 1988) and Hightower et al. (1986) and a Parent–Child Rating Scale adaptation of the T-CARS (Juvonen, Keogh, Ratekin, & Bernheimer, 1992; Keogh, Juvonen, & Bernheimer, 1989). Both scales tap competence factors of Frustration Tolerance, Assertive Social Skills, Task Orientation, and Peer Social Skills, and three clusters of behavior problems: Acting out, Shy/Anxious, and Learning. Mothers and teachers also completed a checklist assessing children's status in areas of independence, conduct, social skills, and health. In general there were few differences between mothers' and teachers' ratings of competencies and problems, although teachers rated children higher (better) than did their mothers on the global checklist items. For both mothers and teachers, personal social competencies and behavior problems at age 11 were associated with difficult temperament and DQ in the preschool years. For mothers, difficult temperament at age 3 was associated with acting out, frustration tolerance (negative correlation), and assertive social skills. For teachers, difficult temperament at age 3 was associated with assertive social skills. For both mothers and teachers, DQ at age 3 was associated with assertive social skills and task orientation. Not surprisingly, DQ was also associated negatively with learning problems for teachers.

The findings confirmed that the children had persistent problems in behavior and learning, but that there were differences related to home or school setting. High-frequency behaviors identified by teachers included difficulty in following directions, failure to complete assignments, inattention to task, messy work, and the like. Home-specific behavior problems included loud, disobedient, argues a lot, brags and boasts, bites fingernails, jealous, and temper tantrums (Keogh et al., 1992). The range of *r* between mothers' and teachers' ratings was .18–.57 for the full sample, .19–.57 for boys, .07–.71 for girls. Correlations between the children's cognitive scores and the behavior ratings were for the most part nonsignificant, but were greater for mothers than for teachers, a rather surprising finding. There was also stronger agreement between rater groups in externalizing than internalizing problems. The findings confirmed that children with cognitive delays have higher than normative expectancies in behavior problems and are less competent in personal social areas both at home and at school, as compared with the scores reported by Hightower et al. (1986).

Taken as a whole, our findings are consistent with prior literature on cognitive and personal/social outcomes for children with developmental delays, suggesting that early signs of developmental problems are reasonable predictors of subsequent problem status. Examination of patterns over time confirmed considerable variation among individual children in the degree and rate of cognitive change, and in their social/behavioral problems and competencies. We emphasize that cognitive level did not explain variations in personal/social competencies, and that cognitive status did not necessarily predict personal social competence. Further, problems in one personal domain did not always generalize to problems in general. There were differences related to time, setting, and observers, suggesting the need to assess outcomes at different time points and in different settings using a variety of techniques. Based on our findings, we underscore the importance of including a range of child attributes when assessing outcomes for children, especially when outcome data are used as the basis for placement and intervention decisions or for evaluating intervention effects. We also emphasize the importance of considering context when evaluating children's personal and behavioral problems.

IV. FAMILY RESPONSES TO CHILDREN WITH DEVELOPMENTAL DELAYS

A major purpose for undertaking Project CHILD was to expand the scope of REACH's investigations of early developmental delays to family responses to rearing such children. Project REACH had documented that many families were actively engaged in proactive strategies that were not well represented in a research literature focused mainly on stress and psychopathology. In 1983, for example, a lead article in the *American Journal of Mental Deficiency* concluded no theory presently "exists through which one can develop an empirical understanding of families of retarded children. Rather, investigators have seemed to rally around the concept of anticipated pathology in these families" (Crnic, Friedrich, & Greenberg, 1983, p. 126). Our goal in CHILD was to document and understand the functional nature of family adaptations to children with developmental problems.

In CHILD we augmented standard procedures and measures with a more exploratory, open-ended approach that might discover new categories of family response to developmental delay. Project CHILD families were visited either at home or at a location of their choice by an experienced fieldworker who conducted a 2–3-h semistructured interview with the principal caretaker (mothers, with few exceptions). These interviews were conducted three times, at child ages 3, 7, and 11. Parents were asked to talk about their experiences with the child with delays, the family's daily routines, and how their child affected everyday life. This interview approach was designed to provide each family the opportunity to "tell their story" in accord with evidence that adults organize and recall personal experiences and knowledge in narrative form (Bruner, 1989; Coles, 1989).

To insure uniform coverage of topics, interviewers were provided open-ended questions and topics to be covered. In addition, they were trained to use probes to ensure that equivalent material was obtained for all families on all key topics. The same protocol was followed in the interviews at 3, 7, and 11. For the interviews when the children were 7 and 11 some topics no longer relevant were deleted and new topics were added as appropriate. All interviews were audio recorded, and later transcribed for more systematic analysis. Parents were in general enthusiastic for the "story" interview approach, and many commented that they felt for the first time someone had been willing to listen to their account of their child's disabilities and related issues. Using materials from the "story-interview" we explored several lines of investigation, including the three summarized here: ambiguity of child status and parental expectations, family adaptations to developmental delay, and family outcomes.

A. Ambiguity of Child Status and Parental Expectations[1]

Except for the most profound handicapping conditions, young children with developmental disabilities or delays often present a highly ambiguous diagnostic and prognostic picture. As Bernheimer and Keogh (1986) noted, even though parents and professionals usually recognize that "something is wrong" by the first or second year of life, it may take several months or years to identify autism, cerebral

[1]Portions of this section adapted from Clare, Garnier, and Gallimore (1998).

palsy, and visual, hearing, or speech disorders. Even Down syndrome which may be less ambiguous to diagnose has an uncertain prognosis, with the degree of retardation ranging from mild to severe. For parents of children with delays of uncertain or unknown etiology and prognosis, case materials suggest a substantial impact of the ambiguity of children's status.

Ambiguity of child status is a potentially significant factor for parents since it puts in doubt what might be realistic expectations for their child's development. This effect has raised concern given the correlational evidence that parents' developmental expectations are associated with outcomes for all children with and without developmental delays (Duran & Weffer, 1992; Entwistle & Hayduk, 1981; Hunt & Paraskevopoulos, 1980). Such findings reinforce the idea that parents' expectations can create a "self-fulfilling prophecy" (Merton, 1948) that may determine or at least affect the level of functioning a child ultimately achieves. Extended to parents of children with delays and disabilities, the assumption that parents' expectations for their children may create self-fulfilling prophecies has raised concerns about possible inaccurate expectations due to ambiguity of the child's status. Some have suggested that parents may underestimate their children with delays, and do not challenge them enough (Schneider & Gearhart, 1988). Others have suggested the opposite effect, that parents may overestimate their children's future development, and thus not adequately prepare children to cope if their disabilities persist into adulthood (Zetlin & Turner, 1984).

However, strong claims that parents' expectations have causal effects on children's development are undercut in many studies by the limitations of correlational and cross-sectional designs. In most cases, it is equally plausible to propose an opposite direction of influence between parents and children (Bell, 1968). Parents may adjust their expectations over time as a child's abilities and functioning level become more apparent. This may be especially true of parents with children with developmental delays of unknown etiology whose future developmental status is frequently ambiguous early on, but becomes more certain in subsequent years (Bernheimer & Keogh, 1982). Indeed, parents generally get more accurate in their estimations of children's abilities as children mature (Anton & Dindia, 1984; Jensen & Kogan, 1962), and adjust their developmental goals for children over time in response to children's abilities (Clare, 1998).

When their children were preschoolers, a majority of REACH and CHILD parents initially expressed strong hopes of a "catch-up" to age norms. Except for about 8% of the children in both cohorts who did "catch up," this was not the case. To explore the impact "not catching up" had on the parents and their children, Clare et al. (1998) used data from the CHILD cohort to examine relationships between parents' developmental expectations and child characteristics for children at ages 3, 7, and 11. At each of these age periods, part of the "story interview" described above was devoted to a conversation about parents' "developmental expectations" using parents' personal semantic frames. Using interview materials, parents were reliably assigned to one of four categories: (1) Parents who thought that their children would definitely be permanently handicapped or "mentally retarded" as adults; (2) parents who were uncertain about their children's future functioning and handicapping conditions; (3) those who believed that their children would be only marginally handicapped (i.e., that the handicap would be present in some form, but not salient); and (4) parents who believed that their children would outgrow their developmental delays (i.e.,"catch-up") and have no residual handicaps.

Clare et al. (1998) found that parents' developmental expectations were moderately stable over time, but tending to decline as children matured. As hypothesized, parents' developmental expectations were associated with children's characteristics at age 3, and, over time, became increasingly correlated with cognitive functioning, daily living competence, child hassle, and total number of child problems. The results of regression analyses generally supported the hypothesis that early child characteristics, but not early parent expectations, were the best predictors of parents' developmental expectations and child outcomes at child age 11. The one exception was the children's daily living competence, which was predicted by a combination of early parent expectations and children's Gesell DQ scores. Path analysis revealed a transactional relationship between parents' expectations and children's daily living competence. Although parents may not be completely accurate in assessment of 3-year-olds, over time they adjust their expectations in response to children's developmental status and functioning.

The CHILD case materials indicated that the ambiguity of diagnosis is early on a source of great concern to most families, but in time some parents began to discount its importance. By the time children were 11 or older, most families were more focused on finding programs that fit the needs at hand. Although they still were concerned with the long-term, many had come to recognize and accept that they may never know why their child was delayed in development. Almost all had also come to terms with the recognition that the delays would continue, despite the fact that the diagnoses became more specific and changed over time. As example, at age 3, the most frequent diagnoses were language or communication disorder (65%); developmental delay (58%); cerebral palsy (33%); and mental retardation (30%). By age 11, 7% were identified with language/communication disorders; 15% with developmental delay; 23% with cerebral palsy; and 19% with mental retardation. Other diagnoses reported at age 11 included ADD/hyperactivity (22%), learning disabilities (13%), and other neurological conditions (11%).

B. Family Adaptation to Developmental Delay

One purpose of Project CHILD was to explore alternatives to the historic focus of researchers on stress and coping (Beresford, 1994). The stress and coping focus had many good effects: it helped justify services for parents dealing with childhood disability, documented that these families needed assistance, and called attention to the need for more funding. However, so exclusive a focus on crises, stress, and psychological reactions also perpetuated the notion "that a family with a child who has a disability is a family with a disability" (Glidden, 1993, p. 482).

During the period in which Project CHILD was conducted, there were many calls to broaden research perspectives on families of children with disabilities to include adaptation and adjustment. One impetus has been new legislation mandating that services for children with developmental delays and disabilities are to build family capacity. Another press has come from families themselves. For example, a recent volume included numerous first-person accounts of coping with childhood disabilities, many of which suggested families are concerned with more than crises and their management (Turnbull et al., 1993). Some parents of children with disabilities have forcefully objected to researcher and practitioner focus on stress and coping (Vohs, 1993). Some suggest researchers ask additional questions.

> Professionals kept asking me what my "needs" were. I didn't know what to say. I finally told them, "Look, I'm not sure what you're talking about. So let me just tell you what happens from the time I get up in the morning until I go to sleep at night. Maybe that will help." (Remark made by parent panelist at a 1989 HCEEP conference on Parent-Professional Partnerships, reported in Bernheimer, Gallimore, & Kaufman, 1993, p. 267)

This mother's comment about her daily routine echoes the approach taken in Project CHILD to examine what accommodations families made to establish a daily routine that included a child with significant delays. We started with the assumption that except for a pathological few, all families try to construct a sustainable daily routine (Gallimore, Bernheimer, & Weisner, in press). To achieve a sustainable routine, families must balance the needs and characteristics of its members with the ecological constraints with which they must live in a way that matches as close as possible their values and goals. When we began to interview the Project CHILD families using the "story interview" we quickly discovered that in fact the "accommodations" they made to sustain daily routines were a familiar topic, and one that they readily and, in some cases, eagerly discussed.

Using "story interview" materials, we successfully coded accommodations and tracked changes from children age 3 to 11 (Gallimore et al., 1989; Gallimore, Goldenberg, & Weisner, 1993; Gallimore, Coots, Weisner, Garnier, & Guthrie, 1996). Accommodation was defined as a family's functional responses or adaptations to the demands of daily life with a child with delays. Family accommodation is presumed to occur in response to both serious concerns and mundane problems of daily life, and does not require individual or family stress to be activated. There is no presumption that accommodation is intentional, or that families are conscious of their activities, or that they see themselves as dramatically different or special. We emphasize that this approach to family functioning is not limited to families with children with developmental problems. All families construct daily routines, some of which appear to be orderly, others somewhat haphazard, even chaotic. The daily routine captures the common "stuff" of family life and is an expression of how families organize their lives, what is done and what is not done (Bernheimer & Keogh, 1995). The content of the daily routine reflects the nature of the accommodations made in order to ensure some continuity of everyday family life and reflects both the cultural code and the family code as proposed by Sameroff (1994).

Every accommodation is presumed to have costs as well as benefits to each individual in the family and to the family as a whole. To illustrate, intense and daily language therapy may improve a delayed child's speech, but may intrude upon parents' time with other siblings. Such an accommodation could be judged "positive" for the child, but both "positive" and "negative" for the parents or siblings. Developing and maintaining a workable daily routine of family life depends on parents making accommodations to sometimes competing pressures, such as getting a child to inconveniently located or scheduled services when both parents work full-time, distributing care of a child who requires constant monitoring, balancing needs of a child with behavior problems against religious or social obligations. Accommodation is not assumed to be positive or negative in its effects on the family or child, as the "valence" of an accommodation must be determined by its correlation with other variables. The "goodness" of accommodations depends on long-term outcomes for parents and siblings as well as for children with delays.

In our work on family accommodations to childhood disability we have documented accommodations in ten different ecological and cultural domains, including those pertaining to health and safety, family subsistence, domestic chores, and social and emotional relationships. The accommodation domains are listed in Table II. The cross-cultural evidence of the universality of most of these domains can be found in Weisner (1984). As example of an accommodation, to incorporate a long commute to a special needs program into a family routine, a mother might cut her paid work to part-time but strike a deal with her employer to keep on a valued career path. The father might arrange to leave his job early to pick up a sibling from day care. Each of these functional trade-offs and adjustments represents a family accommodation to childhood disability (Gallimore, Coots, Weisner, Garnier, & Guthrie, 1996).

From preschool to late childhood, 93 families reported a statistically significant increase in the number of accommodations made: 749, 891, and 1,388 at child ages 3, 7, and 11, respectively. Ratings of intensity, or how much effort families put into their accommodations, on the other hand, showed little change over the same period. The discrepancy between increased frequency and stable effort suggested that by late childhood families were spreading their adaptive efforts and energies across more domains (Gallimore et al., 1996). The findings are consistent with the expectation that significant forms of family adaptation to childhood disability continue into early and late childhood and are not simply a function of an early stage of parental grieving and adjustment or a feature of specific developmental periods. Accommodation continues because sustaining a daily routine is an enduring fam-

TABLE II
ACCOMMODATION DOMAINS AND EXAMPLES[a]

Family subsistence: Hours worked; flexibility of work schedule; adequacy of financial resouces; amount of coverage provided by medical insurance
Services: Availability of services; eligibility for services; sources of transportation; amount of parent involvement required
Home/neighborhood safety and convenience: Safety and accessibility of play area; alterations in home (installation of locks, fences related to safety concerns); choice of particular neighborhood
Domestic workload: Amount of work which needs to be done; persons available to do it; amount of time spent by different family members
Child care tasks: complexity of child care tasks; presence of extraordinary child care demands (medical problems, behavior problems); number and availability of caregivers
Child peer groups: Child's playgroups (children with disabilities versus typically developing children); amount of parent supervision needed; role of siblings as playmates
Marital roles: Amount of shared decision making regarding child with delays; degree to which child care and household tasks are shared
Instrumental/emotional support: Availability and use of formal (church, parent groups) and informal (friends, relatives) sources of support; costs of using support
Father/spouse role: Amount of involvement with child with delays; amount of emotional support provided
Parent information: Reliance on professional versus nonprofessional sources of information; amount of time and effort spent accessing information

[a]From Bernheimer & Keogh, 1995. (Copyright 1995 by PRO-ED. Reprinted by permission.)

ily project, not a transient stage in family life or child development (Gallimore et al., in press; Weisner, 1998).

The accommodations identified in Project CHILD are consistent with findings from other researchers who have studied families' functional responses to children with problems. Based on their work with physically disabled children and their families, Sloper and Turner (1993) suggested that parent resources and coping strategies include: material resources, employment, housing, social and family resources, social networks and support systems, family environment, marital relationship; psychological resources such as personality, control orientation, and problem-solving and help-seeking skills and strategies. In a comprehensive review of relevant literature, Beresford (1994) identified "socio-ecological coping resources," which included social support, support from spouse, extended family, and formal agencies, marital status, socioeconomic circumstances, and the family environment. These categories are consistent with the domains of accommodations reported by the CHILD families.

1. HOW DO FAMILY ACCOMMODATIONS RELATE TO CHILD CHARACTERISTICS?

To examine this, Keogh, Bernheimer, Garnier, and Gallimore (1998) used path analytic techniques to compare the fit of child-driven and transactional models. In these analyses children's status in cognitive, personal social, behavior competencies and problems, and "hassle" domains were assessed at ages 3, 7, and 11. Family accommodations and adjustments to the children were collected at the same time points. Results of path analytic techniques indicated that the longitudinal relationships between children's cognitive and daily living competencies and family accommodations were best explained by a child-driven model. The direction of effects for both intensity and types of accommodation activities was from child to family. Children's hassle levels were both child-driven and transactional, suggesting that family accommodations influenced children's behavioral characteristics, and that child characteristics in turn influenced accommodations. Thus, for cognitive and daily living competencies, family accommodations are in part a response to the child, and there is no reason to think that one or the other type of family accommodation produces a better outcome for the child. For behavior characteristics the relationships are both more interesting and more complex with accommodations having an effect on behavior, and subsequently the behavior affecting accommodations—a dynamic pattern of adaptation from child ages 3 to 11. The two hypothesized path models representing child-driven and transactional models are shown in Figure 1.

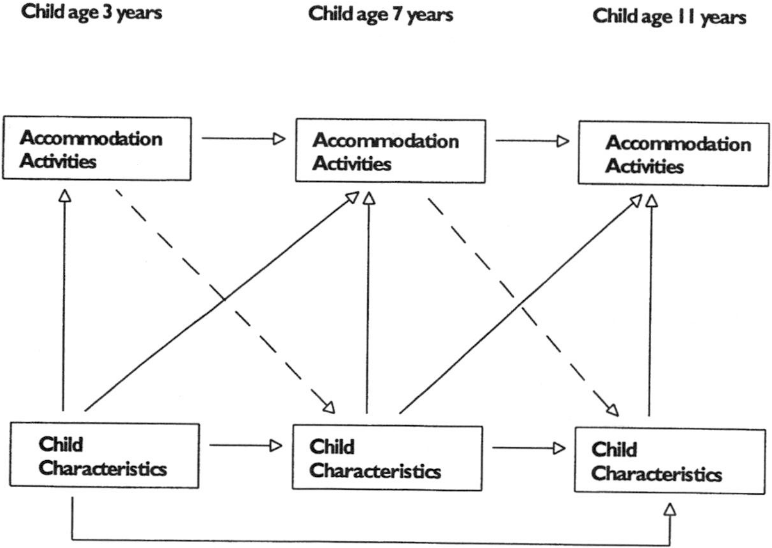

FIG. 1. Two theoretical models of parent accommodation activities and child characteristics, child age 3 to 11 years. The transactional model specifies a reciprocal direction of effects between child characteristics to parent accommodation activities. The child-driven model specifies a one direction of effects from child characteristics to parent accommodation activities. The cross-domain paths from ages 3 to 7 and ages 7 to 11 are indicated by a dashed line (— —) for the transactional model and a solid line for the child-driven model (———).

At all child ages, the frequency and intensity of family accommodations were not strongly tied to the family status variables such as SES or mothers' education. Rather, they were most consistently associated with child characteristics that directly impact the daily routine. Families who reported more accommodations were adapting to high "hassle" children who had many behavioral and emotional problems and relatively poor everyday competencies. For example, one family's accommodations were related primarily to the behavior of an extremely difficult child who required constant monitoring because he was capable of injuring himself or wreaking serious destruction. His mother commented when he was age 3: "Our house is set up around Michael. We still have a gate in here and there's a smaller area for him and he can function better, and it isn't that he's ever been destructive, its just that he can't control himself." By late childhood, although he was still a high hassle child, the deadbolts and gates required at age 3 were no longer needed. Parents reported he was now capable of many more things—he was more competent but also more troublesome. For example, he became so competent at using a computer the family bought for him that he managed to purchase a car through the Internet. His family still needed to monitor closely his activities, but the nature of their accommodations had changed—less intense, more varied.

2. CLINICAL IMPLICATIONS OF FAMILY ACCOMMODATION[2]

Michael and his family illustrate the generalization that different accommodations emerge in response to children's changing developmental competencies and problems. Our findings concur with the literature describing changing parental concerns over time (Dyson, 1993; Orr, Cameron, Dyson, & Day, 1993) and underscore the importance of designing interventions that are sensitive to family changes in response to developmental transitions. For example, the restructuring of child–family relationships in adolescence for normally developing children is well documented in the developmental literature. It seems likely that the influence of children's characteristics on family accommodations will be especially strong as children with delays enter adolescence and new issues of autonomy and independence become salient. Thus the indices of family outcome will vary as a function of children's developmental age.

Perhaps as much or more than strategies for coping with stress, family accommodations to sustain their daily routine should be factored into planning interventions. Since the inception of Part H of IDEA (currently referred to as Part C in the Amendments to the Individuals with Disabilities Education Act), the focus in early intervention has shifted from child-centered to family-centered care (Bernheimer & Keogh, 1995). The Individualized Family Service Plan (IFSP), developed by professionals in collaboration with families, identifies family as well as

[2]Portions of this section adapted from Gallimore et al. (1998).

child strengths and needs, and identifies priorities for intervention. Given dynamic contexts into which interventions are to be inserted, it is not surprising the shift to IFSP sometimes encounter difficulties. Many IFSP plans fail to be fully implemented or to be sustained by parents (Meyer & Bailey, 1993). Clinicians frequently complain that parents do not follow through on what seem to be well thought-out intervention plans. Bernheimer and Keogh (1995) observed that the gap between professional advice and parental practice is common and gives pause—why aren't well-designed plans always implemented and sustained? Family-focused interventions may not always be consistent with accommodations families are already making and thus are not well "fitted" into the everyday routines of family life. This possibility is clearly indicated in recent literature emphasizing the importance to parents of professionals who "consider unique family environments and routines" (Brotherson & Goldstein, 1992, p. 519; see also Affleck & Tennen, 1993; Bosch, 1996; Herman, Marcenko, & Hazel, 1996).

Does knowledge about accommodations being made to sustain a daily routine insure that professional interventions will be successfully implemented in all families? Clearly, no. Some families faced with overwhelming external pressures will always challenge the professionals who plan interventions. The daily routine in these families is likely to be composed of activities and accommodations which seem unrelated to the child (e.g., keeping up with the rent, making food stamps stretch until the end of the month, coping with substance abuse) (Bernheimer & Keogh, 1995; Gallimore et al., in press). Yet making "a sensitive examination of the . . . context . . . that receives an intervention" (Gallimore et al., 1993, p. 553) should help practitioners understand what needs to happen in order for an intervention to be implemented and maintained. It should also prevent practitioners from introducing additional stress to a multiply challenged family by adding to their adaptive burden.

C. Family Outcomes

With a few exceptions, by child age 13 Project CHILD families are doing relatively well. Like all families, there are ups and downs, but 10+ years of case materials suggest that about 90% of the Project CHILD families are managing "good enough" if not as well as they'd like (Weisner, Matheson, Coots, & Gallimore, 1997). Except for a troubled few, the families included those with stable daily routines, those who were vulnerable but resilient, and those who were described as "hanging on" (Weisner et al., 1997). Some of the variations in accommodation among families in these different circumstances were predictably related to income, availability of instrumental support, and other resources. These variations aside, whatever their circumstances families were actively making accommodations to incorporate the child with delays into their daily routine.

An important point, however, is that contrary to some literature on families adapting to early childhood delay, Weisner et al. (1997) found no indication that Project CHILD families were suffering from exceptionally high levels of stress, emotional problems, or family difficulties. Most of the major problems were not related specifically to children's developmental delays: Death of a grandparent, spouse or a child, loss of a job, or housing, and other such major events loomed larger than childhood delays in most cases. We do not mean to minimize the stresses, strains, and problems the families have faced. Indeed, some families have carried and some still carry great burdens, but the overall impression is that these families are not that much different from others and we are wise to heed Glidden's challenge of the assumption that a child disability inevitably means the family itself has a disability (Glidden, 1993, p. 426). That is certainly not true of 90+% of the families in the CHILD and REACH cohorts.

V. GENERALIZATIONS AND OBSERVATIONS FROM TWO LONGITUDINAL STUDIES

Our work in REACH and CHILD has documented that early signs of developmental delays signal the likelihood of continuing cognitive delays. We have also identified a broad range of developmental and personal/social outcomes for children with delays and their families, and we have shown that children's status and family status are only loosely linked. Said directly, a child with problems does not necessarily mean a family with problems. Just as outcomes for children cannot be assumed to be an index of the outcomes for families, family outcomes do not necessarily provide information about child status. Successful outcomes for families may not be the optimal outcomes for a single family member. Similarly, intense parental focus on a single family member may be disruptive to the family as a whole. In addition, from preschool to late childhood we watched the proactive and positive adaptations families made to children with delays, our observations challenging the mental health model of family pathology. We acknowledge that the generalizations from our findings are tempered by the selective nature of our samples, but we argue that the functional accommodations comprising family life are not limited to families of children with delays, but rather are inherent in every culture (Weisner, 1998). While there may be differences in specifics, the kinds of adaptive problems faced by families with children with delays occur in all families with children (Keogh, Bernheimer, Gallimore, & Weisner, 1998).

The theoretical as well as the practical issue has to do with the nature of family–child relationships and the effects on children's development (Caldwell & Bradley, 1994; Sameroff, 1994). The accommodations by families are driven by the children's cognitive status, but personal/social outcomes for children are, in part at least, a function of transactions between families and children. The findings of limited influence of family practices on the cognitive development of children with delays does not negate the importance of family environments. It does underscore the need to expand the scope and content of research on families' adaptations to children with special needs and draws attention to the need to consider a range of child outcomes.

What are appropriate goals for children with developmental delays? What should be emphasized in early intervention? What child outcomes should be considered in program evaluation? These questions have both clinical and research implications, and the answers are not certain. Our findings confirm the stability of early cognitive delays, but underscore the variability among children in social/behavioral outcomes. This raises questions of the emphasis and content of intervention programs, including the possibility that the focus should be on personal/social and behavioral competencies, rather than on cognitive change. This is not to argue that enhancing cognitive development should be ignored, but rather that personal/social characteristics and behavior may deserve to be the central focus of interventions.

An emphasis on personal/social competencies of children with delays also has implications for assessment and diagnosis. The emphasis on cognitive/language delays has produced a number of well-designed and well-tested measures for identification and diagnostic purposes (Bailey & Wolery, 1989). There are fewer differentiated and reliable approaches for assessing children's social, affective, and behavioral status (Harbin, Gallagher, & Terry, 1991). Thus, diagnosticians and clinicians who work with young children with delays often must rely on observation and on adults' reports, data sources that may contain threats to validity and reliability (Keogh & Bernheimer, 1998). Similarly, there are few well-developed systems for describing families and for determining family outcomes. A consequence is to rely on summarizing demographic markers (e.g., SES, parents level of education) to describe families. Yet our findings document wide variations in the functioning of families within demographically defined family groups. Income level does not determine how families function. This, of course, implies the need for clinicians and researchers to get beyond demographics to the functional level of family life.

From a policy perspective, our findings of cognitive stability, and of continuing need for special education services through school, may seem discouraging. However, we argue that these findings should not be construed as indicating a "failure" of early intervention. We underscore the variability in personal social outcomes, and note that these outcomes were unrelated to cognitive status. Another interpretation of the placement findings is that the children were appropriately identified early on (e.g., that the delays signaled long-term problems that required ongoing educational intervention). We find it encouraging that the term, *developmental delay*, although still not a precise diagnostic category, now provides opportunities for intervention from birth to 8 years of age. We also find encouraging the fact that the majority of our families are doing well. The divorce rate in both samples is well below the average for the state. In addition, while few children have "caught up," most of our families have been able to construct and maintain a daily routine of life that balances the needs of the child with those of other family members.

Finally, from a research perspective we underscore the benefits and the problems in conducting longitudinal studies. Our experience in both REACH and CHILD has increased our sensitivity to and understanding of methodological pitfalls and ethical considerations. Like other longitudinal researchers (Bergman & Magnusson, 1990; Egeland, 1991; Nesselroade & Reese, 1973; Nunnally, 1973; Werner & Smith, 1982, 1992), we faced questions of sampling criteria, of the validity, reliability, and appropriateness of measures and assessment techniques in different developmental periods, of possible effects of repeated testing, and of investigator bias in interpretation of interview data. We also were aware of possible cohort effects, given the policy and legislative changes affecting services in the 10 years between studies. A serious problem had to do with the use of standardized tests with children with significant developmental delays, as many of the usual measures have heavy language demands, and the majority of children in both studies were delayed in language development. We also note the practical and analytic problems of dealing with increasingly large data sets over time, at the same time recognizing that there were additional or different data that should have been collected. The "why didn't we" question appeared and reappeared with some regularity.

In addition to methodological issues, over time we became aware of the changing nature of researcher–parent relationships, and of the impact of our research on parents and families (Keogh & Bernheimer, 1998). In initiating both of our studies, we made it explicitly clear that these were research efforts, not interventions. Yet over the years it was apparent that the lines between research and interventions were increasingly blurred. Although we provided only occasional referrals or referral information, something unfolded over the years that we did not anticipate. Despite our continuing efforts to define our work as research, over time more and more parents viewed us as advocates, resources, and friends. One mother in the REACH study said that the project was the most effective intervention she and her child had experienced. We interpret this as evidence of the importance of stable and ongoing professional–parent relationships, the significance of letting parents tell their stories, and the value of listening to them.

We also became aware of the impact of our research on the families themselves. For example, our policy was to test the children in their homes, encouraging parents to be present, on the assumption that the setting would "demystify" the assessment process. Over time we found that fewer and fewer parents participated in the assessment, as for many this documented the discrepancies between their child's status and "normal" expectancies. The repeated testings appeared to have little effect on the children, but became increasingly painful for parents. Closely related, we were concerned about negative feedback to parents, given the possible effects on their expectations for their children's futures. Similar questions arose in regard to information given to teachers and other professionals.

We conclude with the observation that our research in these two projects has changed our views and enhanced our understanding of children with developmental problems and their families. We have been impressed with the range of personal and social outcomes of the children, with the resilience and commitment of the families, and with the positive adaptations and accommodations they have made. As we came to know these children and their families we were increasingly aware of the effects of being good listeners, rather than dispensers of information or advice. Despite the many problems and pitfalls in longitudinal research, we are convinced that it was the continuing research effort over time that allowed us to understand the course of development for both children and families.

ACKNOWLEDGMENTS

This research was supported by National Institute of Child Health and Human Development Grants Nos. HD19124 and HD11944. The assistance of the Statistical Core (D. Guthrie, Director & G. Gordon, Senior Statistician) was provided with the support of a Mental Retardation Center Grant (HD04612) to the Mental Retardation Research Center (MRRC) at UCLA. The authors appreciate the cooperation and contributions of the participating families. We gratefully acknowledge the contributions of our collaborator Tom Weisner to the projects on which this chapter is based. Many and diverse additional contributions were made to the longitudinal studies by Kazuo Nihira, Iris Mink, Donald Guthrie, Sandra Z. Kaufman, Lori Stolze, Catherine Matheson, Gwen Gordon, Mary Note, Sue Sears, Monique DeCicco, Rhodora Maliksi-Farmer, Phyllis Schneider, Jennifer Furin, and Lindsay Clare. The authors acknowledge the support of Robert B. Edgerton and their other colleagues in the Sociobehavioral Research Group of UCLA's Mental Retardation Research Center, the Division of Social and Community Psychiatry, and the Neuropsychiatric Institute.

REFERENCES

Achenbach, T. M. (1981). *Child Behavior Checklist.* Burlington, VT: University of Vermont.

Affleck, G., & Tennen, H. (1993). Cognitive adaptation to adversity: Insights from parents of medically fragile infants. In A. P. Turnbull, J. M. Patterson, S. K. Behr, D. L. Murphy, J. G. Marquis, & M. J. Blue-Banning (Eds.), *Cognitive coping, families, and disability* (pp. 135–150). Baltimore: Paul H. Brookes.

Alpern, G. D., & Boll, T. J. (1972). The developmental profile. Aspen, CO: Psychological Development Publications.

Anton, B. S., & Dindia, G. (1984). Parental perceptions of cognitive abilities of children with cerebral palsy. *Psychological Reports, 54,* 987–990.

Bailey, D., & Wolery, M. (1989). *Assessing infants and preschoolers with handicaps.* Columbus, OH: Merrill Publishing Co.

Batshaw, M. L., & Perrett, Y. M. (1981). *Children with handicaps: A medical primer.* Baltimore: Paul H. Brookes Publishing Co.

Bell, R. Q. (1968). A reinterpretation of the direction of effects in studies of socialization. *Psychological Review, 75,* 81–95.

Bergman, L. R., & Magnusson, D. (1990). General issues about data quality in longitudinal research. In D. Magnusson & L. R. Berman (Eds.), *Data quality in longitudinal research* (pp. 1–31). Cambridge: Cambridge University.

Beresford, B. A. (1994). Resources and strategies: How parents cope with the care of a disabled child. *Journal of Child Psychology and Psychiatry, 35*, 171–209.

Bernheimer, L. P., Gallimore, R., & Kaufman, S. (1993). Clinical child assessment in a family context: A four group typology of family experiments with young children with developmental delays. *Journal of Early Intervention, 17*, 253–269.

Bernheimer, L. P., & Keogh, B. K. (1982). *Research on early abilities of children with handicaps*. (Final report, longitudinal sample). Los Angeles: University of California.

Bernheimer, L. P., & Keogh, B. K. (1986). Developmental disabilities in preschool children. In B. K. Keogh (Ed.), *Advances in special education Vol. 5* (pp. 61–94). Greenwich, CT: JAI.

Bernheimer, L. P., & Keogh, B. K. (1988). Stability of cognitive performance of children with developmental delays. *American Journal on Mental Retardation, 92*, 539–542.

Bernheimer, L. P., & Keogh, B. K. (1995). Weaving interventions into the fabric of everyday life: An approach to family assessment. *Topics in Early Childhood Special Education, 15*, 415–433.

Bernheimer, L. P., & Keogh, B. K. (1996). *Project REACH follow-up report*. Los Angeles: University of California.

Bosch, L. A. (1996). Needs of parents of young children with developmental delays: Implications for social work practice. *Families in Society: The Journal of Contemporary Human Services, 77*, 477–487.

Brotherson, M. J., & Goldstein, B. L. (1992). Time as a resource and constraint for parents of young children with disabilities: Implications for early intervention services. *Topics in Early Childhood Special Education, 12*, 508–527.

Bruner, J. (1989, April). *Culture and human development*. Paper presented at the biennial meeting of the Society for Research in Child Development, Kansas City.

Caldwell, B. M., & Bradley, R. H. (1994). Environmental issues in developmental follow-up research. In S. L. Friedman & H. C. Haywood (Eds.), *Developmental follow-up* (pp. 235–285). San Diego: Academic Press.

Clare, L. (1998). *The relationship of child characteristics and parents' developmental goals for children from preschool to adolescence*. Unpublished dissertation, University of California, Los Angeles.

Clare, L., Garnier, H., & Gallimore, R. (1998). Parent developmental expectations and child characteristics: A longitudinal study of children with developmental delays and their families. *American Journal on Mental Retardation*.

Crnic, K. A., Friedrich, W. N., & Greenberg, M. T. (1983). Adaptation of families with mentally retarded children: A model of stress, coping and family ecology. *American Journal of Mental Deficiency, 88*, 125–138.

Coles, R. (1989). *The call of stories: Teaching and the moral imagination*. Boston: Houghton Mifflin.

DeVries, M. W. (1984). Temperament and infant mortality among the Masai of East Africa. *American Journal of Psychiatry, 10*, 141.

Drillien, C. M., Pickering, R. M., & Drummond, M. B. (1988). Predictive value of screening for difficult areas of development. *Developmental Medicine and Child Neurology, 30*, 294–305.

Duran, B. J., & Weffer, R. E. (1992). Immigrants' aspirations, high school process, and academic outcomes. *American Educational Research Journal, 29*, 163–181.

Dyson, L. (1993). Response to the presence of a child with disabilities: parental stress and family functioning over time. *American Journal on Mental Retardation, 98*, 207–218.

Edgar, E., Heggelund, M., & Fischer, M. (1988). A longitudinal study of graduates of special education preschools: Educational placement after preschool. *Topics in Early Childhood Special Education, 8*(3), 61–74.

Edgar, E., McNulty, B., Gaetz, J., & Maddox, M. (1984). Educational placement of graduates of preschool programs for handicapped children. *Topics in Early Childhood Special Education, 4*(3), 19–29.

Egeland, B. (1991). A longitudinal study of high-risk families: Issues and findings. In R. H. Starr & D. A. Wolfe (Eds.), *The effects of child abuse and neglect: issues and research* (pp. 33–55). New York: Guilford Press.

Entwistle, D. R., & Hayduk, L. A. (1981). Academic expectations and the school attainment of young children. *Sociology of Education, 54*, 34–50.

Erikson, E. H. (1959). Identity and the life cycle: Selected papers. *Psychological Issues*, 1–171.

First, L. R., & Palfrey, J. S. (1994). The infant or young child with developmental delay. *The New England Journal of Medicine*, 478–483.

Gallimore, R., Bernheimer, L. P., & Weisner, T. S. (in press). Family life is more than managing crisis: Broadening the agenda of research on families adapting to childhood disability. In R. Gallimore, L. Bernheimer, D. MacMillan, D. Speece, & S. Vaughn (Eds.), *Developmental perspectives on high incidence handicapping conditions*. New Jersey: Erlbaum & Associates.

Gallimore, R., Coots, J. J., Weisner, T. S., Garnier, H. E., & Guthrie, D. (1996). Family responses to children with early developmental delays II: Accommodation intensity and activity in early and middle childhood. *American Journal on Mental Retardation, 101*, 215–232.

Gallimore, R., Goldenberg, C. N., & Weisner, T. S. (1993). The social construction and subjective reality of activity settings: Implications for community psychology. *American Journal of Community Psychology, 21*, 537–559.

Gallimore, R., Weisner, T. S., Kaufman, S. Z., & Bernheimer, L. P. (1989). The social construction of ecocultural niches: Family accommodation of developmentally delayed children. *American Journal of Mental Retardation, 94*, 216–230.

Glidden, L. M. (1993). What we do *not* know about families with children who have developmental disabilities: Questionnaire on resources and stress as a case study. *American Journal on Mental Retardation, 97*, 481–495.

Goodman, J. F. (1977). Medical diagnosis and intelligence levels in young mentally retarded children: A follow-up study. *Journal of Mental Deficiency Research, 21*, 205–212.

Harbin, G. L., Gallagher, J. J., & Terry, D. V. (1991). Defining the eligible population: Policy issues and challenges. *Journal of Early Intervention, 15*, 13–20.

Havighurst, R. J. (1972). *Developmental tasks and education* (3rd ed.). New York: David MacKay.

Hayden, A. H., & Beck, G. R. (1982). The epidemiology of high-risk and handicapped infants. In C. T. Ramsey & D. L. Trohanis (Eds.), *Finding and educating high-risk and handicapped infants* (pp. 19–52). Baltimore: University Park Press.

Herman, S. E., Marcenko, M. O., & Hazel, K. L. (1996). Parents' perspectives on quality in family support programs. *Journal of Mental Health Administration, 23*, 156–169.

Hightower, A. D., Spinell, A., & Lotyczewski, B. S. (1988). *Teacher-Child Rating Scale (T-CRS) Guidelines*. Rochester, MN: University of Rochester, Primary Mental Health Project, Inc.

Hightower, A. D., Work, W. C., Cowen, E. L., Lotyczewski, B. S., Spinell, A. P., Guare, J. C., & Rohrbeck, C. A. (1986). The Teacher-child rating scale: A brief objective measure of elementary children's school problem behaviors and competencies. *School Psychology Review, 15*, 393–409.

Hunt, J. M., & Paraskevopoulos, J. (1980). Children's psychological development as a function of the inaccuracy of their mothers' knowledge of their abilities. *Journal of Genetic Psychology, 136*, 285–298.

Jensen, G., & Kogan, K. L. (1962). Parental estimates of the future achievement of children with cerebral palsy. *Journal of Mental Deficiency Research, 6*, 56–64.

Juvonen, J., Keogh, B. K., Ratekin, C., & Bernheimer, L. P. (1992). Children's and teachers' views of school-based competencies and their relation to children's peer status. *School Psychology Review, 21*, 410–442.

Keogh, B. K., & Bernheimer, L. P. (1995). Etiologic conditions as predictors of children's problems and competencies in elementary school. *Journal of Child Neurology, 10*, S100–S105.

Keogh, B. K., & Bernheimer, L. P. (1998). Concordance between mothers' and teachers' perceptions of behavior problems of children with developmental delays. *Journal of Emotional and Behavioral Disorders, 6*, 33–41.

Keogh, B. K., & Bernheimer, L. P. (1998). Issues and dilemmas in longitudinal research: A tale of two studies. *Thalamus, 16*, 5–13.

Keogh, B. K., Bernheimer, L. P., Gallimore, R., & Weisner, T. S. (1998). Child and family outcomes over time: A longitudinal perspective on developmental delays. In M. Lewis & C. Feiring (Eds.), *Families, risk, & competence* (pp. 269–288). New Jersey: Lawrence Erlbaum.

Keogh, B. K., Bernheimer, L. P., Garnier, H., & Gallimore, R. (1998). *Models of change for children with developmental delays: Child-driven or transactional?* Unpublished manuscript.

Keogh, B. K., Bernheimer, L. P., & Guthrie, D. G. (1997). Stability and change over time in cognitive level of children with delays. *American Journal on Mental Retardation, 101*, 365–372.

Keogh, B. K., Bernheimer, L. P., Haney, M. P., & Daley, S. (1989). Behaviour and adjustment problems of young developmentally delayed children. *European Journal of Special Needs Education, 4*, 79–90.

Keogh, B. K., Coots, J. J., & Bernheimer, L. P. (1995). School placement of children with nonspecific developmental delays. *Journal of Early Intervention, 20*, 65–78.

Keogh, B. K., Juvonen, J., & Bernheimer, L. P. (1989). Assessing children's competence: Mothers' and teachers' ratings of competent behavior. *Psychological Assessment: A Journal of Consulting and Clinical Psychology, 1*(3), 224–229.

Keogh, B. K., & Kopp, C. B. (1982). *Project REACH Final Report*, Los Angeles, CA: University of California.

Keogh, B. K., Pullis, M. E., & Cadwell, J. (1979). *Parent temperament questionnaire. Project REACH.* Los Angeles, CA: University of California.

Keogh, B. K., Pullis, M. E., & Cadwell, J. (1982). A short form of the Teacher Temperament Questionnaire. *Journal of Educational Measurement, 19*, 323–329.

Keogh, B. K., Ratekin, C. B., & Bernheimer, L. P. (1992). *Behavior problems of developmentally delayed children: Stability over time.* Project CHILD Technical Report, University of California, Los Angeles.

Kopp, C. B., Krakow, J. B., & Johnson, K. L. (1983). Strategy production in young Down syndrome children. *American Journal on Mental Retardation, 88*, 164–169.

Krakow, J. B., & Kopp, C. B. (1982). Sustained attention in young Down syndrome children. *Topics in Early Childhood Special Education, 2*, 32–42.

Masten, A. S., Best, K. M., & Garmezy, N. (1990). Resilience and development: Contributions from the study of children who overcome adversity. *Development and Psychopathology, 2*, 425–444.

Maziade, M., Cote, R., Boutin, P., Bernier, H., & Thivierge, J. (1987). Temperament and intellectual development: A longitudinal study from infancy to four years. *American Journal of Psychiatry, 144*, 144–150.

Merton, R. (1948). The self-fulfilling prophecy. *Antioch Review, 8*, 193–210.

Meyer, E. C., & Bailey, D. B. (1993). Family-centered care in early intervention: Community and hospital settings. In J. L. Paul & R. J. Simeonsson (Eds.), *Children with special needs: Family culture, and society* (pp. 181–209). Orlando, FL: Harcourt Brace Jovanovich.

Nesselroade, J. R., & Reese, H. W. (1973). (Eds.). *Life-span developmental psychology: methodological issues.* New York: Academic Press.

Nunnally, J. C. (1973). Research strategies and measurement methods for investigating human development. In J. R. Nesselroade & H. W. Reese (Eds.), *Life-span developmental psychology* (pp. 87–109). New York: Academic Press.

Orr, R. R., Cameron, S. J., Dyson, L. A., & Day, D. M. (1993). Age-related changes in stress experienced by families with a child who has developmental delays. *Mental Retardation, 31*, 171–176.

Palfrey, J. S., Singer, J. D., Walker, D. K., & Butler, J. A. (1987). Early identification of children's special needs: a study in five metropolitan communities. *Journal of Pediatrics, 111*, 651–659.

Sameroff, A. (1994). Ecological perspectives on longitudinal follow-up studies. In S. L. Friedman & H. C. Haywood (Eds.), *Developmental Follow-up* (pp. 45–66). New York: Academic Press.

Schneider, P., & Gearhart, M. (1988). The ecocultural niche of families with mentally retarded children: Evidence from mother-child interaction studies. *Journal of Applied Developmental Psychology, 9*, 85–106.

Shonkoff, J. P., Hauser-Cram, P., Krauss, M. W., & Upshur, C. C. (1992). Development of infants with disabilities and their families. *Monographs of the Society for Research in Child Development*, 57 (6, Serial No. 230).

Sloper, P., & Turner, S. (1993). Risk and resistance factors in the adaptation of parents of children with severe physical disability. *Journal of Child Psychology and Psychiatry, 34*, 167–189.

Stavrou, E. (1990). The long-term stability of WISC-R scores in mildly retarded and learning disabled children. *Psychology in the Schools, 27*, 101–110.

Stayton, V. D., & Karnes, M. B. (1994). Model programs for infants and toddlers with disabilities and their families. In L. J. Johnson, R. G. Gallagher, M. J. Montagne, J. B. Jordan, J. J. Gallagher, P. L. Hutinger, and M. B. Karnes (Eds.), *Meeting early intervention challenges* (pp. 33–58). Baltimore: P. H. Brookes.

Truscott, S. D., Narrett, C. M., & Smith, S. E. (1994). WISC-R reliability over time: Implications for practice and research. *Psychological Reports, 74*, 147–156.

Turnbull, A. P., Patterson, J. M., Behr, S. K., Murphy, D. L., Marquis, J. G., & Blue-Banning, M. J. (1993). (Eds.). *Cognitive coping, families, and disability*. Baltimore: Paul H. Brooks.

Vanderveer, B., & Schweid, E. (1974). Infant assessment: Stability of mental functioning in young retarded children. *American Journal of Mental Deficiency, 79*, 1–4.

Vohs, J. (1993). On belonging. In A. P. Turnbull, J. M. Patterson, S. K. Behr, D. L. Murphy, J. G. Marquis, & M. J. Blue-Banning (Eds.), *Cognitive coping, families, and disability* (pp. 51–66). Baltimore: Paul H. Brookes.

Volkmar, F. R. (1991). Autism and the pervasive developmental disorders. In M. Lewis (Ed.), *Child and adolescent psychiatry* (2nd ed., pp. 489–497). Baltimore, MD: Williams and Wilkins.

Walker, D. K., Singer, J. D., Palfrey, J. S., Orza, M., Wenger, M., & Butler, J. A. (1988). Who leaves and who stays in special education: A 2-year follow-up study. *Exceptional Children, 54*, 393–402.

Weisner, T. S. (1984). Ecocultural niches of middle childhood: A cross-cultural perspective. In W. A. Collins (Ed.), *Development during middle childhood: The years from six to twelve* (pp. 335–369). Washington, DC: National Academy of Sciences.

Weisner, T. S. (1998). Human development as a culturally organized adaptive project. In D. Sharma & K. Fischer (Eds.), *Socio-emotional development across cultures. New directions in child development* (pp. 69–85). San Francisco: Jossey Bass.

Weisner, T. S., Matheson, C., Coots, J. J., & Gallimore, R. (1997, April). *Sustainability of daily routines as a family outcome*. Paper presented at Society for Research in Child Development, Washington, D.C.

Werner, E. E., & Smith, R. S. (1982). *Vulnerable but invincible: A longitudinal study of resilient children and youth*. New York: McGraw-Hill.

Werner, E. E., & Smith, R. S. (1992). *Overcoming the odds. High risk children from birth to adulthood.* Ithaca, NY: Cornell University Press.

Zetlin, A. G., & Turner, J. L. (1984). Self-perspectives on being handicapped: Stigma and adjustment. In R. B. Edgerton (Ed.), *Lives in process: Mildly retarded adults in a large city*, (pp. 93–120). Washington, DC: American Association on Mental Deficiency.

Savant Syndrome

TED NETTELBECK

DEPARTMENT OF PSYCHOLOGY
UNIVERSITY OF ADELAIDE
ADELAIDE, SOUTH AUSTRALIA

ROBYN YOUNG

DEPARTMENT OF PSYCHOLOGY
FLINDERS UNIVERSITY OF SOUTH AUSTRALIA
ADELAIDE, SOUTH AUSTRALIA

I. INTRODUCTION

What is savant syndrome? How do savants do the extraordinary things that they do? What implications does savant syndrome have for improving our understanding of human intelligence? In what follows, we address these questions, in the light of research undertaken predominantly during the past 20 years. Although interest in this topic has a very long history (Foerstl, 1989), attempts to develop a theoretical account for savant syndrome are relatively recent, with two reviews appearing in 1978 (Hill, 1978; Rimland, 1978a). Rimland's overview focused on incidence, a possible relationship between autism and giftedness, and provided descriptions of the accomplishments of individual savants. Hill's review comprehensively surveyed literature from the late 1890s to the mid-1970s and discussed various explanations for how savants achieve their feats. He found more than 60 reports and publications involving over 100 savants, with several of these sources in languages other than English. Hill drew attention to the largely anecdotal nature of much of this literature but substantially based his conclusions on the small body of scientific research then available.

The past two decades have seen a significant expansion to published research into the nature of psychological processes underpinning savant skills, with more than 100 publications appearing between 1978 and the present, including five books (Howe, 1989; Miller, 1989; Sacks, 1995a; Smith & Tsimpli, 1995; Treffert,

INTERNATIONAL REVIEW OF RESEARCH IN
MENTAL RETARDATION, Vol. 22
0074-7750/99 $30.00

1989). Miller (1989), Sacks (1995a), and Smith and Tsimpli (1995) were primarily concerned with the remarkable accomplishments of single individuals—a musician, an artist, and a linguist, respectively—although all three considered a wider theoretical context. Howe (1989) covered a range of savant skills, with particular attention to feats of memory and calendar calculation. Treffert (1989) followed and expanded on his earlier review (Treffert, 1988), providing a detailed account of the accomplishments and personal histories of the most famous savants, past and present, together with his theory about the nature of putative modified brain structures that might result in savant syndrome. These five books and two brief overviews that have considered the implications of savant syndrome for the education of children with intellectual and developmental disabilities (Cheatham, Rucker, Polloway, Smith, & Lewis, 1995; Wehmeyer, 1992) are all valuable additions to the literature, but none set out to provide a comprehensive review of research in the field.

This chapter takes as its starting point Hill's (1978) review, the most comprehensive to that time. Generally, we have not reviewed sources covered by Hill, and his chapter remains essential for newcomers to the field. Instead we expand on the issues that he raised, especially about the nature of memory and of motivational processes involved in savant skills. In doing so we have reviewed all published research during the period 1978–1998 and, following Hill, we have included in the bibliography those articles and reports not cited in this chapter. We present a testable theoretical explanation for savant syndrome and our assumption, drawn from others, is that savant skills, although highly developed, are accomplished without the degree of thought necessary to regard them as "intelligent." This assertion is therefore the antithesis of the viewpoint that savant syndrome establishes the existence of different kinds of intelligence. Nonetheless, because savant skills must at some level require cognitive processes that also can contribute to intelligent behavior, savant syndrome does need to be accommodated within a theory of intelligence. In attempting to formulate a solution to this problem we acknowledge the extent to which we have drawn on the work of others, particularly Miller (1989), Treffert (1989), and on the systematic, empirical research of O'Connor and Hermelin, to which we will refer in section IV.

II. DEFINITION AND INCIDENCE

Hill's (1978) analysis of definition and nomenclature drew attention to concern about the inadequacy of the earlier term *idiot savant*.[1] ("Idiot" is now widely regarded as pejorative and in any case, as Tredgold [1923] first noted, it implies a

[1]The English physician J. Langdon Down (1887) has been credited with inventing this term, presumed to derive from the French words *idiot* and *savoir*, although both *idiot* and *savant* have long existed in English usage. Spitz (1995) has raised doubts about this attribution, and there has been debate about the appropriateness of savant (Hill, 1978).

significantly lower level of general mental functioning than commonly characterizes savants). Instead, Hill preferred the term *savant*. This view has largely prevailed, although the older terminology is still in use.

Hill (1978) defined a savant as "a mentally retarded person demonstrating one or more skills above the level expected of nonretarded individuals" (p. 281). With the caveat that such skills are invariably limited to relatively narrowly defined areas, Hill's definition has satisfactorily stood the test of time. Despite considerable discussion of definitional matters, there is no clearly better alternative to Hill's suggestion. Debate will probably continue about preferable alternative terminology (see, for example, correspondence between Frey [1995] and Sacks [1995b]); but the major direction of research during the past two decades has been towards improving theory about how savant abilities develop.

There would be advantage in being able to quantify more precisely levels of exceptionality. Savants differ considerably in proficiencies, and Treffert (1989) has proposed that "prodigious" and "talented" levels be distinguished from each other and from "splinter skills." He suggested reserving the first term for skills so exceptional that only few nondisabled people can match them. Among rare individuals, these cases would, by Treffert's reckoning, be very rare indeed; only about 100 over the past century (Treffert, 1989, p. 217). The second term, on the other hand, identified those relatively more frequent individuals whose skills, while clearly inconsistent with an otherwise general low level of functioning, would not be beyond the capabilities of many nondisabled persons. This distinction excluded splinter skills that are fairly common among persons with autism—i.e., the same kinds of activities performed by savants but at levels that would be unremarkable but for the presence of an intellectual disability. However, there are difficulties with this category system. At present there are no reliable means for quantifying such skills. Interested experts could probably agree about relative rankings within a given area of skill, and may agree that rare cases of artistic achievement are somehow more remarkable than relatively more frequent calendrical calculators. However, experts probably could not make reliable comparisons across different kinds of skill without first setting arbitrary rules.[2] Moreover, although Treffert (1989) implied otherwise, it is not clear that "prodigious" skills are not more developed "talented" skills. We agree with Treffert that some achievements may be categorically different from others. However, we will suggest in section VI that skill domains rather than levels of accomplishments may in part define boundaries.

Treffert (1989) also suggested *savant syndrome* as the generic term. Doubts

[2]The authors achieved a highly significant correlation of .89 when independently ranking the skills of 31 savants observed directly by Young (1995), with Nettelbeck working from videos, examples of savants' works, and written reports. Nonetheless, it is doubtful that this high level of correspondence could have been reached had there not been substantial broad agreement between the two raters beforehand that domains like music, art, and mathematics were generally somehow more remarkable than memory for facts or calendar skills and that IQ should be disregarded.

have been expressed about the suitability of *syndrome* because concurrent defining characteristics are no more than exceptionally high skill and markedly subaverage general intellectual functioning, the latter inevitably representing a wide diversity of diagnostic classifications (Wehmeyer, 1992). Although, as Treffert has suggested, the incidence for visual impairments and autistic characteristics may be higher among savants than among others with an intellectual disability, (see also Rimland, 1978a), these do not provide suitable definitional symptoms. All savants are not visually impaired; not all autistic persons are savants, and nor are all savants autistic. However, despite doubts about the term, *savant syndrome* has been widely adopted during the past decade. We agree with Wehmeyer that the term is acceptable, providing that these limitations are recognized. In summary then, problems of definition as identified by Hill (1978) have remained on the agenda, but the main aims of research have been to explain how exceptional skills develop when general intellectual functioning is deficient, and thereby to reveal more about the nature of intelligence.

Hill's (1978) estimate for incidence (<1% among persons with an intellectual disability) has been widely accepted, although Bergman and DePue (1986) have argued for high numbers of musical savants, and Hill did allow that his estimate might be marginally low. However, no published account since 1978 has seriously challenged Hill's conclusion that savants are rare. Hill's observation that males significantly outnumber females (approximately 6:1) still stands. In part this high ratio must reflect the higher ratio of males to females (4:1) among the autistic population. The only extension to Hill's estimates comes from Rimland (1978a), who concluded that incidence of savant skills among persons with autism is considerably higher than is found for the mentally retarded population, at about 10%. This estimate, based on parental observations, may be exaggerated by an unreliable definition for savant syndrome. Treffert (1989) has observed that about half of all savants have autism.

III. THE SKILLS OF SAVANTS

A remarkable characteristic of savant and splinter skills is that they develop within only a narrow range of activities. Hill (1974) first made this observation, identifying seven categories. *Calendar calculating* involves at least naming the day of the week on which a given date has fallen or will fall, although it may extend to even more complicated feats, like nominating in which years during the next century Good Friday will fall on a given date; or in which years New Year's Day will be a Wednesday. Several investigations of this ability have been published in the past 20 years (Burling, Sappington, & Mead, 1983; Casey, Gordon, Mannheim, & Rumsay, 1993; Dorman, 1991; Hermelin & O'Connor, 1986; Ho, Tsang, & Ho, 1991; Howe & Smith, 1988; Moriarty, Ring, & Robertson, 1993;

O'Connor & Hermelin, 1984, 1992; Ohtsuka, Miyasaka, & Kamizono, 1991; Rosen, 1981; Smith & Howe, 1985; Stevens & Moffitt, 1988; Young & Nettelbeck, 1994). Another relatively frequent category is *memory* for relatively obscure and trivial facts (always narrowly prescribed but with individual interests in a range of topics—post codes, telephone numbers, public transport routes and timetables, sports results, capital cities, street names, sundry geographical statistics, etc.) (Gordon, Valentine, & Wilding, 1984; O'Connor & Hermelin, 1989). *Musical ability* is also a relatively frequent category (Hermelin & O'Connor, 1989; Hermelin, O'Connor, & Lee, 1987; Hermelin, O'Connor, Lee, Treffert, 1989; Miller, 1987a, 1987b, 1995; Miller & Monroe, 1990; Sloboda, Hermelin, & O'Connor, 1985; Young & Nettelbeck, 1995). *Artistic ability* (generally drawing and painting although there is one well-publicised case of a sculptor; see Treffert, 1989, pp. 123–127) has attracted research interest (Anwar & Hermelin, 1982; Hermelin & O'Connor, 1990a; Hermelin, Pring, & Heavey, 1994; Mottron & Belleville, 1993, 1995; O'Connor & Hermelin, 1987a, 1987b, 1990; Pring & Hermelin, 1993; Pring, Hermelin, & Heavey, 1995). *Mathematical skills* (most commonly arithmetic but occasionally more complex mathematics like the identification of prime numbers) have also been investigated (Anderson, O'Connor, & Hermelin, in press; Hermelin & O'Connor, 1990b; Kelly, Macaruso, & Sokel, 1997). *Mechanical dexterity skills* involve preoccupation with mechanical objects and generally reflect the widespread availability of appliances like washing machines, vacuum cleaners, televisions, and radios. However, there has been no research in this area, other than the presentation of psychometric profiles and anecdotal accounts of these abilities (Brink, 1980; Hoffman & Reeves, 1979).

Hill expressed reservations about including the seventh category, *fine sensory discriminations.* Acute smell, vision, or hearing and extremely fine tactile ability have occasionally been reported in persons with mental retardation, and particularly among persons with autism. However, accounts have been anecdotal; the only quantitative test (for abnormally sensitive smell by Horwitz, Kestenbaum, Person, & Jarvik, 1965) failed to confirm superior ability. No one has since researched this category and, in view of Hill's cautiousness about its validity, we will not include this skill in further discussion.

The other six categories have been widely accepted as providing a near complete description of savant activities. However, two further categories should now be added to Hill's list: linguistic representations and sporting skills. The first has generally been termed *hyperlexia* or *pseudoverbal* skill (Rimland, 1978a; Rimland & Fein, 1988). This involves the superior recall or reproduction of language, either written, spoken, or reading ability, but with only poor comprehension of content (Cobrinik, 1982; Dowker, Hermelin, & Pring, 1996; Fontenelle & Alarcon, 1982; Healy, Aram, Horwitz, & Kessler, 1982; Kistner, Robbins, & Haskett, 1988; Mottron, Belleville, & Stip, 1996; O'Connor & Hermelin, 1994). There is also one case in the literature of exceptional linguistic skills together with remarkably good understanding, yet otherwise low levels of abilities (O'Connor & Hermelin, 1991; Smith & Tsimpli, 1995). The subject communicates and translates fluently in 12 or more languages, including some in different alphabets from English (his primary language).

Sixteen of the 119 "autistic-type" individuals were reported by Rimland (1978a) as having superior "coordination" skills in swimming, skating, and balance. Rimland (1978a; Rimland & Fein, 1988; Rimland & Hill, 1984) described children with skills for balancing objects or who could walk around the edge of their cribs or along rails at elevation. Treffert (1988) provided an example of a man who never missed when making free throws in basketball. Similarly, although Young (1995) was not seeking evidence for precocious athletic skills, parents of nine subjects (from 39), previously identified as demonstrating skills in other areas, reported athletic prowess. Skills included basketball shooting, volleyball serving, bicycle riding, cross-country skiing, running, swimming, ten-pin bowling, and unspecified ball skills. All of these athletic skills can be developed through solo practice, independently from interactions with others because teamwork is not involved, a characteristic of other savant skills.

That savant skills are only found within such a small range of activities is important. As Anderson (1992) has pointed out, this confirms that these skills are not random occurrences. They cannot be ignored as idiosyncratic—no more than freak accidents of no theoretical relevance. As Gardner (1983) has noted, these eight or nine categories describe broad, universal human activities that are generally highly valued. (Calendar calculating is an exception in so far as it is not developed by persons without an intellectual disability except rarely, and it seems a somewhat pointless activity. Yet, as argued below, it shares with the other categories psychological processes that presumably also are universal).

IV. SAVANT SKILLS AND INTELLIGENCE

The fact that savants exist has been widely held to challenge current theories about the nature of intelligence. Most people with average, or even appreciably above-average IQ, do not seem able to do the kinds of things that savants can do. Yet in order for savant skills to emerge, they must in some way be supported by mental processes responsible for accumulating knowledge, establishing rules for organizing it and retrieving it efficiently as required—in other words, mental activities consistent with age-old intuitions about what constitutes intelligence. There appears to be a contradiction about extraordinary abilities that few can match coexisting with low levels of general intellectual functioning that define mental retardation.

Gardner (1983) has argued that this contradiction is more apparent than real because savant accomplishments prove that intelligence is not a single entity. Gardner's point is that human abilities encompass a much broader range than the linguistic, spatial, and logical problem-solving activities sampled by most IQ tests. Injury to the brain can impair some areas of cognitive functioning, yet leave others intact. Human abilities are therefore better theoretically defined in terms of a number of independent intelligences that are supported by specific regions of the brain. Gardner (1983) has provided an account of six: musical, bodily-kinesthetic, personal and social, linguistic, logical-mathematical, and spatial intelligences. Only the last three are sampled by the most widely used IQ tests. Howe (1990) has extended this argument, insisting that a general intelligence factor (for which IQ is widely regarded as a proxy) lacks theoretical relevance; the core of Howe's position is that although the term *intelligence* can serve a useful descriptive function, it is not an explanatory construct.

However, whereas most modern psychometricians would support Gardner's conclusion that intelligence is multifaceted, many would disagree with his interpretation that each of the abilities introduced by his theory constitutes a separate "intelligence." We hold that this term, which is embedded in the language to refer to general adaptive capacities as applied to a very wide variety of circumstances, is inappropriate if referring to a relatively narrow range of cognitive performance. We acknowledge the importance of the six abilities emphasized by Gardner; but it serves no purpose to diminish the relevance of intellectual deficiencies that, in fact, mean that most savants do not function independently because they do not develop the life skills and common sense required to do so. We disagree with Gardner (1983) and Howe (1990) because they downplay the importance of general intelligence (Nettelbeck & Young, 1996).

The most detailed analysis yet available of the psychometric structure of intelligence has been provided by Carroll (1993), based on a meta-analysis of 461 large sets of data, published between about 1930 and 1985. Consistent with Gardner's view, Carroll has confirmed that a much more complex account for intelligence is required than a single test like the Wechsler scales can provide where, typically, factor analysis finds only three or four underlying factors (McGrew, 1997). However, beyond this point of agreement, Carroll's account of intelligence is very different from Gardner's. His "three-stratum theory of cognitive abilities" conceptualizes intelligence as a hierarchical structure involving three levels (see Carroll, 1993, Figure 15.1). The three strata have been identified by factor analysis, with the first application to a very broad battery of ability tests defining some 69 relatively narrow primary mental abilities. Correlations among these have defined a second stratum of eight broad abilities that are essentially those identified by Gf-Gc theory (Horn & Knoll, 1997).[3] In turn, correlations among these have resulted

[3]The current extended Gf-Gc theory has been developed, principally by J. L. Horn, from the distinction that Cattell (1941) first drew between fluid (i.e., abstract reasoning) and crystallized (acquired knowledge) intelligences. The theory describes human cognitive abilities in terms of 8–10 broad factors, including fluid and crystallized abilities and various memory, sensory processing, and speed dimensions.

in the third stratum, occupied by a single general factor. Carroll (1993) equates this factor with Spearman's *g*—"the apprehension of experience (what might now be called *metacognition* [italics in the original]) and the eduction of relations and correlates" (p. 637). Clearly, this definition encapsulates the notion of broad adaptiveness, and there is abundant evidence that *g* predicts not only academic achievement but also other real-life accomplishments that, by common consensus, require intelligence (Kline, 1991; Neisser et al., 1996). To accept this does not require that one supports highly publicized opinions that *g* is entirely or even almost entirely responsible for academic achievement, work success, and social competence (Brand, 1996; Herrnstein & Murray, 1994). Our position is that *g* is one of many personal and sociocultural factors that can shape social outcome—but it is too important to be set aside.

Savant skills do not pose a challenge to a theory that holds general intelligence to be an important commodity, because they do not constitute intelligent behaviors. Nonetheless, these skills do challenge current theories about the nature of intelligence to provide an adequate explanation for how savant syndrome remains independent from general intelligence because, in some way, savant skills must be supported by processes that contribute to general intelligence.

By asserting that savant performance is not intelligent, we do not mean that these behaviors are not important. On the contrary, as Gardner (1983) has noted, high achievement in music, the graphic arts, dance and sport, and interpersonal activities are generally highly valued in all cultures. Such skills certainly require considerable dedication to master and their investigation has the potential to enhance understanding of how intelligent functioning is organized.

This line of theorizing is consistent with Hill's (1978) tentative conclusion that savant skills may be relatively independent from IQ. However, we have been influenced predominantly by O'Connor who, in long-term collaboration with Hermelin, and together with other colleagues, was the first to apply formal experiments to investigate most of the range of savant skills. As already detailed in section III, this research has covered calendar calculating, music, art, linguistic proficiencies, mathematics, and memory. Their 30 articles provide the largest and most comprehensive single body of research on the topic of savant syndrome.

On the basis of comparisons between savants and appropriate controls without mental retardation, O'Connor and Hermelin established that savant activities are largely independent from IQ. In so far as they regarded an IQ score as an index for general intelligence, the inference to be drawn was that savant skills are distinct from intelligence—although, as discussed further, O'Connor and Hermelin (1987a) also speculated that IQ may play a supporting role in the quality of skills developed. Of course, a conclusion that savant skills and intelligence are relatively independent begs the question as to how this can be so? Spearman's (1927) concept of general intelligence was that it should to some degree influence all mental activities, and this assumption is explicit in theories that conceptualize intelligence as hierarchically organized. This is an issue to which we will return in section VII.

Three tenets provide the basis for our account of savant syndrome; these skills are supported by at least competent long-term memory; in some cases savant accomplishments are associated with a domain-specific talent, and savant skills are automatic. We will expand on these ideas in the sections to follow, beginning with a discussion of memory.

V. MEMORY

A. Rote Memory

Hill's (1978) discussion of possible explanations for savant syndrome did not generate firm conclusions. He tended to discount genetic influences but favored sensorimotor and rote memories as causal mechanisms, together with the capability to concentrate on the task for extended periods of time. (He seemed to assume that the latter is the consequence of environmental influences. Issues of practice and motivation will be addressed in sections VI.A and B).

Sensorimotor memory and *rote memory* are by no means unambiguous terms. If Hill intended nothing more than an inflexible, stable knowledge base that is stored without processing but perhaps maintained by rehearsal (e.g., a rigid, invariant association between sensory input and motor output, or for dates and days, or years and sporting statistics), this does not provide an adequate explanation for most savant skills. Although one might formulate a plausible explanation based on rote memory for learning lists of facts, these skills beyond splinter levels display flexibility (e.g., immediate random access to information and being able to reorder without delay lists of facts according to different defining criteria). Such capabilities suggest a less rigid organization of materials than is implied by a literal definition of rote memory.

B. Rule-Based Memory

Contrary to a literal rote memory explanation, O'Connor and Hermelin have convincingly demonstrated that savant skills are frequently based on the application of rules whereby an extensive body of expert knowledge is organized. For example, O'Connor and Hermelin (1984) found that, consistent with a rule-based system, the reaction times of calendar calculators were slower to remote dates, either past or future, than to proximate dates; and Hermelin and O'Connor (1986) established that calendar calculators were aware of and could use structural regularities within and across calendars when reaching solutions.

Similar findings hold for other kinds of savant skills. Investigations of savant pianists playing previously unknown music "by ear" have found that errors largely conform to musical structures that define style, key center, and rhythmic and harmonic context. So, for example, alterations to melody remain within the prevailing diatonic scale, with rhythm preserved; or an inverted chord, while not a literal rendition, nonetheless maintains harmonic identity (Charness, Clifton, & MacDonald, 1988; Miller, 1989; Sloboda et al., 1985; Young & Nettelbeck, 1995). Even when unfamiliar atonal music was involved, Young and Nettelbeck (1995) found that errors were consistent with that theoretical structure. The case of a musical savant who composes music that is technically complex and expressive directly onto manuscript and without actually performing it (Cameron, 1988) provides compelling evidence that savant skills are built on a comprehensive knowledge of theoretical structures.

Likewise, Selfe (1983) has highlighted that knowledge about perspective among artistic savants is rule-based, depending on depth cues from size–distance scaling and overlapping objects. O'Connor and Hermelin (1987a, 1987b, 1990) have emphasized that, like the skills of artists whose levels of general intelligence are not impaired, the artistic accomplishments of savant artists are supported by relatively complex systems of graphic representation. These authors used the metaphor of a lexicon to capture the sense that relevant knowledge is rule-based.

In the area of mathematics, Kelly, Macaruso, and Sokol (1997) have demonstrated that the mental calculations performed by the savant in their study were solved by applying a left-to-right computational procedure, consistent with methods employed by expert calculators. A clear example of rule-based savant calculation is provided by two elegant experiments by Anderson et al. (in press). These have convincingly demonstrated how a 21-year-old autistic savant, previously investigated by Hermelin and O'Connor (1990b), is able to apply a complex strategy to identify prime numbers. This man's psychometric profile varied widely, but he was diagnosed as autistic when 3 years of age, his communication skills are very poor, and some of his psychometric test scores suggest mild–borderline mental retardation. His performance when distinguishing primes from nonprimes, where both differed in difficulty, was compared to that of a trained mathematician. Although the savant was more accurate and considerably faster, the performance profiles of both subjects relative to difficulty were essentially the same. The control subject confirmed that he was using an algorithm attributed to Erastosthenes (3rd-century Greek mathematician). The second experiment timed mathematics students when dividing target numbers by primes (as required by Erastosthenes' algorithm), thereby providing data with which to generate simulations of the Erastosthenes method. An alternative memory-based strategy was also modeled. The mathematics students were then tested on the same set of primes and nonprimes from the first experiment. Their times were compared with the savant's, and both sets were tested against the two models. Both data sets conformed to the Erastosthenes model, but the memory model did not fit. Anderson et al. therefore concluded that the savant made calculations by using the relatively complex Erastosthenes algorithm based on division.

Finally, in the field of linguistics, a savant with proper name hypermnesia described by Mottron et al. (1996) was shown to use list-learning strategies based on regularity, redundancy, and different categories for grouping objects. Dowker et al. (1996) have demonstrated that their savant poet was able to draw on linguistic knowledge and rules, like the use of similes and metaphors, as well as the poetic device of modified repetition.

These findings therefore establish that more than rote memory is involved in savant skills. Such skills are typically built on decisions made on the basis of a lexicon of well-organized, structurally based knowledge. Nonetheless, even when a detailed knowledge base is available, it does not necessarily follow that flexible strategies will always be applied.

Nettelbeck and Young (1996) have supported O'Connor and Hermelin's conclusions that savants have and can use extensive domain-specific knowledge; but have suggested that the application of this knowledge can still be markedly passive. Young and Nettelbeck (1994; Young, 1995) found no evidence that calendar knowledge (that their subjects demonstrably had) provided the basis for genuine computation using a sophisticated algorithm. Methods applied were invariant because subjects' reaction times were not changed by experimental manipulations of calendar regularities. For each of nine participants (see Young, 1995), speed of responding was fast (2 to 25 sec) and remarkably consistent, irrespective of the recency or distance of the target date and whether repetitions of dates occurred later within trials. Moreover, although these subjects were highly skilled, near-perfect accuracy was restricted to specific but idiosyncratic epochs. In every case limitations to the range of knowledge were readily determined and performance for dates beyond this range deteriorated dramatically. All participants were familiar with perpetual calendars and were highly knowledgeable about the 14 calendar templates that constitute the Gregorian system; and all could match any given year with the correct template, providing that it was within the span of widely available perpetual calendars (most commonly, 1900 to 2100). All savants were also familiar with leap-year rules, identical configurations across certain years, and consistencies across months that produced common date-day relationships. Nettelbeck and Young (1996) therefore concluded that, as Hermelin and O'Connor (1986a) had previously emphasized, calendar calculation does depend on an extensive knowledge of calendar structures. The acquisition of that knowledge has required the assimilation of rules that define template-year relationships, regularities within years, the occurrence of leap years and other appropriate associated adjustments. A plausible procedure would require, first, high familiarity with the 14 templates, enabling the correct template to be matched to any year, then applying memorized rules based on regularities to link a day to a date within that template. Procedures based on these rules would be rigidly applied and rapid, automatic processing achieved and maintained, first, by memorizing the required steps and then practicing them extensively. This suggestion does not address the specific nature of procedures followed; and there probably are individual differences in these. However, the suggestion can accommodate satisfactorily those cases who can make calculations well into the future—instances held to discredit a memory-based method (Anderson, 1998; Hermelin & O'Connor, 1986)—if one assumes that future years *have already been tested* against the 14 templates. Given the keen interest that savants invariably display in their area(s) of expertise, the suggestion that some would practice future dates is plausible—and testable. We therefore predict that, whenever a savant is found to be able to match dates and days within a future year, he or she will also know which template applies to that year.

In light of the foregoing, to claim that some aspects of a savant's memory must be operating at a high level would seem to be stating the obvious. The suggestion that exceptionally good memory is essential if savant skills are to emerge has been made for musical skills (Hermelin et al., 1989; Young & Nettelbeck, 1995), mathematics (Stevens & Moffitt, 1988), artistic ability (O'Connor & Hermelin, 1987a), calendar calculating (Hermelin & O'Connor, 1986; Young & Nettelbeck, 1994), and hyperlexia (Goldberg, 1987). Treffert (1989) argued that exceptionally good memory is the only characteristic shared by all savants, and that superior memory in savants has been confirmed by appropriate memory tests. However, after considering substantially the same research, Hill (1978) was mark-edly circumspect, citing evidence that contradicted this conclusion—even though he finally opted for rote memory as a probable essential candidate.

In fact, despite claims that remarkable memory is critical to the development of savant skills, the role of memory has been discounted by Howe (1989), because savants have been found to perform poorly on standardized memory tests. With the largest single sample of savants obtained so far, Young (1995) found little evidence from standardized tests that savants have exceptional memory abilities. The sample for this study was 51 persons, judged to have prodigious skills (12), talented skills (20), and splinter skills (19). In general, performance on the Wechsler Memory Scale—Revised (WMS-R) was consistent with IQ, irrespective of skill level, and scores for savants recruited for exceptional memory did not differ reliably from the rest of the sample. Word association tests for domain-specific knowledge of calendar calculating, music, and art did not successfully discriminate between those expert in the relevant area and other savants. Savants with memory for facts did not outscore others on the Delayed Memory Quotient, the only subtest from WMS-R that requires longer term recall.

Therefore, despite evidence that *some* savants have good memory, the findings above do not support the hypothesis that this holds for all savants. Yet, despite this unpromising outcome it is possible that Treffert was correct and that, for all savants, some highly effective aspects of memory are preserved. There are four reasons for thinking so.

First, there is direct evidence, considered above, that savants do possess high levels of specialized knowledge about their area(s) of interest; and there are countless references in the literature to the fact that savant skills have long attracted widespread attention, essentially because they appear on the face of it to demonstrate exceptional feats of memory. Second, parents' reports attest to the validity of this impression. Thus, Young (1995) surveyed the parents of 23 diverse savants and 16 subjects with splinter skills about, among other things, memory and other skill areas shown by their children. Thirty seven parents from those 39 reported that their child had demonstrated a precociously good memory from an early age. The reliability of these opinions was supported by Young's observation that details in most responses were consistent with her impressions of individual achievements, formed on the basis of about four hours contact with each of her subjects.

Third, detailed interrogation of memory test performance suggests that, whereas overall profile scores do not discriminate savants from nonsavants with mental retardation, some aspects of savants' results are consistent with the memory hypothesis. For example, the Delayed Memory Quotient from WMS-R is obtained by testing delayed recall from four domains and the final outcome is obviously constrained by the amount of initial learning. Young (1995) noted that her savants (and subjects with splinter skills) had virtually perfect recall for whatever information was encoded initially. Moreover, the performance of these subjects improved with the opportunity, provided by the test, to rehearse across three additional repetitions of these materials. Young therefore raised the possibility that, given sufficient rehearsal opportunity to achieve a high level of initial learning, these subjects could achieve a high level in delayed performance.

The fourth reason relates in part to the third. Current standardized memory tests like WMS-R are not suited to testing savant memory skills adequately. It is likely that difficulties with language and comprehension, and poor semantic encoding, all correlated with low IQ, will confound memory test performance among savants, as among nonsavants with mental retardation. Even more importantly, however, a savant's interest is typically narrowly focused on a single domain and does not necessarily extend to other domains. Unsurprisingly, memory test items do not require recall of information involving calendars, music, or many idiosyncratic domains that interest memory savants. Yet these are precisely the kind of test items required to address adequately the memory functions that, we argue, are preserved among savants. To our knowledge, there is only one example in the literature of a direct attempt to validate the highly selective quality of memory. Valentine and Wilding (1994) have reported that two of their savant subjects scored at the 100th percentile for memory of telephone numbers but were at the bottom of the distribution for story recall. This outcome is consistent with the position advocated here.

To clarify our viewpoint, we assume that, for most cases, low levels of IQ that in part define mental retardation are the consequence of insult to the brain that commonly damages processes responsible for general intelligence and related functions alike, including different memory systems. Savants are individuals who have suffered brain damage but, essential to their exceptional abilities, some aspects of their long-term memory have been spared. For savant skills to develop, aspects of memory processing must be preserved, at least at levels consistent with nonretarded functioning. This position therefore admits the possibility that the achievements of savant mnemonists and calendar calculators could be matched by persons with average memory abilities and without intellectual disabilities who could be persuaded to attempt such accomplishments. On the other hand, the only published attempt to train calendrical calculating skills involved a university postgraduate, who presumably would have possessed above-average mental abilities (Addis, 1968). Thus, whether savant skills are based on average or above-average memory abilities is open to question.

Memory is not a unitary system. It involves many theoretically distinct systems for storing different kinds of information (Badderley, 1997). This conclusion is supported by neurological evidence from investigations into epilepsy (Blaxton, 1992; Samson & Zatorre, 1991), amnesia (Glisky, 1995; Hamann & Squire, 1995; Hamann, Squire, & Schacter, 1995; Kapur, 1988; Schmidtke, Handschu, & Vollmer, 1996), Alzheimer's disease (Squire & Butter, 1992), and other neurological disorders (Soliveri, Brown, Johanshahi, & Marsden, 1992) that demonstrate intact separate memory capacities despite damage to other brain structures. Recent neuroanatomical evidence also suggests that different structures make distinct contributions to memory processing (Eichenbaum, Otto, & Cohen, 1996; Peretz, 1996; Toates, 1996). It is important to note, however, that although memory can be thought of as a number of separate systems, these will interlock and in most situations, processes that traverse these structures must be involved.

C. Declarative Memory

The type of memory demonstrated by savants is narrowly focused, sometimes within a single domain. This is declarative memory (Squire, 1992) (i.e., a long-term system for storing and retrieving distinct factual units of information and for making associations between them). Squire has distinguished episodic (reference to specific time or place) from semantic (more abstract and conceptual) declarative memory. Young (1995) observed that most of her savant cases had good recall for trivia and other memory feats, in addition to their main skill domain. Norris (1990) was able to simulate calendar calculations, using a connectionist model given factual calendar knowledge but without explicit rules or a sophisticated arithmetical algorithm. Low-level processes followed a three-step procedure and, given sufficient learning trials, this network was "trained" to calculate days accurately for past and future dates. Norris's model included procedure, an issue discussed further in the section to follow, but the memory system was essentially declarative. On this basis we propose that a preserved episodic declarative memory provides a minimum structure required to support savant skills. The neuroanatomical substrate responsible for declarative memory is thought to be distinct from other memory structures (Goldberg, 1987).

Although savant skills appear to be diverse, preserved episodic declarative memory should permit development of more than one skill, given appropriate encouragement, opportunity, and perhaps interest and talent, as will be considered in the next section.[4] Although it has often been assumed that most savants develop only one skill, there have been reports of multiple skills (Rimland, 1978a), particularly among autistic savants (Rimland, 1978b). All but one of Young's (1995) parents ($N = 39$) reported more than one skill for their child (with savant or splinter skills). The average was more than four, with six parents reporting eight or nine skills. This outcome suggests the development of multiple skills based on common underlying processes.

D. Procedural Memory

Preserved declarative memory is necessary but will not always be sufficient for savant syndrome to develop. Procedural memory must also be involved in activities (other than memory for facts) whereby declared knowledge is applied according to a sequence of steps. Units of declarative knowledge must be connected by means of a strategy and transformed into procedural knowledge that enables the immediate recall of information, probably through well-organized schemata, with little conscious awareness of the strategy involved. Initially, awareness of procedures may be involved, although some procedural rules may be learned implicitly, without conscious application (Anderson, 1998; Spitz, 1995).[5]

The arithmetic competence of most calendrical calculators has generally been found to be poor (Hill, 1978; Treffert, 1989), which would appear to rule out cal-

[4]Darold Treffert (personal communication, 10 August, 1998) has drawn our attention to musical skills demonstrated by Stephen Wiltshire, an autistic artist whose drawings have attracted considerable publicity and commercial success (Sacks, 1995a; Wiltshire, 1991). Accounts of these accomplishments appeared in *The Times* (London, UK; Hawkes, 1993; Hewson & Taylor, 1993). Stephen's musical capabilities involve perfect pitch, including key recognition and accurate, instant mental analysis of music. Thus, for example, he is able to name correctly a sequence of chords that defines the harmonic structure that underpins a tune.

[5]Savants typically seem unable to account for their accomplishments (Treffert, 1989), although in part this may reflect the common experience for complex behavior long since become automatic, and perhaps in part that no one has yet asked the right question. For example, Young (1995) was the first to report calendar calculators' knowledge about the set of 14 templates covering all years. She has also described a savant's clear account of his method for calendar calculation that starts from an anchor date within any year from which to project forwards or backwards, using rules for regularities and simple addition or subtraction to adjust for regularities.

culation by use of a complex formula. However, as with any ability test for which the standardization sample was predominantly without disabilities, interpretation of a savant's results can be problematical, particularly if autism is involved. Thus, one of Young's (1995) calendar savants could rapidly solve problems embedded in a calendar problem that he apparently could not solve if presented as an arithmetical operation.[6] The declarative and procedural memory structures of some calendar savants may be sufficient to support a procedural algorithm like one of those devised by Lewis Carroll (in 1887 as cited by Spitz, 1995). As Spitz (1995) pointed out, there is probably no single method that all calculators use. Similar diversity of method is likely to apply in all skill domains.

A fuller account of savant syndrome also requires accommodating the impression that development of savant skills only follows considerable practice, a commitment to which may require uncommon personality characteristics. This issue will be discussed further in section VI. Moreover, except for memory for facts and for calendar calculation, other savant skills may involve additional exceptional aptitudes that have been spared the effects of brain damage. Thus some savants with skills in music, mathematics, language, or art may be utilizing memory structures that are qualitatively different, not only from those of others with an intellectual disability, but also from those of many from the normal population. The assumption here is that for these savant activities to develop to the highest levels requires talent.

VI. TALENT

By "talent" we assume a brain capacity specialized for particular knowledge and capable of operating at an unusually high level. Talent is independent from IQ and from emotional and social development. Moreover, a strong motivation to develop the skill may be an integral part of the talent (Feldman, 1993), although it is possible that people gravitate towards those activities that come easier to them.

The assumption that savant skills depend on domain-specific talents has a long and continuing history (Feldman, 1993; Gardner, 1983; Goddard, 1914; Jensen, 1990; O'Connor, 1989; Rife & Snyder, 1931; Sacks, 1985; Spitz, 1995; Treffert, 1989). There is, however, debate about invoking talent as an explanatory construct and whether prodigious accomplishments can instead be explained by motivational characteristics.[7] Howe (1989) and Ericsson and Faivre (1988) have argued

[6]Recent research by Cowan, O'Connor, and Samella finds that some calendar calculators have arithmetical capabilities that are not detected by common standardized tests, and that higher levels of calendar skills reflect better arithmetical skills (R. Cowan, personal communication, 20 May 1998).

[7]This alternative does not rule out the possibility that an extraordinarily high level of motivation is itself a form of talent. However, as our definition makes clear, we hold that potential for a specialized knowledge base is also required.

that practice alone can account for outstanding accomplishment. Retrospective studies of accomplished artists (Sloane & Sosniak, 1985), swimmers (Kalinowski, 1985), and mathematicians (Gustin, 1985) have suggested that such accomplishments are due to practice and parental encouragement, not talent. Nor does existing psychometric evidence reliably identify specific aptitudes for music, art, mathematics, or language (Carroll, 1993). Furthermore, there is evidence that savant-type skills can be developed through persistent, repetitive practice (Addis, 1968; Morishima & Brown, 1977).

Nevertheless, it is unlikely that practice can provide a sufficient explanation. Many individuals with autism typically engage in sustained, repetitious activities but relatively few develop savant proficiencies. Moreover, evidence of a talent is most frequently apparent before there has been prolonged opportunity for rehearsal. (There will be further discussion of practice-related issues below.) The major evidence for this is anecdotal but persuasive. It has widely been observed that exceptional capabilities typically emerge at a very early age, in a manner that seems qualitatively different from the appreciably longer learning curves that the majority of the population display. The drawing abilities of Nadia (Selfe, 1977) were first evident at age $3\frac{1}{2}$. Miller (1989) has reviewed the histories of musical savants, finding evidence of early interest in music. Young (1995) also found that skills were early evident in most of her subjects, although there were large differences in mean emergent ages between different skill domains (for example, music $4\frac{1}{2}$ years, memory 8, calendars 10) and one artistic savant's skills only emerged at age 22 (although he had earlier memory and calendrical skills from an unknown age).

Talent may be genetically determined, with the potential present from birth, or it may be the consequence of very early developmental experiences (Fein & Obler, 1988). However, the argument here requires only that high potential for the skills involved should be obvious from an early age. There is speculation in the literature about the nature of functions that might underpin different specific talents. O'Connor and Hermelin (1990) have suggested that artistic talent depends on long-term memory for visual detail, independent from IQ, that results in an excellent sense of perspective. This, in turn, is thought to underpin drawing ability to a level far beyond what would be predicted by IQ. Because the memory is domain specific, its influence is not manifested in other activities. Thus, as O'Connor and Hermelin reported, savant graphic artists can display exceptional drawing ability, while at the same time demonstrating poor visual recognition for shapes, consistent with their low IQs. An analogous memory system dedicated to tactile detail could explain savant sculpturing skills. O'Connor and Hermelin's proposal is consistent with speculation that artistic talent is supported by specific brain structures (Schweiger, 1988). Nonetheless, there may be some overlap between different domains and the processes involved. Rimland (1978b) observed that certain skills tended to cluster within individuals (for example, music and mathematics) and Young (1995) found some evidence for such grouping.

According to Miller (1989; see also Judd, 1988), the high musical competence by savants, who typically can improvise and "play by ear," requires exceptional working memory for melodic and harmonic relationships, together with exceptional long-term memory for a musical repertoire. All known musical savants appear to have these capacities, and they are apparently automatic—in Miller's terms, "performance is 'mindless'" (p. 116). Short-term span for unfamiliar note rows may be unexceptional, but errors are consistent with structural rules for scales and keys. Thus, in addition to encoding specific notes, the musical savant must be able simultaneously to encode and evaluate information about the structural context from which the note rows have been sampled. Nettelbeck and Young (1996) have speculated that "perfect pitch"[8] is a good candidate for a talent underpinning the exceptional musical memory structures displayed by savants—and commonly by musical prodigies. Perfect pitch does not guarantee musicality and nor is perfect pitch an essential precursor to any accomplished musical performance, but it provides a good start.

As Miller (1989) pointed out, perfect pitch provides the individual with a significant advantage for encoding and retrieving new music. It extends beyond melody to horizontal chord arrangements, including the instant analysis of complex chords that include chromatic notes outside of conventional rules. That musical savants and prodigies alike are stronger in the areas of melodic and harmonic content than with rhythmic content (Miller, 1989) is consistent with our proposal that the basis for the talent is perfect pitch, which relates to the first two elements but not to temporal aspects of music. Absolute pitch has been noted in persons with autism without musical achievements and in savants with other skills but not music. This confirms that, although a talent may provide a basis for the emergence of skill, it does not explain satisfactorily the realization of that potential.

Similarly, Smith and Tsimpli (1995) concluded that a linguistic lexicon is necessary to support the exceptional linguistic accomplishments of their savant case study. Consistent with theory above, they envisage this memory system as modular and independent from central cognitive control and that its operations are automatic, complex, selective, and generative, being based on rules that govern the structures of language. Their descriptions of this man's linguistic capabilities sug-

[8]Perfect or absolute pitch is the ability to identify correctly the pitch of any note without aid from an external source. It is widely believed to be a relatively rare innate capacity (Bachem, 1955), although Takeuchi and Hulse (1993) have argued that it is potentially universal, dependent only on appropriate environmental opportunities during a relatively critical period of early development. These authors are influenced by evidence that accurate absolute pitch perception can be acquired with practice, providing that learning occurs before the child is about 4 to 5 years of age. It is also the case that substantial individual differences in perfect pitch accuracy are found, although this does not invalidate the innate hypothesis. Certainly, whether innate or determined by very early learning, absolute pitch is rarely reported among the normal population, even for musicians, whereas published accounts of musical savants suggest that every one of them has virtually error-free absolute pitch (Charness et al., 1988; Miller, 1989; Sloboda et al., 1995; Young & Nettelbeck, 1995).

gest that the exceptional nature of these was established from about the age of 6, with a precocious interest in technical books evident from about 3 years of age. This account is therefore consistent with what we have defined as a talent. Sacks (1985, 1995a) has also speculated about domain-specific categorical memory that results directly in an intuitive grasp of structures relevant to that domain. This general model is similar to those outlined here for talents in the fields of art, music, and language, and it provides an account of how a talent might work in areas like mathematics or mechanics.

Sacks's suggestion is similar to Anderson's (1998), that some savant abilities are based on implicit inductive processing. Thus, individual differences in a talent may reflect differences in unconscious processing capabilities. Feldman (1993) has observed that child prodigies not only cannot account for their accomplishments but are also surprised that others cannot emulate them.

A common thread running through these various speculations about the nature of savant talent is that, within their areas of expertise, savants operate very much in the same manner as nonretarded experts in those fields. The implications, already explored above, are that memory structures involved are exceptional, and that these have somehow been protected from trauma that has damaged structures elsewhere in the brain. Research into giftedness has generated two different theories about the nature of talent (Fein & Obler, 1988; Feldman, 1993). According to one, what is meant by "exceptional" is that the ability, although at a high level, is still within the range of normal development. This viewpoint is consistent with the observation that talent is not all-or-none and may be represented as a distribution of individual differences. If this is so, highly talented performance should be quantitatively rather than qualitatively different from less talented activities. On the other hand, it has also been widely assumed that talented performance is somehow qualitatively different from activities that are not inspired by talent.

Treffert (1989) has raised an alternative possibility, that savant skills directly result from pathological events. He has outlined a theory (pp. 197–199) about the origins of superior skills deriving from exceptional neural structures that form during prenatal brain development. Following direct injury or abnormal biochemical activity in the left hemisphere, a pathological but compensatory mechanism is held to trigger the migration of neurons from the left to the right hemisphere. Sacks (1995a) has also suggested that some exceptional domain-specific structures might be pathological. Treffert (1989, pp. 158–163) summarized evidence from autopsy reports, electroencephalographic, and computer-assisted tomography (CAT) scan data and neuropsychological tests to support his theory, noting a number of cases with right hemispheric imbalance. However, these cases constitute a very small literature, and there are still too few cases to determine the significance of this observation.

Treffert's proposal raises questions about the nature of talent in the wider nondisabled population. Are the causes of savant talent qualitatively different from those active in the wider population? Or, although he did not suggest so, does Treffert's theory about pathologically different brain structures causing exceptional talent apply to all (i.e., nondisabled) cases with extraordinary abilities? At the present time it seems premature to conclude that savant skills are dissimilar from those of accomplished performers who are not intellectually disabled. These are open questions however. The performance of an exceptionally talented individual can appear to be qualitatively different from that of someone less talented, but this could represent nothing more than a considerable difference between them in level of talent.

To summarize our position, domain-specific talents exist, they probably involve implicit processes, they are available from a very early age, and they reflect individual differences, so that talent is not all-or-none. Motivation to pursue a particular activity may be an integral part of talent. Memory structures that support talents like music and art are domain specific and therefore different from those that support memory for facts and calendar calculation that are declarative and procedural but general purpose, not dedicated. Different talents may require different kinds of memory structures, although for some domains there may be overlap in the processes involved. The levels of accomplishment of a savant in a domain reflecting talent should be only possible for someone with the same talent. However, because the memory structures that support memory for facts and calendar calculation involve general purpose processes, a savant interested in one kind of fact should be capable of developing expertise in other areas, given motivation. Moreover, anyone with the same declarative and procedural memory capacities should be capable of matching savant accomplishments.

A. Practice

The role of practice in the development of savant skills is a complex issue. O'Connor (1989) proposed that talent is innate and that its manifestation is not dependent on rehearsal. Anecdotal evidence about the developmentally precocious appearance of exceptional aptitude in areas of music and art are consistent with O'Connor's suggestion and it seems that development of high levels of skill in exceptional cases follows a different course to that describing common intellectual abilities. A child prodigy will usually learn required techniques more quickly and with less effort than a normal child. Levels of skill achieved early are often well in advance of mental age or social development (Feldman, 1993). O'Connor's suggestion would also explain why the prodigious accomplishments of some individuals develop within a relatively short period of time during late adolescence or very early adulthood, if one assumes that talent lies dormant until opportunity and interest result in its development.

However, even if O'Connor was correct, the development of skill based on talent to a high level almost certainly requires practice (Anastasi & Levee, 1960;

Ericsson & Faivre, 1983; Hoffman & Reeves, 1979; Howe, 1989; Miller, 1989; Treffert, 1989). Anecdotal claims that savant skills suddenly emerge fully developed without much by way of tutoring or practice are probably exaggerated; (see Miller, 1989, p. 16, and Treffert, 1989, pp. 104–107, for background information about a widely publicized musical savant). Observations of savants' behaviors and reports from their parents have shown that considerable practice is typically involved (Charness et al., 1988; Comer, 1985; Hill, 1978; Treffert, 1989; Young, 1995). Nonetheless, as Miller's (1989) discussion of this topic makes clear, it is not certain that such practice necessarily involves the focused, strategic-based rehearsal that characterizes traditional, formal training; for example, many musical savants have been largely self-taught and their practice is equally well described as long periods of performing that is not directed to anything much other than just playing. Such practice would presumably help to overcome technically disadvantageous physical and motor limitations that may accompany intellectual disability (Miller, 1989). It is not established, however, what part such practice plays in the retention or improvement of skill. For example, in the case of the musical savant Eddie, Miller (1989, Chapter 5) found that recall of 23 previously learned preludes—but not played for 12 months—was markedly variable. Yet error rate was remarkably low for some of these pieces, and recall of all of them was far better than that shown by two accomplished pianists who had also learned them but not played them for six months. Of course, it is trivially obvious that had these materials been played regularly, they would have been maintained; but Miller's experiment does suggest that the long-term maintenance of exceptionally high levels of skill does not necessarily depend on rehearsal. One of Young's (1995) results equates with this. From the reports of 39 parents, she found a wide range of different savant skills and that amount of practice did not correlate with level of achievement, despite very wide variations in the amount of practice claimed (from 0 to 84 hours/week).

On the other hand, even given exceptional skill developed over a long period of time, it appears that skill can be lost without sustained practice. Treffert (1989) discusses the case of the autistic artist Nadia whose ability apparently disappeared when she no longer practiced; Young (1995) similarly observed that the calendar-calculating skills of a well-documented savant (Sacks, 1985) were much diminished following separation from his twin and the transfer of his interests to an unrelated area.

B. Motivation

Hill (1978) discussed a number of motivational explanations for savant syndrome. All had in common that the development of savant skills was somehow a form of compensatory adaptation, perhaps reinforced by parental or caregiver encouragement—for example, a reaction to a limited institutional environment, or the adoption of concrete mental processes as a means of coping with the cognitive consequences of brain damage. Hill raised several inadequacies in these ideas, the most telling being that none could explain why, if such factors were causal, many more persons with mental retardation do not develop savant levels of skills. He concluded that an important aspect of savant ability is a capacity to concentrate on the chosen task for very long periods of time, although he recognised that this was not so much a cause as a description of motivation and interest associated with skill development. Although his review included discussion of whether special abilities might be inherited, and pointed to a paucity of research addressing information about family background, Hill considered that the small amount of available research gave little credibility to this suggestion. He seemed, furthermore, inclined to reject the possibility that a capacity to concentrate might be congenital, as a personality trait, or even as an integral aspect of the special ability itself.

Treffert (1989), on the other hand, directly raised this possibility, noting that savants have frequently seemed compelled to engage in their special activities. He acknowledged the likely relevance of encouragement by others but was of the opinion that the talent itself includes a motivating force (see p. 218). Certainly, reports cited previously that many savants do follow extremely demanding practice routines are consistent with the idea that obsessional aspects of personality may contribute to the development of savant skills (Charness et al., 1988).

A small number of studies have followed Hill's (1978) suggestion that the family backgrounds of savants be investigated for evidence of similar interests and talents. Rimland (1978a) reported that abilities among relatives, similar to those of a savant family member, have been noted. Brink's (1980) investigation of a mechanical savant uncovered that the father had similar interests and Hermelin and O'Connor (1990b) found that both parents of their autistic mathematical prodigy had tertiary degrees in mathematics.

Young (1995) questioned the parents, siblings, and other close relatives of participants in her research about their (the relatives') interests and skills. She found substantial evidence of high levels of skills among family members, although not always within the domain of skill exhibited by the savant. This outcome was, of course, consistent with the above-average IQs of parents (16 from 38 had IQs above 130), and their high level of education (more than half had attended college/university). However, some 49 close relatives were documented as demonstrating skills mostly within the discrete range of abilities associated with savants, and 10 savant participants had one or more relatives with the same skill as theirs. All five savants with art as their primary skill had artist relatives, and three of the four musical savants whose parents participated in the study had musically accomplished close relatives. Moreover, the frequency with which skills were reported for other family members correlated significantly (0.5) with Young's ranking of savant expertise. These results contradict earlier reports of no history of similar skills existing among family members (Hill, 1978). They are obviously consistent with a proposition that a family environment can shape and encourage savant interests; but they also raise the possibility that, without discounting the relevance of environmental influences, a talent that includes a capacity to focus on developing the skills involved can be inherited.

VII. Explaining Savant Syndrome

We now outline a tentative psychological explanation for savant syndrome. This is located within a model for intelligence that is capable of accommodating savant skills as essentially nonintelligent activities. In doing so, we have drawn heavily on recent models formulated by Anderson (1992) and by Detterman (1982, 1986; Detterman et al., 1992). To recapitulate what should be accounted for, theory should recognize the importance of both specific domains and a general factor as integral constituents of human intelligence; and savant skills do not constitute alternative, multiple forms of intelligent behavior. Thus, further to the observation that they are independent from IQ, savant skills should be shown logically not to rely on more than low levels of intelligence.

A. Anderson's Theory of the Minimal Cognitive Architecture

Anderson's (1992) theory accounts for two essential aspects of intellectual growth throughout childhood; children become smarter as they get older but individual differences within any age cohort remain remarkably stable across cohorts. A central proposition underpinning the theory is that mental age (MA) and IQ are caused by fundamentally different processes. Discontinuities in MA development reflect the operation of ontogenetically determined modules that come on-line at different ages. Modules are all-or-none; one either has them or, because of brain damage, one does not. Modules may be computationally complex but they deal with highly specific competencies, not abilities. Mark I modules are fast, automatic, and they are innately specified and critically important in an evolutionary sense (for example, three-dimensional visual perception, language acquisition), but they do not generate thought. A second type of module (Mark II) is neither complex nor innate but acquired by rehearsal until the processes involved become automatic (for example, retrieving well-rehearsed materials from long-term memory). Modules therefore contribute to the acquisition of knowledge, but they are not intelligent.

Intelligence requires thought via the implementation of general-purpose computational routines generated by specific processors dedicated to independent knowledge domains (for example, the verbal-spatial distinction). Intelligence also requires the operation of a basic processing mechanism (BPM) that constrains output from the specific processors, whatever their latent capabilities. The BPM does not constrain output from modules. This structure therefore reconciles Spearman's (1927) and Thurstone's (1938) theories with Piagetian theory (Piaget, 1953). Specific abilities contribute to intelligence, but the efficiency of the BPM, which is constant across age, determines the level of *g* and maintains *g*'s stability, while modules account for increasing MA.

In broad terms this model might be made to account for savant syndrome, and Anderson (1992, 1998) has provided a number of case studies to illustrate how. In the case of the prime number calculator described by Anderson et al. (in press), his BPM is thought to be preserved. However, other examples encounter difficulties for two reasons. First, although Anderson assumes that some savant activities, like calendrical skills or memory for facts, are modular, there is no account for how a savant, with a deficient BPM, copes with relevant processing before automaticity is achieved. Second, and most importantly, because he disallows modular activities to reflect individual differences, he is forced to account for abilities like music, mathematics, or art in terms of an intact and highly efficient specific processor—but together with a damaged BPM to explain low IQ. This architecture will not work because output from a specific processor is directly constrained by the BPM, meaning that specific skill and general intelligence will always be correlated, contrary to what has been found with savant syndrome.

Smith and Tsimpli (1995) have raised essentially the same criticism to Anderson's model when developing an account for the remarkable linguistic achievements of their savant. They argue that this man possesses an exceptional lexical memory module that transfers from the first language (English) to a new language on a word-for-word basis. The language module can be isolated from a damaged central system and interaction between the module and higher cognitive processes is necessarily limited. Smith and Tsimpli modified Anderson's model to include direct communication of a "quasi-modular" form from a specific processor to output, without constraint by the BPM, and included an executive function to control the progress of information within the central system.

We agree with Smith and Tsimpli's assessment. Despite the continuing philosophical problem that including an executive function poses, the past 20 years have witnessed considerable progress in clarifying the nature of control processes (Rabbitt, 1997), and it is not possible to avoid invoking some kind of executive function as an essential quality of human intelligence (Sternberg, 1985).

B. Detterman's Model for *g*

Detterman's (1982, 1986) suggestion is that *g* is not a single element, like the BPM, but a statistical composite output from a system of a small number of independent elements. Although each element is responsible for activities independent from the activities of other elements, they must combine to produce output from the system, and the output of any element is influenced by the quality of input from the others. Detterman et al. (1992) tested this model by operationalizing executive and memory constructs in terms of different elementary information-processing tasks. Their modified model for *g* isolated long-term memory from executive control, which is maintained over less permanent memory.

C. An Integration of Anderson's and Detterman's Models

Integrating these two models produces a model wherein independent processes result in a general intelligence factor (Detterman), but which reconciles specific and general aspects within a developmental framework (Anderson); and accommodates savant syndrome by representing the skills as highly specialized modular activities that reflect individual differences and do not require more than low general intelligence. The resulting model is illustrated in Figure 1.

Following Anderson (1992), the model consists of a central system and two different kinds of module. The progress of knowledge generated by different specific processors (SPs) is constrained by the overall efficiency of the processing system which, following Detterman et al. (1992), consists of an initial register and working memory system, both under the control of an executive function, long-term memory (including declarative and procedural systems), and encoding and retrieval mechanisms that handle input and output for the different memory systems. Rehearsal within working memory is controlled by the executive. Anderson's category of specific processors is expanded to include the ability domains identified with savant syndrome; music, art, language, mechanics, mathematics, and physical coordination.

Long-term memory is independent from executive control. This configuration is consistent with Detterman et al.'s results and with Spearman's (1927) speculation that some aspects of long-term memory would prove to be independent from *g*. Psychometric evidence for this is poor, essentially because long-term memory tests are based on retention across minutes or hours and not the longer periods required. However, such as it is, the evidence is supportive (Horn & Knoll, 1997).

Anderson's distinction between adaptable processors and dedicated modules is retained. Mark I modules are as described above but in the current model Mark II modules are "quasimodular"—they can have limited communication with the central system via intact long-term memory. For example, musical or artistic knowledge—or lists of facts—can be processed into long-term declarative and procedural systems that eventually support a module, providing that (a) the executive function has a minimum efficiency required to generate rehearsal in the first place; and (b) there is sufficient motivational input to sustain rehearsal until automatic functioning is achieved. The quasi-module is capable of low-level generative activity.

Although long-term memory is independent from the executive function, it is apparent that the overall general efficiency of Detterman's system relies heavily

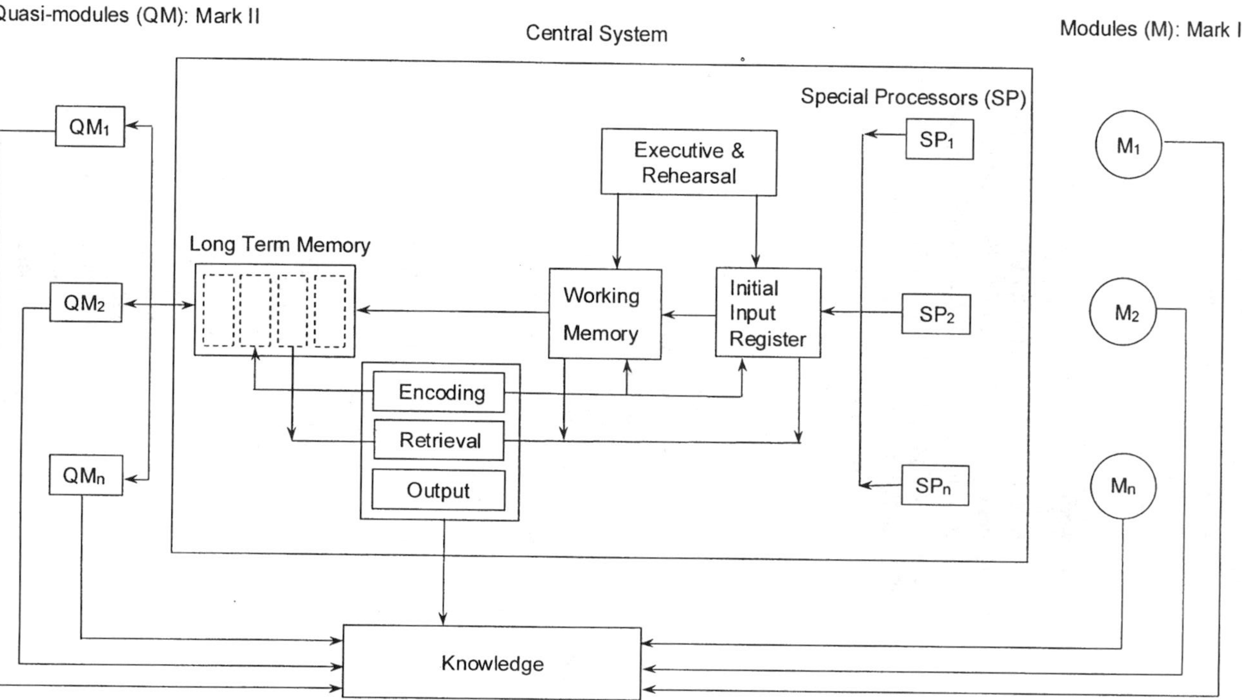

FIG. 1. A model for intelligence that accounts for savant syndrome.

on the executive role. In the event that the executive was deficient, IQ would be low. The first proviso, above, therefore raises the question of how low general intelligence could be, while still supporting savant-level skills. According to Hoffman (1971), the probable answer is about IQ 50 (i.e., in the range defining upper moderate-lower mild mental retardation). Young (1995) has provided confirmatory evidence for this suggestion, finding that among 51 subjects with savant and splinter skills the lowest IQ (Wechsler Scales) was 54. However, there have been cases in the literature where IQ was lower than this (Treffert, 1989). It is unlikely that this manner could be settled in the near future, especially given unreliability of IQ measures when autism is involved.

O'Connor and Hermelin (1988) have similarly speculated that some floor-level IQ is necessary if savant skills are to develop and that the highest levels of achievement may depend on higher general levels of functioning.[9] Again, Young's (1995) results have supported this suggestion. She found significant correlations between skill levels and IQs (0.5, Wechsler; 0.7 Raven's matrices; age controlled) among 32 savants but no suggestion that ability development among 19 subjects with splinter skills was IQ dependent.

D. Creativity

Creativity is a much debated construct, but it has commonly been defined psychologically in terms of flexibility, fluency, originality, and elaborative quality of thought (Torrance, 1974). We consider it here, rather than earlier, because it poses a theoretical problem that is arguably not resolved by the model outlined above. Hill (1978) found little evidence that savants can perform creatively. Young's (1995) results from the Torrance tests of creative thinking supported this conclusion. The scores were consistent with low IQ, including those for savants skilled in art. However, although savant skills commonly reflect imitative and inflexible characteristics, there have been savant artists whose works have been judged by experts to reveal individuality. Nadia's (Selfe, 1977) astonishingly energetic drawing of horseman and rider on the cover of Howe (1989) is a familiar example. The sculptor Alonzo Clemens (Treffert, 1989, chapter 10) and the artist Stephen Wiltshire (Sacks, 1995a; Wiltshire, 1991) have established international reputations and their works fetch high prices. If these accomplishments show originality, then considerable generative thought must be involved—and skills should not be independent from IQ.

Both Treffert (1989) and Sacks (1995a) have concluded that rare savant individuals in music and art do achieve originality in the sense of personal expression

[9]A recent finding by O'Connor, Cowan, and Samella, that differences in quality of calendar skills correlate with Wechsler IQ, predominantly because of Digit Symbol subtest scores, is consistent with this prediction (R. Cowan, personal communication, 20 May, 1998).

by way of a generative ability, but that the quality of this is limited and repetitive. Essentially the argument is that the processes underpinning savant creative performance are similar to those of nondisabled creative persons, but quality of performance is limited by low IQ. Recent research by Hermelin et al. (1987; Hermelin et al., 1989), comparing savant and nonsavant musicians, is consistent with this interpretation. Both Ho et al. (1991) and Young (1995) have found that creativity is correlated with IQ, and O'Connor and Hermelin (1987a) have speculated that higher orders of creativity require a quality of conceptualization that depends on at least average levels of IQ.

In terms of the model in Figure 1, a limited form of inventiveness could be accommodated as an aspect of talent. Any such determination is arbitrary, however. The point of Sack's distinction between high and low levels of creativity is readily appreciated, but whether Stephen Wiltshire's drawings are judged more representational than impressionistic is presently a matter of aesthetic opinion. This matter will remain unresolved until a single agreed definition for creativity is formulated.

VIII. CONCLUSIONS

A. Directions for Future Research

The main challenge remains being able to explain precisely how savants do the things they do. Associated with this, whether savant talents can be influenced by IQ is a question that should be high on a research agenda. If creativity and/or very high levels of skill are established as depending on IQ, the parameters of these relationships should be explored. Our speculation about cognitive processes underlying the development of savant skills is consistent with current theories about how memory develops (Rovee-Collier, 1990), although there has been little exchange to date between experimental and psychometric approaches (Carroll, 1993). Our account can draw on little direct evidence from the psychometric literature and an adequate investigation of individual differences and development aspects of long-term memory is yet to be made. Neuropsychological assessment of the memory processes of savants, compared with those of prodigies among the nondisabled population could prove useful to providing a broader understanding of processes involved in the manifestation of savant skills and of general brain function, providing that currently available tests are equal to the task. If they are not, then new procedures will be required; the potential for brain imaging techniques to be employed to examine structure and function in savants is yet to be explored.

We have argued that savant skills are modular—automatic and independent from executive functioning—but how practice in the presence of low IQ transforms talent into skill remains unknown. Longitudinal research is required to investigate the role of practice in developing the automatization and maintenance of these skills, including the extent to which they can be learned by ordinary persons without a disability. It is certainly possible that savant personality characteristics are responsible for the high motivation to maintain extensive practice that can in some cases become an obsessional preoccupation with an area of interest. Whether savant talents derive from inherited characteristics remains an open question.

Most savants have had exceptional opportunities to develop and maintain their interest(s). This may, however, be at the expense of the development of social skills and other adaptive behaviors. Because savant skills are typically solitary, they reduce opportunities for social interaction (Rubin & Monaghan, 1965). It can be noted, too, that, because module-based competencies are independent from general capabilities, investment in a talent will not generalize to broader areas of functioning. Intense preoccupation with an interest may therefore be detrimental to other areas of functioning. Barnes and Earnshaw (1995) noticed that when their savant participant was forced to abstain from art, his social skills and language abilities improved dramatically.

On the other hand, those associated with savants tend to view their skills as positive and intriguing (Treffert, 1989), and as a result these skills are often encouraged. Sacks (1985) argued that the forced separation of well-known savant twins to further their adaptive development deprived them of their numerical communication with each other, something of great importance in their lives. Howe and Smith (1988) and Goldsmith and Feldman (1988) have also recognized the pleasure that savants derive from their activities.

The best interests of a savant are probably served by a balanced educational approach that includes social skills training, counseling, and opportunities for interaction with others (Shields-Wolfe & Gallagher, 1992), but also encourages savant skills, without permitting them to dominate the individual's life (Barnes & Earnshaw, 1995). A creative educational suggestion worth exploring is that savants be provided with a mentor, a strategy that has been used successfully with gifted children (Zorman, 1993). Moreover, the opportunity to engage in one's skills may prove to be a useful reinforcer for the development of other more adaptive skills. While anecdotal evidence supports this belief, empirical validation is required.

Talented individuals tend to be valued in our society—unless they have an intellectual disability, when respect can be replaced by curiosity. A few well-publicized savants have, however, been able to profit financially from their skills. There is also anecdotal evidence that some savants have used their skills in paid positions within libraries and mechanical workshops. Research is required to determine the longer term prospects for such individuals.

B. Summary

Interest in savant syndrome as one means of furthering understanding of human intelligence has expanded significantly in the 20 years since Hill's (1978) review. This research has established that literal rote memory does not provide an adequate account for savant skills, which have been found to be based on extensive, expert, rule-based knowledge that can support limited generative activity. Savant skills are generally constrained to narrowly defined activities and are most commonly imitative and inflexible. This much is fact; what follows is speculative but plausible. Savant skills do not define separate forms of intelligence and are essentially unintelligent, depending on modular processing, established by rehearsal on the basis of preserved special talents and short-term and/or long-term memory structures that have been spared damage affecting other areas of the brain. Most researchers doubt that very rare savants whose accomplishments reveal personal artistic expression are capable of genuinely inventive originality. The highest levels of achievement by savants, including creative input, are probably IQ dependent.

ACKNOWLEDGMENTS

Our interest in this field was stimulated by the late Dr Neil O'Connor, whose untimely death on 1 October 1997 brought great sorrow to those privileged to have known him. We are grateful to Dr Carlene Wilson and Dr Darold Treffert for many useful suggestions and comments on the first draft.

REFERENCES

Addis, B. (1968). *Resistance to parsimony: The evolution of a system for explaining the calendar calculating abilities of idiot-savant twins.* Paper presented at the meeting of the Southwestern Psychological Association, New Orleans, LA.

Anastasi, A., & Levee, R. (1960). Intellectual defect and musical talent: A case report. *American Journal of Mental Deficiency, 64*, 695–703.

Anderson, M. (1992). *Intelligence and development: A cognitive theory.* Oxford: Blackwell.

Anderson, M. (1998). Individual differences in intelligence. In K. Kirsner, C. Speelman, M. Mayberry, A. O'Brien-Malone, M. Anderson, & C. MacLeod (Eds.), *Implicit and explicit mental processes* (pp. 171–185). Mahwah, NJ: Erlbaum.

Anderson, M., O'Connor, N., & Hermelin, B. (in press). A specific calculating ability. *Intelligence.*

Anwar, F., & Hermelin, B. (1982). An analysis of drawing skills in mental handicap. *Australian and New Zealand Journal of Developmental Disabilities, 8*, 147–155.

Bachem, A. (1955). Absolute pitch. *Journal of the Acoustical Society of America, 27*, 1100–1185.

Baddeley, A. (1997). *Human memory: Theory and practice* (rev. ed.). Exeter, UK: Psychology Press.

Barnes, R. C., & Earnshaw, S. M. (1995). Problems with the savant syndrome: A brief case study. *British Journal of Learning Disabilities, 23*, 124–126.

Bergman, J., & DePue, W. (1986). Musical idiot savants. *Music Educators Journal, 72*, 37–40.

Blaxton, T. A. (1992). Dissociations among memory measures in memory-impaired subjects: Evidence for a processing account of memory. *Memory and Cognition, 20*, 549–562.

Brand, C. (1996). *The g factor: General Intelligence and Its Implications.* Chichester: Wiley.

Brink, T. L. (1980). Idiot savant with unusual mechanical ability: An organic explanation. *American Journal of Psychiatry, 137*, 250–251.

Burling, T. A., Sappington, J. T., & Mead, A. M. (1983). Lateral specialisation of a perpetual calendar task by a moderately mentally retarded adult. *American Journal of Mental Deficiency, 88*, 326–328.

Cameron, L. (1998). *The music of light: The extraordinary story of Hikari and Kenzaburo Oe.* New York: Simon & Schuster.

Carroll, J. B. (1993). *Human cognitive ability: A survey of factor analytic studies.* London: Cambridge University Press.

Casey, B., Gordon, C. T., Mannheim, G. B., & Rumsey, J. M. (1993). Dysfunctional attention in autistic savants. *Journal of Clinical and Experimental Neuropsychology, 15,* 933–946.

Cattell, R. B. (1941). Some theoretical issues in adult intelligence testing. *Psychological Bulletin, 38,* 592.

Charness, N., Clifton, J., & MacDonald, L. (1988). Case study of a musical "mono-savant": A cognitive-psychological focus. In L. Obler & D. A. Fein (Eds.), *The exceptional brain* (pp. 277–293). New York: Guilford.

Cheatham, S. K., Rucker, H. N., Polloway, E. A., Smith, J. D., & Lewis, G. W. (1995). Savant syndrome: Case studies, hypotheses, and implications for special education. *Education and Training in Mental Retardation and Developmental Disabilities, 30,* 243–253.

Cobrinik, L. (1982). The performance of hyperlexic children on an "incomplete words" task. *Neuropsychologia, 20,* 569–578.

Comer, D. (1985, May 16). Musical talent brightens life in a blind severely retarded man. *The Toronto Star,* p. 6.

Detterman, D. K. (1982). Does *g* exist? *Intelligence, 6,* 99–108.

Detterman, D. K. (1986). Human intelligence is a complex system of separate processes. In R. J. Sternberg & D. K. Detterman (Eds.), *What is intelligence? Contemporary viewpoints on its nature and definition* (pp. 57–61). Norwood, N.J.: Ablex.

Detterman, D. K., Mayer, J. D., Caruso, D. R., Legree, P. J., Conners, A., & Taylor, R. (1992). Assessment of basic cognitive deficits. *American Journal of Mental Retardation, 97,* 251–286.

Dorman, C. (1991). Exceptional calendar calculation ability after early left hemispherectomy. *Brain Cognition, 15,* 26–36.

Dowker, A., Hermelin, B., & Pring, L. (1996). A savant poet. *Psychological Medicine, 26,* 913–924.

Down, J. L. (1887). *On some of the mental affections of childhood and youth.* London: Churchill.

Eichenbaum, H., Otto, T., & Cohen, N. J. (1996). The hippocampal system: Dissociating its functional components and recombining them in the service of declarative memory. *Behavioral and Brain Sciences, 19,* 772–776.

Ericsson, K. A., & Faivre, I. (1988). What's exceptional about exceptional abilities? In L. Obler & D. A. Fein (Eds.), *The Exceptional Brain* (pp. 436–473). New York: Guilford Press.

Fein, D., & Obler, L. K. (1988). Neuropsychological study of talent: A developing field. In L. Obler & D. A. Fein (Eds.), *The exceptional brain* (pp. 3–18). New York: Guilford Press.

Feldman, D. (1993). Child Prodigies: A distinctive form of giftedness. *Gifted Child Quarterly, 37,* 188–193.

Foerstl, J. (1989). Early interest in the idiot savant. *American Journal of Psychiatry, 146,* 566.

Fontenelle, S., & Alarcon, M. (1982). Hyperplexia: Precocious word recognition in developmentally delayed children. *Perceptual and Motor Skills, 55,* 247–252.

Frey, H. S. (1995). Musical ability. *Science, 269,* 1498.

Gardner, H. (1983). *Frames of mind: The theory of multiple intelligences.* New York: Harper & Row.

Glisky, E. L. (1995). Acquisition and transfer of word processing skill by an amnesic patient. *Neuropsychological Rehabilitation, 5,* 299–318.

Goddard, H. H. (1914). *Feeble-mindedness.* New York: Macmillan.

Goldberg, T. E. (1987). On hermetic reading abilities. *Journal of Autism and Developmental Disorders, 17,* 29–44.

Goldsmith, L. T., & Feldman, D. H. (1988). Idiots savants—thinking about remembering: A response to White. *New Ideas in Psychology, 6,* 15–23.

Gordon, P., Valentine, E., & Wilding, J. M. (1984). One man's memory: A study of a mnemonist. *British Journal of Psychology*, *75*, 1–14.
Gustin, W. C. (1985). The development of exceptional research mathematicians. In B. S. Bloom (Ed.), *Developing talent in young people* (pp. 270–333). New York: Ballantine Books.
Hamann, S. B., & Squire, L. R. (1995). On the acquisition of new declarative knowledge in amnesia. *Behavioral Neuroscience*, *109*, 1027–1044.
Hamann, S. B., Squire, L. R., & Schacter, D. L. (1995). Perceptual thresholds and priming in amnesia. *Neuropsychology*, *9*, 3–15.
Hawkes, N. (1993, September 13). Autistic youth has the genius of Mozart? *The Times*, p. 1. (See also leading article, p. 17).
Healy, J. M., Aram, D. M., Horwitz, S. J., & Kessler, J. W. (1982). A study of hyperlexia. *Brain and Language*, *9*, 1–23.
Hermelin, B., & O'Connor, N. (1986). Idiot savant calendrical calculators: Rules and regularities. *Psychological Medicine*, *16*, 885–893.
Hermelin, B., & O'Connor, N. (1989). Intelligence and musical improvisation. *Psychological Medicine*, *19*, 497–457.
Hermelin, B., & O'Connor, N. (1990a). Art and accuracy: The drawing ability of idiot-savants. *Journal of Child Psychology and Psychiatry and Allied Disciplines*, *31*, 217–228.
Hermelin, B., & O'Connor, N. (1990b). Factors and primes: A specific numerical ability. *Psychological Medicine*, *20*, 163–169.
Hermelin, B., O'Connor, N., & Lee, S. (1987). Musical inventiveness of five idiot-savants. *Psychological Medicine*, *17*, 79–90.
Hermelin, B., O'Connor, N., Lee, S., & Treffert, D. (1989). Intelligence and musical improvisation. *Psychological Medicine*, *19*, 447–457.
Hermelin, B., Pring, L., & Heavey, L. (1994). Visual and motor functions in graphically gifted savant. *Psychological Medicine*, *24*, 673–680.
Herrnstein, R. J., & Murray, C. (1994). *The bell curve: Intelligence and class structure in American life.* New York: Free Press.
Hewson, M., & Taylor, P. (1993, September 13). Stephen's genuis to amaze. *The Times*, p. 11. (See also leading article, p. 17).
Hill, A. L. (1974). Idiot savants: A categorization of abilities. *Mental Retardation*, December, 12–13.
Hill, A. L. (1978). Savants: mentally retarded individuals with special skills. In N. Ellis (Ed.), *International review of research in mental retardation*, (*Vol. 9*, pp. 277–298). New York: Academic Press.
Ho, E., Tsang, A., & Ho, D. (1991). An investigation of the calendar calculation ability of a Chinese calendar savant. *Journal of Autism and Developmental Disorders*, *21*, 315–327.
Hoffman, E. (1971). The idiot savant: A case report and a review of explanations. *Mental Retardation*, *9*, 18–21.
Hoffman, E., & Reeves, R. (1979). An idiot savant with unusual mechanical ability. *American Journal of Psychiatry*, *136*, 713–714.
Horn, J. L., & Knoll, J. (1997). Human cognitive capabilities: G_f-G_c theory. In D. P. Flanagan, J. L. Genshaft, & P. L. Harrison (Eds.), *Contemporary intellectual assessment: Theories, tests, and issues* (pp. 53–91). New York: Guilford Press.
Horwitz, W. A., Kestenbaum, C., Person, E., & Jarvick, L. (1965). Identical twins—"idiot savants"—calendar calculators. *American Journal of Psychiatry*, *121*, 1075–1079.
Howe, M. J. A. (1989). *Fragments of genius: The strange feats of idiot savants.* London: Routledge.
Howe, M. J. A. (1990). *The origins of exceptional abilities.* Oxford: Blackwell.
Howe, M. J., & Smith, J. (1988). Calendar calculating in "idiots savants": How do they do it? *British Journal of Psychology*, *79*, 371–386.

Jensen, A. R. (1990). Speed of information processing in a calculating prodigy. *Intelligence, 14*, 259–274.

Judd, T. (1988). The varieties of musical talent. In L. Obler & D. A. Fein (Eds.), *The exceptional brain* (pp. 127–152). New York: Guilford Press.

Kalinowski, A. G. (1985). The development of Olympic swimmers. In B. S. Bloom (Ed.), *Developing talent in young people.* New York: Ballantine.

Kapur, N. (1988). Selective sparing of memory functioning in a patient with amnesia following herpes encephalitis. *Brain and Cognition, 8*, 77–90.

Kelly, S. J., Macaruso, P., & Sokol, S. M. (1997). Mental calculation in an autistic savant: A case study. *Journal of Clinical and Experimental Neuropsychology, 19*, 172–184.

Kistner, J., Robbins, F., & Haskett, M. (1988). Assessment and skill remediation of hyperlexic children. *Journal of Autism and Developmental Disorders, 18*, 191–205.

Kline, P. (1991). *Intelligence: The psychometric view.* London: Routledge.

McGrew, K. S. (1997). Analysis of the major intelligence batteries according to a proposed comprehensive G_f-G_c framework. In D. P. Flanagan, J. L. Genshaft, & P. L. Harrison (Eds.), *Contemporary intellectual assessment: Theories, tests, and issues* (pp. 151–179). New York: Guilford Press.

Miller, L. K. (1987a). Determinants of melody span in a developmentally disabled musical savant. *Psychology of Music, 15*, 76–89.

Miller, L. K. (1987b). Developmentally delayed musical savant's sensitivity to tonal structure. *American Journal of Mental Deficiency, 91*, 467–471.

Miller, L. (1989). *Musical savants: Exceptional skill in the mentally retarded.* Hillsdale, NJ: Erlbaum.

Miller, L. K. (1995). Sensitivity to sequential structure in musical savants. *American Journal on Mental Retardation, 99*, 391–398.

Miller, L. K., & Monroe, M. J. (1990). Musical aptitudes and adaptive behaviour of people with mental retardation. *American Journal on Mental Retardation, 95*, 220–227.

Moriarty, J., Ring, H. A., & Robertson, M. M. (1993). An idiot savant calendrical calculator with Gilles de la Tourette syndrome: Implications for an understanding of the savant syndrome. *Psychological Medicine, 23*, 1019–1021.

Morishima, A., & Brown, L. F. (1977). A case report on the artistic talent of an autistic idiot savant. *Mental Retardation, 15*, 33–36.

Mottron, L., & Belleville, S. (1993). A study of perceptual analysis in a high-level autistic subject with exceptional graphic abilities. *Brain and Cognition, 23*, 279–309.

Mottron, L., & Belleville, S. (1995). Perspective production in a savant autistic draughtsman. *Psychological Medicine, 25*, 639–648.

Mottron, L., Belleville, S., & Stip, E. (1996). Propername hypermnesia in an autistic subject. *Brain and Language, 53*, 326–350.

Neisser, U., Boodoo, G., Bouchard, T. J. Jr., Boykin, A. W., Brody, N., Ceci, S. J., Halpern, D. F., Loehlin, J. C., Perloff, R., Sternberg, R. J., & Urbina, S. (1996). Intelligence: Knowns and unknowns. *American Psychologist, 51*, 77–101.

Nettelbeck, T., & Young, R. (1996). Intelligence and savant syndrome: Is the whole greater than the sum of the fragments? *Intelligence, 22*, 49–67.

Norris, D. (1990). How to build a connectionist idiot (savant). *Cognition, 35*, 277–291.

O'Connor, N. (1989). The performance of the "idiot savant": Implicit and explicit. *British Journal of Disorders of Communication, 24*, 1–20.

O'Connor, N., & Hermelin, B. (1984). Idiot savant calendrical calculators: Maths or memory? *Psychological Medicine, 14*, 801–806.

O'Connor, N., & Hermelin, B. (1987a). Visual and graphic abilities of the idiot savant artist. *Psychological Medicine, 17*, 79–90.

O'Connor, N., & Hermelin, B. (1987b). Visual memory and motor programmes. Their use by idiot-savant artists and controls. *British Journal of Psychology, 78*, 307–323.
O'Connor, N., & Hermelin, B. (1988). Low intelligence and special abilities. *Journal of Child Psychology and Psychiatry and Allied Disciplines, 29*, 391–396.
O'Connor, N., & Hermelin, B. (1989). The memory structure of autistic idiot savant mnemonists. *British Journal of Psychology, 80*, 97–111.
O'Connor, N., & Hermelin, B. (1990). The recognition failure and graphic success of idiot savant artists. *Journal of Child Psychology and Psychiatry and Allied Disciplines, 31*, 203–215.
O'Connor, N., & Hermelin, B. (1991). A specific linguistic ability. *American Journal on Mental Retardation, 95*, 673–680.
O'Connor, N., & Hermelin, B. (1992). Do young calendrical calculators improve with age? *Journal of Child Psychology and Psychiatry and Allied Disciplines, 33*, 907–912.
O'Connor, N., & Hermelin, B. (1994). Two autistic savant readers. *Journal of Autism and Developmental Disorders, 24*, 501–515.
Ohtsuka, A., Miyasaka, Y., & Kamizono, S. (1991). The calendar calculating process: "Idiot savant" calendar calculators. *Japanese Journal of Special Education, 29*, 13–22.
Peretz, I. (1996). Can we lose memory for music? A case of music agnosia in a nonmusician. *Journal of Cognitive Neuroscience, 8*, 481–496.
Piaget, J. (1953). *The origin of intelligence in the child.* London: Routledge & Kegan Paul.
Pring, L., & Hermelin, B. (1993). Bottle, tulip and wineglass: Semantic and structural picture processing by savant artists. *Journal of Child Psychology and Psychiatry and Allied Disciplines, 34*, 1365–1385.
Pring, L., Hermelin, B., & Heavey, L. (1995). Savant, segments art and autism. *Journal of Child Psychology and Psychiatry and Allied Disciplines, 36*, 1065–1976.
Rabbitt, P. M. A. (Ed.). (1997). *Methodology of frontal and executive function.* Hove, UK: Psychology Press.
Rife, D., & Snyder, L. (1931). Studies in human inheritance. *Human Biology, 3*, 547–559.
Rimland, B. (1978a). Inside the mind of the autistic savant. *Psychology Today, 12*, 68–80.
Rimland, B. (1978b). Savant capabilities of autistic children and their cognitive implications. In G. Serban (Ed.), *Cognitive defects in the development of mental illness* (pp. 43–65). New York: Brunner/Mazel.
Rimland, B., & Fein, D. (1988). Special talents of autistic savants. In L. Obler & D. A. Fein (Eds.), *The exceptional brain* (pp. 472–492). New York: Guilford Press.
Rimland, B., & Hill, A. L. (1984). Idiot savants. In J. Wortes (Ed.), *Mental retardation and developmental disabilities, 13*, (pp. 155–169). New York: Plenum Press.
Rosen, A. M. (1981). Adult calendar calculators in a psychiatric OPD: A report of two cases and comparative analysis of abilities. *Journal of Autism and Developmental Disorders, 11*, 285–292.
Rovee-Collier, C. K. (1990). The "memory system" of prelinguistic infants. *Annals of the New York Academy of Sciences, 608*, 517–542.
Rubin, E. J., & Monaghan, S. (1965). Calendar calculation in a multiple-handicapped blind person. *American Journal of Mental Deficiency, 70*, 478–485.
Sacks, O. (1985). The twins. *The New York Review of Books, 32*, 16–20.
Sacks, O. (1995a). *Anthropologist on Mars.* Sydney: Pan Macmillan.
Sacks, O. (1995b). Musical ability "Comment." *Science, 269*, 1498.
Samson, S., & Zatorre, R. J. (1991). Recognition memory for text and melody of songs after unilateral temporal lobe lesion: Evidence for dual encoding. *Journal of Experimental Psychology Learning, Memory, and Cognition, 17*, 793–804.
Schmidtke, K., Handschu, R., & Vollmer, H. (1996). Cognitive procedural learning in amnesia. *Brain and Cognition, 32*, 441–467.

Schweiger, A. (1988). A portrait of the artist as a brain-damaged patient. In L. Obler & D. A. Fein (Eds.), *The exceptional brain* (pp. 303–309). New York: Guilford Press.
Selfe, L. (1977). *Nadia: A case of extraordinary ability in an autistic child.* New York: Harcourt Brace Jovanovich.
Selfe, L. (1983). *Normal and anomalous representational drawing ability in children.* London: Academic Press.
Shields-Wolfe, J., & Gallagher, P. A. (1992). Functional utilization of splinter skills for the employment of a young adult with autism. *Focus on Autistic Behavior, 7,* 1–16.
Sloane, K. D., & Sosniak, L. A. (1985). The development of accomplished sculptures. In B. S. Bloom (Ed.), *Developing talent in young people.* New York: Ballantine.
Sloboda, J., Hermelin, B., & O'Connor, N. (1985). An exceptional musical memory. *Musical Perception, 3,* 155–170.
Smith, J., & Howe, M. J. (1985). An investigation of calendar calculating skills in an "idiot savant." *International Journal of Rehabilitation Research, 8,* 77–79.
Smith, N., & Tsimpli, I. (1995). *The mind of a savant: Language, learning and modularity.* Oxford: Blackwell.
Soliveri, P., Brown, R. G., Jahanshahi, M., & Marsden, C. D. (1992). Effect of practice on performance of a skilled motor task in patients with Parkinson's disease. *Journal of Neurology, Neurosurgery and Psychiatry, 55,* 454–460.
Spearman, C. (1927). *The abilities of man.* London: Macmillan.
Spitz, H. H. (1995). Calendar calculating idiots savants and the smart unconscious. *New Ideas in Psychology, 13,* 167–182.
Squire, L. (1992). Declarative and nondeclarative memory: Multiple brain systems supporting learning and memory. *Journal of Cognitive Neuroscience, 4,* 232–243.
Squire, L. R., & Butter, N. (Eds.). (1992). *Neuropsychology of memory* (2nd ed.). New York: Guilford Press.
Sternberg (1985). *Beyond IQ: A triarchic theory of human intelligence.* New York: Cambridge University Press.
Stevens, D. E., & Moffitt, T. E. (1988). Neuropsychological profile of an Asperger's syndrome case with exceptional calculating ability. *Clinical Neuropsychologist, 2,* 228–238.
Takeuchi, A. H., & Hulse, S. H. (1993). Absolute pitch. *Psychological Bulletin, 13,* 345–361.
Thurstone, L. L. (1938). *Primary mental abilities.* Chicago: University of Chicago Press.
Toates, F. (1996). The hippocampus seen in the context of declarative and procedural control. *Behavioral and Brain Sciences, 19,* 771–772, 775–776.
Torrance, E. P. (1974). *Torrance Tests of Creative Thinking.* Bensenville, IL: Scholastic Testing Service, Inc.
Tredgold, A. F. (1923). *Mental deficiency (Amentia)* (3rd ed.). Bailliere, Tindall & Cox: London.
Treffert, D. A. (1988). The idiot savant: A review of the syndrome. *American Journal of Psychiatry, 145,* 563–572.
Treffert, D. A. (1989). *Extraordinary people.* London: Bantam Press.
Valentine, E. R., & Wilding, J. M. (1994). Memory expertise. *The Psychologist, 7,* 405–408.
Wehmeyer, M. L. (1992). Developmental and psychological aspects of the savant syndrome. *International Journal of Disability, Development and Education, 39,* 153–163.
Wiltshire, S. (1991). *Floating cities: Venice, Amsterdam, Leningrad, and Moscow.* London: Michael Joseph.
Young, R. (1995). *Savant syndrome: Processes underlying extraordinary abilities.* Unpublished doctoral dissertation, University of Adelaide, South Australia.
Young, R. L., & Nettelbeck, T. (1994). The "intelligence" of calendrical calculators. *American Journal of Mental Retardation, 99,* 186–200.

Young, R. L., & Nettelbeck, T. (1995). The abilities of a musical savant and his family. *Journal of Autism and Developmental Disorders*, *25*, 231–248.

Zorman, R. (1993). Mentoring and role modeling programs for the gifted. In K. A. Heller, F. J. Moenks, & A. H. Passow (Eds.), *International handbook of research and development of giftedness and talent,* (*Vol. 16,* pp. 727–741). Oxford UK: Pergamon Press.

BIBLIOGRAPHY

Bloom, B. S. (1982). The role of gifts and markers in the development of talent. *Exceptional-Children*, *48*, 510–522.

Conners, F. A. (1992). Special abilities of idiots savants, hyperlexic children, and phenomenal memorizers: Implications for intelligence theory. In D. K. Detterman (Ed.), *Current topics in human intelligence*, 2 (pp. 187–227). Norwood, NJ: Ablex.

Dalphonse, S. (1993, February). *The mysterious powers of Peter Guthrie.* The Readers Digest, 119–123.

Donnelly, J., & Altman, R. (1994). The autistic savant: Recognizing and serving the gifted student with autism. *Roeper Review*, *16*, 252–256.

Hermelin, B., & O'Connor, N. (1982). Naming and classifying: Intelligence and frequency effects. *British Journal of Psychology*, *73*, 361–370.

Hermelin, B., & O'Connor, N. (1983). The idiot savant: Flawed genius or clever Hans? *Psychological Medicine*, *13*, 479–481.

Hermelin, B., & O'Connor, N. (1986). Spatial representations in mathematically and in artistically gifted children. *British Journal of Educational Psychology*, *56*, 150–157.

Hope, J. A. (1987). A case study of a highly skilled mental calculator. *Journal of Research in Mathematics Education*, *18*, 331–342.

Howe, M. J. A. (1989). Separate skills or general intelligence: The autonomy of human abilities. *British Journal of Educational Psychology*, *59*, 351–360.

Hunt, E., & Love, T. (1982). The second mnemonist. In U. Neisser (Ed.), *Memory observed* (pp. 390–398). San Francisco: Freeman.

Hurst, L. C., & Mulhall, D. J. (1988). Another calendar savant. *British Journal of Psychiatry*, *152*, 274–277.

Kehrer, H. E. (1992). Savant capabilities of autistic persons. *Acta Paedopsychiatrica International Journal of Child and Adolescent Psychiatry*, *55*, 151–155.

Laber, E. (1992, January 21). Autism's mysterious links with intelligence. *The Advocate.*

Lauerman, C., & Fryer, M. (1988, August 28). Extraordinary people: The mystery of the savant syndrome. *The Chicago Tribune Magazine*, Section 10.

Lebrun, Y., Van Endert, C., & Szliwowski, H. (1988). Trilingual hyperlexia. In L. Obler & D. A. Fein (Eds.), *The exceptional brain* (pp. 253–264). New York: Guilford Press.

Lucci, D., Fein, D., Holevas, A., & Kaplan, E. (1988). Paul: A musically gifted autistic boy. In L. Obler & D. A. Fein (Eds.), *The exceptional brain* (pp. 310–324). New York: Guilford Press.

Milbrath, C., & Siegel, B. (1996). Perspective taking in the drawings of a talented autistic child. *Visual Arts Research*, *22*, 56–75.

Monty, S. (1981). *May's Boy.* Nashville, TN: Thomas Nelson.

Morelock, M. J., & Feldman, D. H. (1993). Prodigies and savants. In K. A. Heller, F. J. Monks, & A. H. Passow (Eds.), *International handbook of research and development of giftedness and talent* (pp. 161–181). Oxford: Pergamon.

Nelson, E. C., & Pribor, E. F. (1993). A calendar savant with autism and Tourette syndrome: Response to treatment and thoughts on the interrelationships of these conditions. *Annals of Clinical Psychiatry*, *5*, 135–140.

Obler, L., & Fein, D. A. (Eds.). (1988). *The exceptional brain.* New York: Guilford Press.

O'Connor, N. (1978). General and specific handicap in cognitive development. *Mental Retardation Bulletin, 6,* 135–143.

O'Connor, N. (1987a). Cognitive psychology and mental handicap. *Journal of Mental Deficiency Research, 31,* 329–336.

O'Connor, N. (1987b). Intelligence, handicaps and talents. *Mental Retardation and Learning Disability Bulletin, 15,* 41–56.

O'Connor, N., & Hermelin, B. (1982). The comparative judgements of generally and specifically gifted children. *Quarterly Journal of Experimental Psychology Human Experimental Psychology, 34,* 443–457.

O'Connor, N., & Hermelin, B. (1983). The role of general ability and specific talents in information processing. *British Journal of Developmental Psychology, 4,* 389–403.

O'Connor, N., & Hermelin, B. (1991). Talents and preoccupations in idiot-savants. *Psychological Medicine, 21,* 959–964.

Patti, P. J., & Lupinetti, L. (1993). Brief report: Implications of hyperlexia in an autistic savant. *Journal of Autism and Developmental Disorders, 23,* 397–405.

Rattey, J. J., Grandin, T., & Miller, A. (1992). Defense behavior and coping in an autistic savant: The story of Temple Grandin, PhD. *Psychiatry Interpersonal and Biological Processes, 55,* 382–391.

Rovet, J., Krekewich, K., Perlman, K., & Weksberg, Holland, J., & Feigenbaum, A. (1995). Savant characteristics in a child with developmental delay and deletion in the short arm of chromosome 20. *Developmental Medicine and Child Neurology, 37,* 637–644.

Sloboda, J. (1991). *Musical expertise.* In K. A. Ericsson & J. Smith (Eds.), *Toward a general theory of expertise* (pp. 153–171). New York: Cambridge.

Sloboda, J. A., & Howe, M. J. (1991). Biographical precursors of musical excellence: An interview study. *Psychology of Music, 19,* 3–21.

Southall, G. (1979). *Blind Tom: The Post-Civil War enslavement of a black musical genius.* Minneapolis, MN: Challenge Productions.

Southall, G. (1983). *The continuing enslavement of Blind Tom, the pianist composer* (1868–1887). Minneapolis, MN: Challenge Productions.

Spitz, H. H. (1993). The role of the unconscious in thinking and problem solving. *Educational Psychology, 13,* 229–244.

Spitz, H. H. (1996). Commentary on Vandervert's "From *idiots savants* to Albert Einstein." *New Ideas in Psychology, 14,* 93–96.

Steel, J. G., Gorman, R., & Flexman, J. E. (1984). Neuropsychiatric testing in an autistic mathematical idiot-savant: Evidence for nonverbal abstract capacity. *Journal of American Academy of Child Psychiatry, 23,* 704–707.

Vandervert, L. R. (1996). From *idiots savants* to Albert Einstein: A brain algorithm explanation of savant and everyday performance. *New Ideas in Psychology, 14,* 81–92.

White, P. (1988). The structured representation of information in long term memory: A possible explanation for the accomplishments of "idiot savants." *New Ideas in Psychology, 6,* 3–14.

The Cost-Efficiency of Supported Employment Programs: A Review of the Literature

ROBERT E. CIMERA

INSTITUTE ON RESEARCH ON DISABILITY AND HUMAN DEVELOPMENT
UNIVERSITY OF ILLINOIS AT CHICAGO
CHICAGO, ILLINOIS

FRANK R. RUSCH

COLLEGE OF EDUCATION
UNIVERSITY OF ILLINOIS AT URBANA-CHAMPAIGN
CHAMPAIGN, ILLINOIS

I. INTRODUCTION

With the growing acceptance of inclusion and other normalization principles, the importance of vocational options for individuals with mental retardation cannot be understated. The primary vocational options currently available for individuals with mental retardation include supported employment and sheltered workshops. Supported employment programs are characterized as having paid competitive positions within the community where the supports needed by the individual worker are provided by job coaches (Rusch, 1990). Sheltered workshops, on the other hand, are programs that provide individuals with disabilities opportunities to learn work-related skills while often earning below minimum wage in segregated adult rehabilitation facilities (Wehman, 1981).

Although the differences between supported and sheltered employment programs are numerous, operators of these two programs compete against one another for the limited funds allocated by the government for disability services. Because of this competition, it is important to determine which program is the best investment for individuals with disabilities as well as the taxpayer; that is, it must

INTERNATIONAL REVIEW OF RESEARCH IN MENTAL RETARDATION, Vol. 22
0074-7750/99 $30.00

be determined which program returns more money in the form of benefits than the program's costs (i.e., cost-efficient). Thus far, at least 20 studies have investigated the cost-efficiency of supported employment in relation to sheltered workshops. This chapter reviews each of these benefit–cost studies and summarizes their combined findings. Suggestions for additional research are also made.

II. OVERVIEW OF BENEFIT–COST ANALYSES

Benefit–cost analyses seek to answer the question: "Does a program[1] produce benefits that justify the resulting costs?" (Johnston, 1987; Thornton, 1992; Thornton & Will, 1988). This question is answered by using a structured accounting procedure that converts all of the program's benefits and costs into monetary units (Thompson, 1980). For example, one of the effects that may be produced by employment programs could be workers who are less likely to be dependent upon governmental subsidies. The monetary value of this program effect can be approximated by examining the amount of subsidies received by workers prior to entering the employment program and the amount of subsidies received by workers after being enrolled in the employment program.

Once monetary values are placed upon all program benefits and costs, a benefit–cost ratio is formulated. Benefit-cost ratios are typically calculated by dividing gross benefits by gross costs (Kee, 1994). When this formula is utilized, a ratio exceeding 1.00 indicates that the program is economically efficient, or "cost-efficient" (Prest & Turvey, 1965). Conversely, if gross costs exceed gross benefits, the resulting benefit–cost ratio is below 1.00, and the program is said to be economically inefficient.

Prior to formulating and computing benefit–cost ratios, analysts must determine the perspective (e.g., the taxpayer) from which the analyses will occur (Layard, 1972; Thornton, 1984). This is imperative, because a program effect (e.g., taxes withheld) can be a benefit to some and at the same time a cost to others. For example, from the perspective of a worker, taxes withheld is a cost of being employed since income lost to taxes is no longer available for the worker to spend. Yet, from the perspective of a taxpayer, taxes withheld is a benefit since this money increases the revenue base from which the government can attempt to improve the community.

Each program outcome may be perceived from several analytical viewpoints. In the present study, outcomes of supported employment programs are examined from three distinct perspectives. The first is from the perspective of the supported

[1]The word *program* here is meant as an example. Benefit–cost research can be done on anything requiring a decision, such as determining which intervention to use in the classroom (Levin, 1983; Worthen & Sanders, 1987).

employee, or the worker employed within the community. This is also called "private return." The second involves taxpayers, as discussed briefly above. This perspective is often called "state/government return." The third perspective utilized within the present study is that of society in general or "public return."

However, benefit–cost ratios have weaknesses that should be noted. For instance, benefit–cost ratios only indicate whether or not programs are economically efficient. They do not denote the level of investment that should be undertaken in order to optimize monetary returns. For example, even if all studies agreed that supported employment programs are cost-efficient from the taxpayer's perspective, the question of how much revenue should be devoted to such programs would still remain. In other words, should taxpayers double their current investment in supported employment programs? Triple? At some point the amount of revenue earmarked for supported employment programs would experience dwindling returns; that is, the amount of returns from the next dollar invested would gain less benefits than the previous dollar.

Further, benefit–cost ratios are not as useful as internal rates of return when comparing the net benefits of various investment opportunities. For example, if Program A had an internal rate of return equaling 13%, it easily could be determined that it produces monetary returns 8.5% higher than an alternative investment that is producing gains of 4.5% (e.g., a savings bond). However, if Program A's benefit–cost ratio were 1.13, direct comparisons to an alternative investment generating returns of 4.5% are less obvious. As a result, calculations featuring internal rates of return are often preferred to benefit–cost ratios, which are deemed less versatile.

Unfortunately, none of the studies that have investigated supported employment have utilized methods for calculating internal rates of return. Consequently, the conceptual framework of this chapter will revolve around the three analytical perspectives common in the benefit–cost literature. Specifically, this chapter will define the perspectives of the worker, taxpayer, and society. The methodological differences between analyses from these different perspectives will then be delineated.

After the methods utilized to derive each perspective have been outlined, 20 studies examining the benefits and costs of employment programs will be grouped into the following three categories: (a) nine studies that examined program outcomes from all three perspectives (i.e., worker, taxpayer, and society); (b) five studies that examined supported employment outcomes from the perspectives of the worker and the taxpayer; and (c) six studies that examined supported employment program outcomes solely from the perspective of the worker (see Table I). These studies were identified after a comprehensive search of the supported employment literature; each will be discussed individually with respect to their methodology and results.

After all of the studies have been discussed, their findings will be summarized

TABLE I
STUDIES EXPLORING THE BENEFITS AND COSTS OF SUPPORTED EMPLOYMENT REVIEWED IN THIS CHAPTER BY PERSPECTIVE

Worker, taxpayer, and society perspectives	Worker and taxpayer perspectives	Worker perspective
Schneider et al. (1981)	Hill & Wehman (1983)	Cho & Schuermann (1980)
Conley et al. (1989)	Wehman et al. (1985)	Brickey & Campbell (1981)
Tines et al. (1990)	Hill, Banks, et al. (1987)	Lam (1986)
Noble et al. (1991)	Hill, Wehman, et al. (1987)	Schloss et al. (1987)
McCaughrin et al. (1991)	McCaughrin (1988)	Kregel et al. (1989)
Lewis et al. (1992)		Thompson et al. (1992)
McCaughrin et al. (1993)		
Rusch et al. (1993)		
Cimera (1997)		

and presented with regard to the three analytical perspectives found within the literature (i.e., the worker, taxpayer, and society).

A. Worker's Perspective

Workers are the direct beneficiaries of employment programs, as they are the principal consumers of services. Without workers, as well as hiring businesses, supported employment programs could not produce program outcomes impacting taxpayers or society (cf. Cho & Schuermann, 1980). As a result, workers are considered the primary beneficiaries.

B. Taxpayer's Perspective

Supported employment programs are funded by state agencies, such as the Department of Vocational Rehabilitation (Wehman, 1996a). These agencies, in turn, are funded by taxpayers. Consequently, taxpayers are seen as the prominent funders of employment programs for individuals with disabilities. Benefits to taxpayers, such as reduced governmental subsidies, are ancillary to the benefits and costs accrued by the worker as well as to the operation of supported employment programs. For this reason, taxpayers are considered secondary beneficiaries of supported employment programs.

C. Society's Perspective

For the purposes of the present study, society is characterized as an amalgamation of workers and taxpayers. Specifically, the societal perspective includes the sum benefits and costs generated from the previous two perspectives. In this role, society cannot acquire a positive net benefit without the benefits acquired by workers and taxpayers. In summary, everybody (e.g., from newborns to the elderly) who lives in a community comprises the societal perspective. As a result, society is considered a tertiary beneficiary of supported employment programs.

III. METHODOLOGICAL DIFFERENCES

As previously mentioned, each program outcome can be seen as either a benefit or cost from different perspectives (e.g., worker, taxpayer, and society). Therefore, several methodological differences are evident in the computation of benefit–cost ratios from the perspectives of the worker, the taxpayer, and society. In the following sections, each of these perspectives is reviewed with regard to the principal accounting variables traditionally utilized in the literature (e.g., alternative program expenditures) (see Table II).

A. Worker's Perspective

Workers employed via supported employment programs generate numerous benefits while also incurring various costs. Throughout the literature, two prominent benefits to workers were identified: gross earnings and fringe benefits. Similarly, several costs were common. These include forgone wages (i.e., wages that would have been earned had it not been for supported employment), taxes with-

TABLE II
TYPICAL COSTS AND BENEFITS OF SUPPORTED EMPLOYMENT PROGRAMS FROM THREE PERSPECTIVES

Cost-accounting variables	Worker	Taxpayer	Society
Gross earnings	Benefit	—	Benefit[a]
Fringe benefits	Benefit	—	Benefit
Taxes withheld	Cost	Benefit	—
Forgone wages	Cost	—	Cost[a]
Reduction in subsidies	Cost	Benefit	—
Savings in alternative program costs	—	Benefit	Benefit
Supported employment operating costs	—	Cost	Cost
Reduction in taxes due to TJTC[b]	—	Cost	Cost

[a]The primary benefit to society is "increased earnings" (gross earnings minus forgone wages). Forgone wages, technically, is not a cost to society but is included here as such.

[b]TJTC, targeted job tax credits.

held, and reductions in governmental subsidies received (e.g., Supplemental Security Income [SSI]).

B. Taxpayer's Perspective

As with workers, taxpayers experience certain benefits and costs as a result of funding supported employment programs. The benefits to taxpayers that were specified in most of the literature included the taxes withheld from workers, reductions in governmental subsidies, and savings from alternative employment programs (e.g., sheltered workshops). Costs to taxpayers included the operating expenditures for supported employment programs and the reductions in taxes resulting from such tax credits (e.g., Targeted Job Tax Credits [TJIC]) offered to businesses that hire individuals with disabilities.

C. Society's Perspective

The benefits and costs assessed to society are a combination of those assessed to workers and taxpayers. Specifically, increased earnings of the supported employee, fringe benefits, and decreases in operating expenditures of alternative employment programs were seen to comprise benefits to society, according to the majority of studies within the literature. Increased earnings entail gross wages minus forgone wages. Costs to society involved the operating expenditures of supported employment programs and lost revenue resulting from TJTCs.

IV. STUDIES EXAMINING THE PERSPECTIVES OF THE WORKER, THE TAXPAYER, AND SOCIETY

Of the 20 studies examining the benefits and costs of supported employment, nine investigated these benefits and costs from the perspectives of the worker, the taxpayer, and society. Generally, if a study examined only the perspective from society, it also, by definition, furnished most of the accounting variables associated to the worker and taxpayer perspectives. For this reason, Schneider, Rusch, Henderson, and Geske (1981) was included within this section.

A. Schneider, Rusch, Henderson, and Geske (1981)

Schneider et al. (1981) studied the monetary benefits and costs associated with employing 22 individuals with mental retardation via an Illinois-based transitional employment project. The method of training used by the employment program was termed "train-place-train." That is, individuals were trained for positions likely to be found in the community (e.g., kitchen workers), where they were later placed and provided additional support services (Rubin & Roessler, 1995). Though described as "transitional employment," the training model could be considered a precursor of supported employment since supported employment had yet to be formally defined at the time of this study. Further, the program investigated by Schneider et al. provided support for as long as the employees held their positions within the community, which is a characteristic of supported employment (Rusch, 1990), not transitional employment (Wehman, 1996b).

In this study, the authors accounted for the costs and benefits of employment services between July 1978 and June 1980 from a societal perspective. Direct costs were those involved with personal services, contractual, commodities, and travel, whereas indirect costs included agency, administrative, and business office expenses. Benefits, in turn, included the gross earnings of each program participant. These yearly earnings were then subtracted from the cumulative costs, resulting in a cumulative net cost or net benefit. This number was then divided by the number of "person months"; that is, the number of months worked by the program participants.

Using sheltered workshops as the alternative placement, Schneider et al. (1981) then calculated the net cost to society if the participants had not been employed via the transitional training program. Net costs for workshops were calculated by subtracting the dollar amount of contracts acquired from local businesses from total operating expenditures. The resulting figure was then divided by the number of individuals enrolled in the workshop.

Schneider and colleagues (1981) made projections as to the net benefits and costs of transitional training programs and sheltered workshops over a 10-, 15-, and 20-year period. The authors assumed that the level of training provided through both options would remain constant over these durations. Further, the authors accounted for participant attrition, something rarely done in other studies. Specifically, Schneider and colleagues found that one out of every seven persons trained, and two out of those already placed, would separate from the transitional training program. These individuals were no longer entered into the benefit–cost analysis.

Schneider et al. (1981) determined that the yearly benefits of the transition program began to exceed yearly costs after the fifth year of operation. Further, a downward trend of cumulative net costs to society was noted so that, by the eighth year, the transition project would have resulted in positive cumulative benefit. By the end of the twentieth year of program operation, Schneider et al. predicted that cumulative net benefit to society resulting from supported employment would exceed $2 million. Conversely, Schneider et al. predicted that cumulative costs to society resulting from sheltered workshops would exceed $5 million.

Schneider et al. (1981) was the first study to project the costs and benefits associated with employment programs over an extended period as well as to compare these programs to an alternative placement (i.e., sheltered workshops). Further, their sample, though small compared to other studies (cf. Lewis, Johnson, Bruininks, Kallsen, & Guillery, 1992), clearly resembled populations currently being served via supported employment programs. Some methodological shortcomings of this study, however, should be taken into account when examining their findings.

First, forgone benefits (e.g., wages) of being employed in workshops were not figured into the calculations (cf. Tines, Rusch, McCaughrin, & Conley, 1990). As a result, the transitional employment program was compared to alternative programs whose net costs are artificially high, thereby increasing the overall benefits of utilizing community-based programs in relation to sheltered workshops.

Second, the transition program's costs included in this analysis pertained only to the placement and follow-up services provided to program participants. No costs associated with the initial training prior to placement were assessed. As a result, the findings are further skewed to benefit the community-based employment program.

B. Conley, Rusch, McCaughrin, and Tines (1989) and Tines, Rusch, McCaughrin, and Conley (1990)

Using information from the same database (i.e., the Illinois Supported Employment Project database), Conley et al. (1989) and Tines et al. (1990) provided benefit–cost analyses involving 25 supported employment programs in Illinois after their first year of operation. The authors viewed costs and benefits from the perspectives of society, taxpayers, and supported employees.

The benefits and costs of employing 394 individuals with various disabilities in three types of supported employment models were explored: (a) individual placements, (b) enclaves, and (c) mobile work crews. Fifty percent of the participants were employed through individual placements. Another 42% were receiving services in cluster or enclave approaches, while the remaining 8% worked in mobile crews.

Conley et al. (1989) and Tines et al. (1990) found that from the perspective of taxpayers, \$0.66 was gained for every \$1.00 of supported employment cost. From the society's perspective, the return was \$0.75 per \$1.00 of cost. Finally, supported employees received a 37% increase in wages earned over their previous placements (e.g., work evaluation, sheltered workshops, adult day care).

Conley et al. (1989) and Tines et al. (1990) extended the literature in several ways. Not only did they view supported employment from three different perspectives, they included individuals placed via distinct approaches. Unfortunately, no comparisons were made of the cost-effectiveness of different supported employment approaches. Consequently, it is unknown whether the placement approaches included in this study varied in terms of their cost and benefits.

Other issues with Conley et al. (1989) and Tines et al. (1990) also need to be considered. First, these studies examined supported employment during its first year in Illinois. Previous literature has documented that cost initially exceeded benefits before declining (cf. Hill, Banks, et al., 1987; Hill & Wehman, 1983; Hill, Wehman, et al., 1987). It is also logical to assume that agency staff initially were not as effective, and thus cost-efficient, as they would be with more experience (Noble, Conley, Banjerjee, & Goodman, 1991). Consequently, the results provided by Conley et al. and Tines et al. may not reflect results obtained for well-established supported employment programs.

Second, the authors only considered funds specifically earmarked for supported employment services (e.g., grants), rather than the total operating costs needed to run these programs. As a result, the actual program costs may be underestimated, and the benefit–cost ratio inflated.

Third, according to Kregel et al. (1989), persons in individual placements tend to earn higher hourly and monthly wages than workers employed through enclaves or mobile work crews. With half of the sample in the two studies employed via the individual approach, benefits may be biased in favor of supported employment compared to a sample that was more evenly distributed between group placements.

Finally, Conley et al. (1989) and Tines et al. (1990) used the supported employees' last placement (e.g., school programs, evaluation, sheltered workshops, etc.) to calculate forgone wages and costs for alternative programs. Although this may be appropriate in the cases where supported employees were last placed in adult day care or sheltered workshops, it is inappropriate to apply evaluation or school-based programs in this manner, because they are not viable alternatives for supported employment.

For example, once out of high school, a supported employee would not be able to reenter school-based programs. Furthermore, individuals are only enrolled in evaluation programs for a limited amount of time (e.g., 18 months). To presume that they would be in evaluation indefinitely, had it not been for supported employment, is inaccurate. Additionally, the costs of evaluation and school-based programs are higher than more likely alternatives, such as regular work or work activity programs (Tines et al., 1990). Consequently, calculations using evaluation and school-based programs exaggerate the benefits of supported employment.

C. Noble, Conley, Banjerjee, and Goodman (1991)

Noble et al. (1991) examined the cost-efficiency of supported employment programs in the state of New York over a 21-month period. Analyses were conducted from the perspective of taxpayers and society, as well as the worker. Unlike any other study, Noble et al. included job seekers who were referred to supported employment but who were not yet placed in the community. Also unlike previous studies, the authors inspected benefit–cost ratios in relation to type of disability.

Noble et al. (1991) found that both monetary benefits and costs differed widely across disabilities. Specifically, supported employees with cerebral palsy, deafness, or autism generated the highest benefits from the perspective of taxpayers and society, whereas individuals with mild mental retardation and a secondary disability as well as persons with blindness accrued the lowest monetary benefits to society and taxpayers. Individuals with cerebral palsy, deafness, epilepsy, or specific learning disabilities were the most costly populations to serve. The least expensive participants had diagnoses of psychotic mental illness, blindness, or traumatic brain injury. When monetary benefits were subtracted from costs, every disability category had a mean net loss (see Table III).

For the sample as a whole, Noble et al. (1991) found that persons placed in supported employment earned 2.15 times what they were expected to generate in alternative placements. Similar to conclusions in Illinois by Conley and Noble (1990), Conley et al. (1989), and Tines et al. (1990), Noble et al. determined that the benefit–cost ratio of supported employment was roughly \$0.70 and \$0.60 from the perspectives of society and taxpayers, respectively. According to Noble et al., the primary reason costs exceeded benefits was that supported employment programs required 83–91% more funding to operate than other noncommunity-based, employment options. This finding is contradictory to results obtained by Intagliata, White, and Cooley (1979) and Tines et al. (1990), who concluded that community-based programs had lower operating costs than segregated programs.

As Noble and colleagues (1991) noted, results from their study need to be viewed with some caution. First, the results were based upon small sample sizes, and data were gathered when most participants had been working for a brief time (e.g., 6 months). (Noble and his colleagues suggested that a sample be examined

TABLE III

MEAN NET LOSS BY DISABILITY TO NOBLE ET AL. (1991)

Disability	Net loss (\$)
Mentally ill, psychotic	\$2,722
Traumatic brain injury	3,949
Mentally ill, nonpsychotic	4,150
Mild mental retardation, no secondary disabilities	4,178
Moderate/severe retardation	4,574
Other	4,942
Blind	5,238
Autism	5,440
Deaf	5,959
Mild mental retardation with secondary disabilities	6,141
Cerebral palsy	6,548
Specific learning disability	6,568
Epilepsy or other developmental disabilities	6,876

after several years of employment in the community in order to determine the longitudinal impact of disabilities on benefit–cost ratios.) Second, approximately 45% of the subjects were still waiting for positions within the community during the analysis. Though this is probably indicative of the long waiting lists often experienced, inclusion of job seekers underestimates the benefits achieved by those individuals who are actually employed (Hayden & Depaepe, 1994). Also, less than half of the sample had primary diagnoses of mental retardation, the remainder possessing disabilities (e.g., blindness, deafness, learning disabilities) that may not require ongoing supports and thus might have been inappropriate for supported employment. Finally, nearly 30% of the sample were receiving earnings from alternative programs. Although the reason for this is unclear, it may be the result of being placed in other day activities in addition to supported employment.

D. McCaughrin, Rusch, Conley, and Tines (1991)

McCaughrin et al. (1991) extended the benefit–cost analyses conducted by Conley et al. (1989) and Tines et al. (1990) by examining supported employment programs in Illinois through their second year of operation. The costs and benefits resulting from the placement of 588 individuals with various disabilities in mobile work crews, enclaves, and individual placements were evaluated. McCaughrin and colleagues examined supported employment from the same three perspectives as Conley et al. and Tines et al. (i.e., the worker, the taxpayer, and society).

Program benefits were found to increase during the 2 years of the study. These results are corroborated by findings from Hill and Wehman (1983), Hill, Banks, et al. (1987), and Hill, Wehman, et al. (1987), which will be reviewed later. Specifically, McCaughrin et al. concluded that for every $1.00 invested in supported employment over the 2-year period, society received a return of $0.82, with taxpayers receiving $0.73. Further, supported employees earned 67% more in the second year working in the community than they would have in alternative placements.

Although this study exhibits the same methodological shortcomings as Tines et al. (1990) and Conley et al. (1989), McCaughrin and her colleagues elaborated on the knowledge in the field in many ways. First, they replicated Hill, Banks, and colleagues' (1987) results, which indicated that increases in benefit–cost ratios were attributed primarily to savings from alternative programs, rather than increases in supported employment program benefits. Second, the costs incurred by supported employment programs were higher in the second year of the program, which was also noted by Noble et al. (1991). McCaughrin and her colleagues theorized that the increase in program costs was due to the lack of job coach fading after initial placement and training, which was demonstrated by Johnson and Rusch (1990) and Cimera, Rusch, and Heal (1997). Finally, increases in earnings from the first to the second year were the result of less taxes being withheld from supported employees, rather than increases in hourly wages or hours worked. Supported employees who worked throughout both years saw an increase of disposable income due to greater earnings, however.

E. Lewis, Johnson, Bruininks, Kallsen, and Guillery (1992)

Lewis et al. (1992) investigated the cost-effectiveness of supported employment in Minnesota from the perspectives of taxpayers, society, and workers. In their analyses, Lewis and colleagues examined the costs and benefits resulting from services provided to 856 workers with disabilities. Unlike other studies, Lewis et al. compared benefits and costs from five different program approaches: (a) habilitation training (i.e., where no wages are earned); (b) on-site employment (i.e., sheltered workshops); (c) group employment with support (i.e., enclaves and mobile work crews); (d) individual employment with support (i.e., supported work model or individual placement); and (e) competitive employment (i.e., employment in the community without support). Also unlike other studies, Lewis et al. accounted for costs and benefits that occur when individuals are placed in several programs at the same time or during the course of the year. For instance, a supported employee placed individually in the community for 3 hours a day may also be served through a workshop for an additional 5 hours a day.

From analyzing data collected from 11 agencies in Minnesota, Lewis et al. (1992) concluded that over a 1-year period each supported employment approach was more cost-efficient than habilitation training from all perspectives examined. Further, when supported employment programs (i.e., both group and individual placements) were compared to on-site programs (i.e., sheltered workshops), the resulting ratios exceeded 1.00 (i.e., were cost-efficient) in 7 out of 11 agencies (64%) from the societal and taxpayer perspectives. These positive ratios ranged from 1.30 to 4.00.

When compared to all other supported employment approaches, individual placements were found to have positive benefit–cost ratios in 82% of the cases. Further, individual placements facilitated higher wages and more work hours at a generally lower cost to service providers than group placements (e.g., enclaves). These findings conflict with those from Lam (1986), who found that workshops were more cost-efficient and provided more hours worked than supported employment for persons with moderate or severe disabilities. The average hourly wages earned by community-based employees in Lewis and colleagues' study were higher than by sheltered workshops employees. Much like Lam, however, in four instances on-site programs provided employees with earnings greater than supported employees, due primarily to the longer hours sometimes available in workshops.

One of the principal findings offered by Lewis et al. (1992) was that, within Minnesota, cost-effectiveness of programs varied widely between agencies. This is most likely evident within other states as well as across the nation. Further, Lewis and colleagues determined that even in a 1-year analysis, many of the supported employment programs produced benefits that exceeded their costs. Several limitations of this study, however, should be kept in mind.

First, although the authors indicated that the majority of the sample were within the moderate-to-severe range of disability, no other information was presented on the demographics of the employees. Second, agencies were selected based on their size and willingness to participate, which may lead to questions about generalizability (Joint Committee on Standards for Educational Evaluation, 1994). Third, several of the employees in the supported employment analyses were placed in the community via competitive employment, which does not furnish supports and cannot be truly considered a model of supported employment. The inclusion of these individuals could have had the effect of increasing benefits and decreasing costs, thus skewing the study's findings in favor of supported employment. Finally, little information was provided on how costs were determined for each program. When information was presented, it was often based on assumptions, such as calculating fringe benefits as 13% of gross pay or withholding taxes as 14% of gross pay. The accuracy of these assumptions are unknown, however.

F. McCaughrin, Ellis, Rusch, and Heal (1993)

In this study, two different analyses were performed. The first was a benefit–cost analysis similar to that of McCaughrin et al. (1991). The second analyzed the cost-effectiveness of supported employment in terms of the quality of the supported employee's life.

Twenty individuals with developmental disabilities were randomly selected from two Illinois-based adult service agencies. Using a matched-pair design, the authors compared five individuals from each agency who were competitively employed for at least 6 months with five employees who were working in sheltered settings. The two samples were then analyzed based upon their costs, benefits, and quality of life, as assessed by four behavioral assessment instruments.

The authors determined that, during the first year in the community, supported employees with mild mental retardation earned $4,607 more than sheltered employees with mild mental retardation. Further, supported employees with severe mental retardation exceeded the earnings of sheltered employees with severe mental retardation by $1,027. This is contrary to Lam (1986), who found that persons with severe mental retardation earned more in segregated settings than in the community.

According to McCaughrin et al. (1993), supported employees with all levels of mental retardation had negative net benefits from the perspectives of taxpayers and society during the first year of employment. By the fifth year in the community, however, supported employees with all levels of mental retardation had positive net benefits from the perspectives of taxpayers and society. Further, from the perspective of the supported employees, all individuals had positive net benefits in both year 1 and year 5 (see Table IV).

TABLE IV
MEAN NET BENEFIT PER SUPPORTED EMPLOYEE BY SEVERITY OF MENTAL RETARDATION[a]

	Supported employee		Taxpayer		Society	
	High IQ	Low IQ	High IQ	Low IQ	High IQ	Low IQ
Year 1	$4,607	$1,027	($3,841)	($6,126)	($766)	($5,099)
Year 5	$4,607	$1,027	$ 398	$ 105	$5,003	$1,132
Net increase	0	0	$4,239	$6,231	$5,769	$6,141

[a]High IQ group consisted of individuals with mild mental retardation. Low IQ group consisted of individuals with moderate and severe mental retardation.

Results of McCaughrin et al.'s (1993) benefit–cost analysis mirror findings obtained by Hill and Wehman (1983), Hill, Banks, et al. (1987), and Hill, Wehman, et al. (1987), both in terms of benefit–cost ratios and length of time needed for benefits to surpass costs. Interestingly, McCaughrin and colleagues were the only authors reviewed in this chapter who did not factor in taxes withheld as a benefit to taxpayers. Instead, the authors theorized that since most of the withholdings would have been refunded at the end of the year, it would not be a benefit or cost from any perspective. Additionally, changes in the amount of governmental subsidies received by employees were not included in the analysis of benefits and costs. The authors determined that not only were these savings "minimal" (McCaughrin et al., 1993, p. 44), but several supported employees started acquiring public aid for the first time when they entered community employment. This would have increased the costs of supported employment from the perspective of taxpayers.

In addition to the monetary outcomes, McCaughrin et al. (1993) found that competitively employed individuals with moderate to severe mental retardation obtained higher scores on all four quality-of-life indexes than sheltered employees with moderate and severe mental retardation. Supported employees with mild mental retardation obtained higher scores than sheltered employees on two out of four measures (see Table V).

By using the average program cost per person in both sheltered workshops and community-based employment, the authors then calculated the dollar value per point scored on the quality-of-life indexes by individuals in each sample. Supported employees experienced a savings of +\$487 to −\$26/per point on these indexes compared to sheltered employees, indicating that supported employment is cost-effective in ways not previously considered. Surprisingly, the only measurement that was more costly for supported employees than sheltered workers was

TABLE V
MEAN SCORES ON QUALITY-OF-LIFE INDEXES FOR SHELTERED AND SUPPORTED EMPLOYEES ACCORDING TO MCCAUGHRIN ET AL. (1993)[a]

Index	Sheltered		Supported		Gains for SE[b]	
	High IQ	Low IQ	High IQ	Low IQ	High IQ	Low IQ
Employment integration	13	8	35	21	22	13
Co-worker involvement	7	8	16	13	9	5
Worker loneliness	27	17	21	25	−6	8
Quality of life	69	49	67	54	−2	5

[a]High IQ groups consisted of individuals with mild mental retardation. Low IQ groups consisted of individuals with moderate and severe mental retardation.
[b]SE, supported employees.

degree of loneliness (see Table VI). The conclusion that physical integration within the community does not necessarily lead to social integration has stimulated additional research in the social relationships between supported employees and their nondisabled co-workers (cf. Chadsey-Rusch, 1992).

One concern regarding this study is that 3 of the 20 participants did not have mental retardation, but a learning disability and mental illness. Had the study included a larger sample, even more credence could be given to these findings.

G. Rusch, Conley, and McCaughrin (1993)

Rusch et al. (1993) investigated the benefits and costs of 729 supported employees in Illinois programs from 1987 through 1990, thus extending Conley et al.

TABLE VI
AVERAGE COSTS PER POINT ON QUALITY-OF-LIFE INDEXES ACCORDING TO MCCAUGHRIN ET AL. (1993)[a]

Index	Sheltered		Supported		Gains for SE	
	High IQ	Low IQ	High IQ	Low IQ	High IQ	Low IQ
Employment integration	$326	$779	$110	$292	$216	$487
Co-worker involvement	$605	$779	$240	$471	$365	$308
Worker loneliness	$157	$367	$183	$245	($26)	$122
Quality of life	$ 61	$127	$ 57	$113	$ 4	$ 14

[a]"High IQ" groups consisted of individuals with mild mental retardation. "Low IQ" groups consisted of individuals with moderate and severe mental retardation.

TABLE VII

BENEFIT–COST RATIOS OVER A 4-YEAR PERIOD FROM THE PERSPECTIVE OF SOCIETY ACCORDING TO RUSCH ET AL. (1993)

	1987	1988	1989	1990	Total
Benefits					
Gross increased earnings	$279,412	$351,084	$524,766	$616,444	$1,771,706
Alternative program	975,075	1,577,197	1,652,913	1,717,499	5,922,684
Total	$1,254,487	$1,928,281	$2,177,679	$2,333,943	$7,694,390
Costs					
Supported employment	$1,632,229	$2,142,004	$2,367,409	$2,071,170	$8,212,812
TJTC[a]	36,523	49,090	53,195	66,828	205,636
Total	$1,668,752	$2,191,094	$2,420,604	$2,137,998	$8,418,448
Net benefits	($414,265)	($262,813)	($242,925)	$195,945	($724,058)
Benefit–cost ratio	.75	.88	.90	1.09	.91

[a]TJTC, targeted job tax credits.

(1989), Tines et al. (1990), and McCaughrin et al. (1991). From the societal perspective, the average return over the 4-year period was $0.91 per $1.00 of costs (see Table VII). From the perspective of the taxpayer, supported employment returned an average of $0.77, with the government actually paying $5,066 more in subsidies the third year than the second (see Table VIII). Over the 4-year period, supported employees increased their earnings by an average of 42% over what they would have made in sheltered workshops. Further, gross benefits to society and the taxpayer were shown to increase each year as gross costs decreased 3 out of 4 years.

TABLE VIII

BENEFIT–COST RATIOS OVER A 4-YEAR PERIOD FROM THE PERSPECTIVE OF TAXPAYERS ACCORDING TO RUSCH ET AL. (1993)

	1987	1988	1989	1990	Total
Benefits					
Taxes withheld	$98,457	$114,029	$151,348	$179,906	$543,740
Reduced subsidies	26,138	23,611	($50,366)	5,754	5,147
Alternative program savings	975,075	1,577,197	1,652,913	1,717,499	5,922,684
Total	$1,099,671	$1,714,837	$1,753,905	$1,903,159	$6,471,571
Costs					
Supported employment	$1,632,229	$2,142,004	$2,367,409	$2,071,170	$8,212,812
TJTC[a]	36,523	49,090	53,195	66,828	205,636
Total	$1,668,752	$2,191,094	$2,420,604	$2,137,998	$8,418,448
Net benefits	($569,082)	($476,257)	($666,699)	($234,839)	($1,946,877)
Benefit–cost ratio	.66	.78	.75	.89	.77

[a]TJTC, targeted job tax credits.

Several variables were not taken into consideration by Rusch et al. (1993) when conducting their analyses. First, fringe benefits were not factored into the equation when calculating benefits to supported employees. This may have underestimated the net benefit of supported employment to workers. Second, figures were not adjusted to reflect when supported employees lost their jobs and returned to alternative placements. As a result, benefits of supported employment to taxpayers and society may be inflated. Third, over half of the subjects (383) were placed in individual placements, which have been shown by Lewis et al. (1992) and L. Thompson, Powers, and Houchard (1992) to be more cost-efficient than other approaches. This could have biased the results in favor of supported employment as a whole. Finally, the cumulative costs and benefits reported throughout the 4-year period were not discounted to reflect changes in the value of the dollar as advised by Layard and Glaister (1994). Consequently, the authors' findings may not be accurate.

H. Cimera (1997)

Much like Rusch et al. (1993) and several other previous studies reviewed in this chapter, Cimera (1997) used data from the Illinois Supported Employment Project database. Unlike prior studies, however, Cimera sought to determine the impact of nine demographic variables (i.e., age, ethnicity, IQ, level of mental retardation, previous placement approach, gender, co-worker involvement, length of employment, and multiple disabilities) on cost-efficiency achieved by individual supported employees, rather than supported employment programs. To do this, Cimera calculated three sets of benefit–cost ratios for 57 supported employees with mental retardation, each including perspectives of the worker, taxpayer, and society.

The first set of benefit–cost ratios were based upon 1990 data; the second from 1994 data. The third set of benefit–cost ratios utilized data from 1990 and 1994 to project what the supported employees' cost-efficiency would be if they were to work in the community until age 65 (i.e., a life-long benefit–cost ratio). With these benefit–cost ratios, Cimera analyzed the relationships between demographics and cost-efficiency.

Cimera (1997) found that from the perspective of the worker, individuals with high IQs and less severe mental retardation were more cost-efficient than individuals with lower IQs and more severe mental retardation. This affirms results obtained by Lam (1986), Kregel, Wehman, and Banks (1989), and McCaughrin et al. (1993); however, unlike Lam, Cimera found that, regardless of IQ and level of mental retardation, all supported employees were cost-efficient from the worker's perspective. Further, Cimera found that the effects of IQ and mental retardation on worker cost-efficiency decreased the longer supported employees retained their positions. Additionally, length of employment itself was not related to worker cost-efficiency.

From the taxpayer's and societal perspectives, Cimera (1997) found that IQ and level of mental retardation were not significantly related to cost-efficiency, nor was the presence of a secondary disability or length of employment. In fact, none of the nine variables examined by Cimera predicted long-term cost-efficiency from the taxpayer's and societal perspectives.

Unlike any previous study, Cimera (1997) examined cost-efficiency of supported employees in relation to employment outcomes (e.g., remaining employed) and training strategies (i.e., utilizing nondisabled co-workers to train supported employees). He found that individuals who generated high benefit–cost ratios in 1990 were more likely to be employed in 1994. Further, these individuals were more likely to keep the same job for more than 4 years.

With respect to utilizing nondisabled co-workers to aid in training supported employees, Cimera (1997) found that this procedure did not impact cost-efficiency from any cost-accounting perspective. Rather, utilizing nondisabled co-workers frequently increased to the costs of providing supported employment services from the perspectives of the taxpayers and society.

Cimera's (1997) results enhance the literature on the monetary benefits and costs of supported employment programs in several ways. For example, his findings related to cost-efficiency and job retention add valuable insights as to why supported employees separate from their jobs as well as what variables may reduce the likelihood of recidivism. Further, the inclusion of training strategies (e.g., use of nondisabled workers) sheds important light on the current "natural supports" debate. Lastly, Cimera extended the evidence indicating that supported employees with all levels of mental retardation, as well as those with multiple disabilities, can be served cost-efficiently via supported employment programs.

Like prior studies, however, Cimera (1997) did not factor out potential effects of different placement approaches. As a result, it is unclear if results were influenced by an excess of highly efficient approaches (e.g., individual placements). Further, Cimera's data came only from Illinois. Data from other regions of the country may have produced different results. Still, with the inclusion of a life-long benefit–cost ratio per supported employee, Cimera makes unique additions to the benefit–cost methodology.

V. SUMMARY OF SOCIETY'S PERSPECTIVE

A. Net Benefits

Nine studies examined the benefits and costs of supported employment from the perspective of society. As with the studies on supported employment from the perspective of taxpayers, there appears to be a consensus in the literature that *eventually* society receives a positive net benefit from supported employment programs. This conclusion is supported by trends of increasing gross benefits and decreasing gross costs to society identified by five studies conducted in Illinois (i.e., Cimera, 1997; McCaughrin et al., 1991, 1993; Rusch et al., 1993; Schneider et al., 1981). Further, one study in Minnesota (i.e., Lewis et al., 1992) found that some supported employment programs had positive net benefits from the perspective of society during the first year of operation.

Specifically, Schneider et al. (1981) projected that annual net benefits would surpass annual net costs in Illinois during the fifth year of program operation. These researchers further predicted that cumulative benefits would exceed cumulative costs after 8 years—predictions that were supported by Rusch et al. (1993) and McCaughrin et al. (1991, 1993).

Rusch et al. (1993) found that the annual benefit–cost ratio of supported employment programs in Illinois exceeded 1.00 (i.e., 1.09) by the fourth year of program operation. McCaughrin et al. (1991) found that society earned \$0.66 for every \$1.00 of costs the first year and \$0.73 for every \$1.00 of costs over the first 2 years of program operation. By the fifth year, supported employment in Illinois was returning a positive net benefit to society (McCaughrin et al., 1993).

Lewis et al. (1992) examined 11 agencies in Minnesota that provided supported employment services and found that 7 (i.e., 64%) incurred a positive net benefit to society in 1 year. The benefit–cost ratios generated by these seven agencies ranged from 1.30 to 4.00.

In summary, all five studies that explored the benefits and costs of supported employment programs from the perspective of society over at least a 2-year period came to the same conclusion. That is, the net benefits of supported employment programs increase annually. Further, these studies determined that within the first 5 years of program operation supported employment was cost-efficient from the societal perspective.

Lastly, there is some question in the literature as to why the benefits of supported employment exceed costs over time. For instance, Lewis et al. (1992) found that the positive benefit–cost ratios were largely influenced by higher hourly wages and more hours of work by supported employees compared to sheltered employees. Lam (1986), however, stated that sheltered employees worked more hours than supported employees, and in some cases, earned higher gross wages than supported employees. Lewis et al. also found that supported employment programs had generally lower operating costs compared to alternative programs (e.g., sheltered workshops).

Conversely, Noble et al. (1991) found that supported employment programs cost 83%–91% more to operate than sheltered workshops. However, more studies (e.g., Conley et al., 1989; Hill et al., 1987; McCaughrin et al., 1991, 1993; Rusch et al., 1993) support the findings of Lewis et al. (1992), rather than Noble et al., regarding the costs of supported employment programs. Still, the primary contributing factors to the long-term net benefits of supported employment from the perspective of society are still in question within the literature.

B. Variation in Methodology

It is surprising that the literature is in relative agreement on these issues given the wide variety of methods used to formulate benefits and cost from the societal perspective. For instance, McCaughrin (1988) considered wages earned by supported employees to be a *cost* to society, whereas Schneider et al. (1981) considered gross earnings a *benefit* to society.

Instead of gross earnings, McCaughrin et al. (1991, 1993) and Rusch et al. (1993) calculated increased earnings (i.e., gross earnings minus forgone wages) as being a benefit to society. These authors also included reduction in alternative program operating expenditures as a benefit to society. Noble et al. (1991), on the other hand, considered supported employee earnings *and* taxes paid a benefit to society.

Further, Rusch et al. (1993) and McCaughrin et al. (1991) included taxes lost via targeted job tax credits given to employers as a cost to society. McCaughrin et al. (1993) and Schneider et al. (1981), on the other hand, did not. Costs to society according to Schneider and colleagues included the operating costs of supported employment programs.

Lastly, only four studies (i.e., Cimera, 1997; Hill, Banks, et al., 1987; Hill, Wehman et al., 1987; McCaughrin, 1988) accounted for changes in the value of the dollar over time. Further, of the 12 studies reviewed that extended their analyses over 2 or more years, only these four studies made such discounts as advised by Layard (1972). Without discounting, longitudinal studies may be regarded as invalid.

C. Impact of Mental Retardation

Of the studies reviewed in this section, three examined the impact of mental retardation upon the costs and benefits of supported employment from the societal perspective (viz., Cimera, 1997; McCaughrin et al., 1993; Noble et al., 1991).

Cimera found that IQ and level of mental retardation were not related to cost-efficiency from society's perspective. Noble et al. (1991), on the other hand, found that supported employees with no secondary disabilities had the greatest net benefit to society (i.e., \$4,488), followed by supported employees with moderate or severe mental retardation (i.e., \$4,368), and supported employees with mild mental retardation and a secondary disability (i.e., \$3,925). According to Noble and colleagues, all individuals with mental retardation generated a net loss to society over a 27-month period. Specifically, the authors determined that supported employees with mild mental retardation with and without secondary disabilities averaged a mean loss of \$6,141 and \$4,178, respectively. By comparison, supported employees with moderate and severe mental retardation averaged a mean loss of \$4,574.

Although McCaughrin and her colleagues (1993) found that society earned a net benefit regardless of the degree of mental retardation, these authors also determined that degree of mental retardation impacted the net benefits of supported employment. Specifically, McCaughrin et al. estimated that society received a return of $5,003 and $1,132 per supported employee with mild and moderate or severe mental retardation, respectively. These figures were calculated over a 5-year period.

VI. STUDIES EXAMINING THE PERSPECTIVES OF THE WORKER AND THE TAXPAYER

Of the 20 studies that examined the benefits and costs of supported employment programs, 5 did so from the perspectives of the worker and the taxpayer (see Table I). Four of these were based upon the same data set (cf. Hill & Wehman, 1983; Hill, Banks, et al., 1987; Hill, Wehman, et al., 1987; Wehman et al., 1985). The fifth was an unpublished dissertation (McCaughrin, 1988). Each is reviewed below.

A. Hill and Wehman (1983)

Hill and Wehman (1983) analyzed the employment patterns of 90 individuals with disabilities who were individually placed within the community over a 47-month period (September 1978 through August 1982). The authors determined that cumulative earnings of supported employees exceeded $500,000. Further, after 4 years, the benefits to the public surpassed costs by over $90,000. Annual program benefits outpaced annual program expenditures during the third year of the study. This finding complements similar findings obtained by Rusch and colleagues (1993).

Although Hill and Wehman (1983) included job coach travel time, other non-training expenditures utilized by Cho and Schuermann (1980), such as evaluation and counseling, were not appraised. By neglecting these necessary functions of job coaches, Hill and Wehman may have underestimated the true monetary disbursement of supplying services to supported employees. Further, Hill and Wehman did not consider the effects of inflation, as advised by Arrow and Lind (1994), Feldstein (1972), Hill, Banks, et al. (1987), and Stiglitz (1994).

By neglecting the effects of inflation, the actual dollar values of costs and benefits become distorted over time (Layard & Glaister, 1994). For example, $1 of benefits earned at the beginning of Hill and Wehman's (1983) study (i.e., September 1978) is not equivalent to $1 of benefits earned at the end of the study (i.e., August 1982). Changes in the worth of currency resulting from inflation influence the dollar values of benefits and costs generated by employment programs over time. As a result, longitudinal studies must have a common unit of comparison across the time of the study. This can be accomplished by discounting or by adjusting the value of 1978 dollars to equal the value of 1982 dollars. If authors do not adjust for inflation, monetary values obtained in 1 year cannot be accurately compared to values obtained in other years.

Additionally, Hill and Wehman (1983) used gross income, rather than net income minus forgone wages, when calculating the benefits to supported employees. By including just gross wages, the authors did not consider the earnings lost to taxes or forgone wages that could have been made in alternative placements. Earnings lost to taxes have been estimated as being 15% of gross income (Noble et al., 1991). Consequently, by neglecting this cost to the employee, the net benefits of being employed may be exaggerated.

The authors also did not take into consideration money withheld for Social Security or losses in governmental subsidies. As a result, the costs of obtaining supported employment services may have been underestimated from the perspectives of employees. Finally, the supported employment program studied by Hill and Wehman may have had more resources and skilled staff than typical adult service facilities since it was associated with a research and training center at a major university. For these reasons, results from Hill and Wehman (1983), although important, may not be generalizable to other supported employment programs utilized in other studies (Cimera et al., 1997).

B. Wehman et al. (1985)

Wehman et al. (1985) is the second of four studies by researchers from the Virginia Commonwealth University. Wehman and colleagues presented a descriptive summary of a supported employment program (then called "supported work") over a 6-year period (October 1978 through December 1984). A portion of the article discusses the monetary costs of placing 167 individuals with mental retardation (mean IQ of 50) in a total of 252 positions. The authors also discussed the cumulative wages and taxes generated as a result of these placements.

The authors found that the 167 supported employees in their study earned a total of $1,069,309 in wages over a 75-month period. Further, these individuals paid a total of $245,941 in taxes. The mean cost per supported employee was reported to be $5,255; the mean cost per placement was $3,483.

Wehman et al. (1985) also compared the average cost per supported employment placement ($3,483) with the average costs of placing an individual with mental retardation in adult day program in Virginia ($4,000). Not only was it cheaper to place people with mental retardation in the community, but the costs of adult day programs were for a 12-month period whereas community placements were maintained for an average of 19 months.

Some essential information was missing from this article. For example, Wehman et al. (1985) did not disclose how costs were calculated or how data were gathered. Further, the authors did not disclose from which perspective costs were regarded, or whether the costs were calculated over a 12- or 19-month (i.e., average length of placement) period. Lastly, no citation or reference is made regarding how the cost of adult day programs (i.e., $4,000) was determined.

One of the primary contributions of this study is that the authors compared the average job tenure of supported employees (19 months) with the average job tenure for nondisabled co-workers (less than 5 months), as reported by a study by the National Hotel and Restaurant Association (1983). Although not a benefit–cost analysis, this information complements the data provided by other studies (e.g., Brickey & Campbell, 1981; Cho & Schuermann, 1980) on the costs of hiring supported employees from the perspective of businesses, a topic presently missing in the literature.

C. Hill, Banks, et al. (1987) and Hill, Wehman, Kregel, Banks, and Metzler (1987)

Hill, Banks et al. (1987) and Hill, Wehman, et al. (1987) are continuations of Hill and Wehman (1983). These two studies present findings from the same sample of 214 supported employees roughly 8 years after being individually placed within the community. Hill et al. offered a broad overview of supported employment and benefit–cost analysis, whereas, Hill, Wehman, et al. furnished information focusing specifically on 117 supported employees with moderate or severe disabilities.

According to Hill, Banks et al. (1987), over a 94-month period, the average annual net benefit per individual from the perspective of the supported employee was $6,815; $7,111 from the perspective of the taxpayer. Further, for every $1.00 forgone or spent on supported employment, taxpayers received $1.87 in benefits and workers earned $1.97 in wages.

Hill, Wehman, et al. (1987), however, found that supported employees as a group earned $1.43 for every $1.00 relinquished in forgone wages and public assistance. It is unclear why there is a difference of $0.54 between the benefit–cost ratio indicated for the total samples reported by Hill, Banks, et al. and Hill, Wehman, et al. if they are utilizing the same data.

Further, Hill, Wehman, et al. (1987) indicated that supported employees with moderate and severe mental retardation had longer tenures, saved the taxpayers more money in reduced public assistance and alternative placement costs, and paid more in taxes per person than supported employees with mild or no mental retardation. The moderate-severe subgroup, however, incurred more than twice the supported employment program costs than the higher IQ subgroup. Consequently, the higher IQ subgroup was more cost-efficient from the perspective of taxpayers.

According to Hill and Wehman (1983), benefits did not begin to exceed costs from the perspective of society until the third year of the study. Hill, Banks, et al.

(1987) and Hill, Wehman, et al. (1987) demonstrated that the trends of declining program costs and increasing program benefits continued well after the third year following placement. Further, Hill, Wehman et al. specifically concentrated on the population for which supported employment was created; that is, persons with moderate to severe disabilities (Will, 1984).

The studies by Hill, Banks et al. (1987) and Hill, Wehman, et al. (1987) have methodological shortcomings that must be taken into consideration when interpreting their results. First, although both of these studies used primarily factual, rather than prediction-oriented data (cf. Schneider et al., 1981), several costs and benefits were approximated throughout both studies (i.e., fringe benefits and taxes withheld), with sensitivity tests conducted to determine the impact of these estimations. Second, the authors estimated withheld taxes as being 23% of gross income. This is 7.8% higher than taxes approximated by Noble et al. (1991) and 9% higher than taxes predicted by Lewis et al. (1992). In addition, the authors did not consider that most of the taxes withheld from supported employees may be returned at the end of the year, thus lowering costs to the employees and benefits to society (McCaughrin et al., 1993).

Third, in order to determine program operating costs, the authors only measured time that the job coaches spent with the supported employees, without taking into account other time accrued outside of the workplace, such as traveling, conducting meetings, or writing reports. These off-site tasks have been found to be as much as one-third of the total time that job coaches spend working for supported employees (RRTC, n.d.). Consequently, by neglecting these off-site tasks, the costs of supported employment may be significantly underestimated.

Fourth, Hill, Banks, et al. (1987) have been criticized for inflating benefits of supported employment by underestimating earnings forgone from alternative programs (Noble et al., 1991). Hill, Banks, et al. (1987) and Hill, Wehman, et al. (1987) estimated that annual wages for sheltered employees in 1984 was $1,206. Contrary to Noble and colleagues, these numbers are nearly 10 times *higher*, not lower, than the estimate of sheltered employee annual wages provided by the Department of Labor (i.e., $160) for the same year (Heal, McCaughrin, & Tines, 1989; Will, 1984).

Fifth, the authors considered the tax credits to employers (TJTC) as both a benefit and a cost from the perspective of the taxpayers. These tax credits could have been considered a cost to taxpayers because they decreased the overall tax base of the community (Conley et al., 1989; McCaughrin et al., 1991; Tines et al., 1990); however, they could not have been considered a benefit. By counting them as both, they simply cancel each other out, adding nothing to the analyses. Further, TJTCs are only a cost for the first 2 years of employment, since after this point employers are no longer eligible for these tax credits (Burkhauser & Haveman, 1982; Conley & Noble, 1990).

Finally, the authors did not consider that supported employees may receive services in other programs, such as day programming (Heal et al., 1989; Lewis et al., 1992). This would have negated savings accounting for 60% of the benefits supported employment offered to taxpayers (Noble et al., 1991), thus diminishing the benefit–cost ratios presented.

Despite these methodological shortcomings, Hill, Banks, et al. 91987) and Hill, Wehman, et al. (1987) contributed significantly to the field. Specifically, the authors examined the costs and benefits of supported employment over a longer duration than any other published study. Further, they accounted for inflation and discounted for changes in the value of the dollar over time, something also rarely done by other authors (Thornton, 1992).

D. McCaughrin (1988)

McCaughrin (1988) presented an extension of data furnished by Schneider et al. (1981). Specifically, McCaughrin investigated the benefits and costs resulting from the employment of 22 supported employees with developmental disabilities in Illinois over an 8-year period (i.e., July 1978 through June 1986). Of these 22 supported employees, 6 left Illinois, 10 returned to the workshop, and 6 remained employed via supported employment throughout the 8 years of the study. McCaughrin did not indicate whether these latter individuals maintained the same positions over the 8 years or whether they were replaced in the community after separating from their original positions.

Net benefits increased steadily over the 8 years. By the eighth year, the cumulative benefit–cost ratio ranged from $0.28 to $2.21, with an average of $1.24. This variance in ratios depended upon how sheltered workshops costs were calculated. Specifically, McCaughrin varied the estimated amount of costs accrued by workshops and found that, without these savings, economic efficiency of supported employment could not be demonstrated.

McCaughrin's (1988) findings that supported employment is cost-efficient are corroborated by other researchers (e.g., Hill, Banks, et al., 1987; Hill, Wehman, et al., 1987; Schneider et al., 1981). Additionally, her results showing that cost-efficiency is dependent upon the savings from sheltered workshops have also been demonstrated by Noble et al. (1991). Finally, she conducted sensitivity tests to determine the impact of fluctuations in various accounting variables (e.g., alternative program costs). This was rarely done by other authors.

VII. SUMMARY OF THE TAXPAYER'S PERSPECTIVE

A. Net Benefits

Fourteen studies examined the benefits and costs of supported employment programs from the perspective of taxpayers. Of these, seven explored the benefits and costs of supported employment for 2 years or more. Among these seven studies there is general consensus that, *eventually*, taxpayers obtain a positive net benefit from supported employment programs. Specifically, five studies found a positive net benefit to taxpayers (i.e., Cimera, 1997; Hill, Banks, et al., 1987; Hill, Wehman, et al., 1987; McCaughrin, 1988; McCaughrin et al., 1993). The others (i.e., McCaughrin et al., 1991; Rusch et al., 1993) noted that net benefits increased over time.

Hill, Banks, et al. (1987) found that taxpayers experienced an average net benefit of over $7,000 per supported employee over a 94-month period. Per year, this figure amounted to $900 for each supported employee. Hill et al. also determined that taxpayers obtained $1.87 of benefits for every dollar of cost.

Like Hill, Banks, et al. (1987), Hill, Wehman, et al. (1987) found that net benefits to taxpayers increased annually, so that by the third year of program operation gross benefits exceeded gross costs. Further, over the 8 years of program operation, supported employment had a benefit–cost ratio of 2.93.

McCaughrin (1988) calculated the benefit–cost ratio from the taxpayer's perspective generated by 22 supported employees over an 8-year period. The benefit–cost ratio over this period ranged from 0.28 to 2.21, with the variance depending upon how supported employment and sheltered workshop programs costs were calculated. The average benefit–cost ratio, according to McCaughrin, was 1.24, indicating that taxpayers received a return of $1.24 for every $1.00 of costs.

Finally, McCaughrin and colleagues (1993) examined the benefits and costs of 10 supported employees during their first and fifth year working in the community. During the first year supported employment was inefficient from the perspective of the taxpayers. However, by the fifth year, benefits exceeded costs for a positive net gain.

The trend of decreasing costs and increasing benefits identified by Hill, Banks, et al. (1987), Hill, Wehman, et al. (1987), McCaughrin (1988), and McCaughrin et al. (1993) was corroborated by results obtained by McCaughrin et al. (1991) and Rusch et al. (1993). Specifically, Rusch et al. found that the annual benefit–cost ratios increased 3 of 4 years. Further, the benefit–cost ratio obtained by McCaughrin et al. (1991) in the second program year in Illinois (i.e., .73) is nearly identical to the benefit–cost ratio obtained by Hill, Wehman, et al. during the second year of program operation in Virginia (.79). The consensus of these six studies clearly indicates that, eventually, supported employment is cost-efficient from the perspective of the taxpayer.

B. Impact of Mental Retardation

Four studies examined the impact of mental retardation upon the benefits and costs incurred by taxpayers (i.e., Cimera, 1997; Hill, Wehman, et al., 1987; McCaughrin et al., 1993; Noble et al., 1991). With the exception of Cimera, all found that individuals with mild mental retardation generated greater net benefits than those with moderate or severe mental retardation. However, two studies (i.e., Hill, Wehman, et al. and Noble et al.) found that individuals with moderate or severe mental retardation produced greater gross benefits to taxpayers than individuals with mild mental retardation.

Specifically, according to Hill, Wehman, et al. (1987), supported employees with moderate or severe mental retardation worked longer tenures, paid higher taxes, and reduced their reliance upon governmental subsidies more than supported employees with mild mental retardation. However, the authors found that supported employees with moderate or severe mental retardation incurred nearly 70% of program operating costs. As a result, it was more cost-efficient to serve supported employees with mild mental retardation than supported employees with severe disabilities. Lastly, Hill, Wehman et al. reported that supported employees with moderate and severe mental retardation generated a benefit–cost ratio of 1.24 from the perspective of taxpayers over an 8-year period.

McCaughrin et al. (1993) also found that supported employees, regardless of disabilities, generated a positive benefit–cost ratio from the perspective of taxpayers. Specifically, individuals with mild mental retardation had an average net benefit of $398 after 5 years. Supported employees with moderate or severe mental retardation had an average net benefit of $105 after 5 years. It should be noted, however, that the only variables that McCaughrin and colleagues utilized were supported employment operating costs minus alternative program savings. Thus, compared to other studies (cf. Rusch et al., 1993), McCaughrin et al.'s (1993) analyses were rather limited. For example, Rusch et al. also included reductions in governmental subsidies as a benefit and the use of targeted job tax credits as a cost to taxpayers.

Cimera (1997) found that there was a slightly negative correlation between IQ and taxpayer cost-efficiency so that individuals with low IQs were more cost-efficient from the taxpayer's perspective. However, these correlations were not statistically significant. Cimera found similar results between taxpayer cost-efficiency and level of mental retardation.

Finally, Noble et al. (1991) examined the effects of numerous disabilities upon the impact of benefits and costs from the perspective of taxpayers. Like Hill, Wehman, et al. (1987), Noble and colleagues found that supported employees with moderate and severe mental retardation produced greater benefits than supported employees with mild mental retardation. This was true regardless of whether the supported employees with mild mental retardation did or did not possess a secondary disability. Specifically, mean benefits from individuals with moderate or severe mental retardation was $3,424 over a 27-month period. Supported employees with mild mental retardation, with and without secondary disabilities, averaged benefits of $2,985 and $2,842, respectively.

In summary, three out of four studies that examined the role of mental retardation with taxpayer net benefits reached the same conclusion. That is, supported employees with mild mental retardation were more cost-efficient than supported employees with more severe mental retardation. However, it is unclear whether individuals with moderate or severe mental retardation actually generate greater gross benefits than individuals with mild mental retardation, as determined by Hill, Wehman, et al. (1987) and Noble et al. (1991). It is also unclear how significant secondary disabilities or other demographics impact benefit–cost ratios for individuals with moderate or severe mental retardation since Noble et al. did not include this variable in their analyses.

VIII. STUDIES EXAMINING THE PERSPECTIVE OF THE WORKER

Six studies examined the benefits and costs of being employed from the perspective of the worker. Two of these (i.e., Brickey & Campbell, 1981; Cho & Schuerman, 1980) also examined the benefits and costs of hiring workers with disabilities from the perspective of businesses. Each of these six studies is reviewed below.

A. Cho and Schuermann (1980)

Cho and Schuermann's (1980) investigation was the first benefit–cost analysis of community-based employment programs for individuals with disabilities to be published. While the authors did not specifically mention the term *supported employment* as it was not truly coined until the Developmental Disabilities Act of 1984 (PL 98-527), their findings apply directly to the issue of the costs and benefits of supported employment programs.

Cho and Schuermann (1980) considered costs and benefits associated with a community employment approach called "handicap industries" from August 1975 to December 1978. According to Cho and Schuermann, handicap industries were managed by nonprofit foundations (e.g., adult developmental centers) specializing in hiring people with disabilities who worked alongside of nondisabled coworkers. By the brief description provided by the authors, it appears that these work sites were similar to what would now be called "enclaves" or a variation of the "entrepreneurial" supported employment model (Rusch & Hughes, 1990).

According to U.S. Department of Labor (1977/1979) studies cited by Cho and Schuermann (1980), employees in sheltered workshops made an average of $1.54 per hour. This figure was obtained in 1976 when the federal minimum wage was $2.30 per hour. Mean hourly wages for individuals in sheltered workshops increased by 10% between 1973 and 1976. However, during the same period the minimum wage increased 44%. Cho and Schuermann determined that persons working in the community consistently earned at or above the minimum wage, indicating that employment in the community possessed greater financial rewards for workers with disabilities than segregated settings.

Cho and Schuermann (1980) also investigated the costs and benefits of community-based employment from the perspective of businesses for each of the $3\frac{1}{2}$ years of their study. Costs included evaluation, training, placement, transportation, adaptive devices, aides, attendants, doctors, and personal counseling. Benefits included gross earnings of the workers with disabilities plus fringe benefits, which were estimated as 25% of gross pay.

According to Cho and Schuermann (1980), the sample of 34 workers with disabilities did not accumulate higher benefits than costs until the second full year of employment. During the second year, the benefit–cost ratio was reported to be 1.13; that is, for every $1.00 of cost, $1.13 worth of benefits was acquired. This ratio increased to 1.18 the following year.

Cho and Schuermann (1980) included unique variables in their analysis of costs. Of the 19 studies reviewed in this chapter, they were the only researchers who considered such costs as adaptive devices and various medical expenses, including personal counseling and doctor fees. However, since these costs were not defined within their text, it is difficult to determine their impact.

Cho and Schuermann (1980) were the first to examine the costs and benefits of hiring workers with disabilities from the perspective of the hiring industry. Of the 19 studies reviewed, only Cho and Schuermann and Brickey and Campbell (1981) explored this perspective. However, the methods utilized by Cho and Schuermann were not fully disclosed. Further, it is unclear why transportation and medical-related items would be factored into analyses emphasizing the perspective of the employer or why gross earnings and fringe benefits would be considered a benefit to employers rather than a cost.

Additionally, none of their 34 subjects had cognitive disabilities. All possessed various forms of physical disabilities (e.g., cerebral palsy, quadriplegia, muscular dystrophy, etc.) with the possible exception of those who had been involved in industrial and automobile accidents. Because their small sample did not match the populations traditionally served by supported employment (e.g., individuals with mental retardation or mental illness [Revell, Wehman, Kregel, West, & Rayfield, 1994]), little can be generalized by these analyses to current participants of supported employment programs. Nonetheless, Cho and Schuermann helped build a methodological foundation for future research.

B. Brickey and Campbell (1981)

Investigating the employment outcomes of 17 McDonald's employees who had mental retardation (IQ ranged from 37 to 70; mean equaled 57.4), Brickey and Campbell (1981) were the only authors reviewed in this chapter to examine the turnover rates of supported employees. Specifically, they found that the turnover rate of employees with disabilities was 41% after the first year of employment. This was compared to an average annual turnover rate of 175% for McDonald's workers without disabilities. Further, the authors found that there was a 0% turnover rate of workers with disabilities the second year of employment.

It should be noted that three of the employees with disabilities who left McDonald's during the first year did so after obtaining full-time employment elsewhere. Had these individuals been factored out of the analyses, the annual turnover rate for people with disabilities would have been 24% after the first year of employment. Further, employees with disabilities averaged the same number of hours (i.e., 20 hours per week) worked by nondisabled co-workers and made the same hourly wages (i.e., minimum wage).

In addition to analyzing employment outcomes from the perspective of the employer, Brickey and Campbell (1981) also examined the impact of competitive employment from the perspective of the worker with a disability. After losing the majority (i.e., 62%) of their Social Security (SS) and SSI benefits due to being gainfully employed, employees working 20 hours a week for McDonald's would have a net increase in income of $343 a year compared to working 27½ hours a week in sheltered workshops. After losing all of their SS and SSI benefits, competitive employees with disabilities experienced a net loss of $1,015 compared to sheltered employees. Further, after losing all of their SS/SSI benefits, competitive employees netted less income than individuals who were unemployed (see Table IX).

Brickey and Campbell's (1981) findings should be viewed with some caution for two reasons. First, they do not consider monetary benefits received by competitive employees that are associated with fringe benefits, such as vacation time, employee discounts, and insurance. Further, the authors noted that sheltered workshop wages utilized in the analyses were atypical. Specifically, the sheltered employees were paid higher wages than most and received vacation and sick leave. Sheltered employees typically do not receive these fringe benefits (Wehman, 1996b). As a result, the benefits of community employment may have been suppressed, whereas the benefits of sheltered workshops may have been artificially increased.

Second, whether individuals with disabilities will lose all of their governmental subsidies as a result of being gainfully employed is still under question. In 1987, the Social Security Act (PL 99-643) was changed to protect the income of individuals with disabilities who earn less than $14,000 a year (Knapp, 1988). It is unclear how this modification would have impacted Brickey and Campbell's (1981) findings.

C. Lam (1986)

Using two random samples totaling 50 individuals with developmental disabilities, Lam (1986) compared employment outcomes resulting from placements in sheltered workshops and in the community via supported employment programs.

TABLE IX
NET INCOME OF EMPLOYEES WITH DISABILITIES AFTER ONE YEAR OF EMPLOYMENT, ACCORDING TO BRICKEY AND CAMPBELL (1981)

	Employed with partial SS/SSI	Employed with no SS/SSI	Sheltered employee	Unemployed
Income				
Employment income	$3,067[a]	$3,067[a]	$1,430[b]	$0
Social Security/Supplemental Security Income[c]	1,358	0	2,173	2,498
Total Income	$4,425	$3,067	$3,603	$2,498
Expenses				
Federal income tax	$106	$106	$0	$0
State income tax	12	12	4	0
City income tax	46	46	21	0
Social Security tax	188	188	88	0
Bus fare	240	240	0	0
Total expenses	$592	$592	$113	0
Net income	$3,833	$2,475	$3,490	$2,498

[a]McDonald's income is based on $3.00 per hour x 20 hours per week x 51 weeks (allowing 1 week for sick days as there was no sick leave).

[b]Sheltered workshop income was based on $1 per hour x 27-1/2 hours a week x 52 weeks (the workshop had paid sick and vacation leave). This is considerably higher than the workshops' (sheltered workshop/work activities) average. The participants were among the best employees at the workshop.

[c]SS/SSI income varies considerably among individuals. Most participants received a combination of the two. Income is based on the most typical payment of $208.20 per month, with 50% of income more than $65 a month ($780/year) deducted form SS/SSI payments.

These programs were studied with regard to cost-effectiveness, job satisfaction, client characteristics, and program effectiveness. Results from the study were based upon data limited to one quarter of FY 1985.

Lam (1986) found no significant differences between the two samples based upon job satisfaction, IQ, level of education, and scores on a functional assessment test. Though not different based upon mean IQ scores, the supported employment sample consisted of two distinct subgroups: (a) individuals with IQs clustering around 48, and (b) individuals with IQs clustering around 72. The sheltered workshop sample was more evenly distributed, so that no subgroups based upon IQ were identified.

Lam (1986) examined program effectiveness in terms of wages earned and number of hours worked. The average hourly wage of supported employees was $1.79, and $1.17 for those employed in sheltered workshops (see Table X). Curiously, these figures were similar to the findings of Cho and Schuermann (1980) who, nearly 10 years prior to Lam, determined that community-based and sheltered employees made $2.30 and $1.54, respectively.

TABLE X

AVERAGE WAGES AND HOURS WORKED BY SHELTERED AND SUPPORTED EMPLOYEES BY LEVEL OF MENTAL RETARDATION AS REPORTED BY LAM (1986)

	Sheltered employees			Supported employees		
	High IQ[a]	Low IQ[b]	Total	High IQ[a]	Low IQ[b]	Total
Sample size	29	21	50	31	19	50
Quarterly wages	$423.21	$244.38	$348.11	$483.26	$125.37	$347.28
Hourly wages	$1.41	$0.83	$1.17	$2.40	$0.69	$1.79
Quarterly hours	300.15	294.43	297.53	201.36	181.70	194.01
Weekly hours	24.97	24.64	24.83	16.17	16.78	15.18
Projected annual wages	$1,692.84	$997.60	$1,392.44	$1,933.12	$501.56	$1,389.28
Projected annual hours	1,298.44	1,281.28	1,291.16	872.56	789.36	840.84

[a]"High IQ" groups contained persons with borderline or mild mental retardation.

[b]"Low IQ" groups contained persons with moderate or severe mental retardation.

Lam (1986) further indicated that supported employment programs were less effective than sheltered workshops in providing a higher number of working hours. With the exception of the moderate-severe subgroup, employees in the community generally worked less, but earned more per hour, than sheltered employees. The moderate–severe subgroup placed in the community earned less per hour and worked fewer hours than individuals in workshops. Sheltered employees and supported employees, nonetheless, generated roughly the same amount of gross earnings.

Lam (1986) investigated cost-effectiveness of sheltered and supported employment programs by comparing the costs per dollar earned and cost per hour worked by the employees. These data showed that placing individuals in supported employment programs was more cost-effective under both comparisons. However, when examining the subgroups within the community-based program, Lam found that it was more cost-effective to serve persons with moderate–severe disabilities in workshops under both situations (see Table XI).

Lam's (1986) results conflict with a number of other studies (cf. Cho & Schuermann, 1980). Specifically, individuals working in sheltered workshops in Lam's study earned 336% more than those reported by the U.S. Department of Labor 1977/1979 (cited by Cho & Schuermann, 1980). Further, Whitehead (1979) found that the national hourly wage averaged by sheltered employees was approximately $0.34, 71% less than sheltered employees in Lam's study. Schalock (1983), agreeing with Lam, found that sheltered employees with mental retardation made $1.17. However, Schalock also found that sheltered employees averaged only $417 annually, rather than the $1,392 reported by Lam. Therefore, the sheltered employees in Lam's study must have worked many more hours than the sheltered employees in Schalock's study.

In terms of supported employees, Vogelsberg (1986) found that average hourly wages obtained by supported employees ranged from $3.49 to $4.05, nearly twice the amount reported by Lam. Additionally, Moss, Dineen, and Ford (1986) examined the earnings of 70 supported employees and found that the average hourly wage was $4.05, further questioning Lam's figure of $1.79. On the other hand, Lam's findings of wages earned by supported employees are comparable to those of Wehman et al. (1985), if Lam's data were to be calculated over the same duration.

A major difference between Lam (1986) and Wehman et al. (1985), however, is that the latter examined effectiveness of supported employment in relation to number of placements and hourly wage, whereas Lam considered the total wages earned and hours worked. These analyses yield different results. They also raise the issue of whether it is better to work more hours for lower hourly wages than working fewer hours for higher wages per hour.

In response to Lam's (1986) findings, Wehman, Kregel and colleagues (1987) noted that, in Wehman et al. (1985) every $1.00 of supported employee earnings

TABLE XI

COST EFFECTIVENESS OF SHELTERED AND SUPPORTED EMPLOYMENT PROGRAMS BY LEVEL OF MENTAL RETARDATION AS REPORTED BY LAM (1986)[a]

	Sheltered employees			Supported employees		
	High IQ[b]	Low IQ[c]	Total	High IQ[b]	Low IQ[c]	Total
Sample size (n)	29	21	50	31	19	50
Total costs	\$38,339	\$28,935	\$67,274	\$6,662	\$26,059	\$32,721
Total wages	\$12,273	\$5,132	\$17,405	\$14,981	\$2,382	\$17,364
Total hours	8,689	6,209	14,898	6,242	3,460	9,702
Cost/wages	\$3.12/dollar	\$5.64/dollar	\$3.87/dollar	\$0.44/dollar	\$10.94/dollar	\$1.88/dollar
Cost/hours	\$4.41/hour	\$4.66/hour	\$4.52/hour	\$1.07/hour	\$7.53/hour	\$3.37/hour
(Cost/wages)/n	\$0.11	\$0.27	\$0.08	\$0.01	\$0.58	\$0.04
(Cost/hours)/n	\$0.15	\$0.22	\$0.09	\$0.03	\$0.40	\$0.07

[a]All data for the first quarter of 1985.

[b]"High IQ" groups contained persons with borderline or mild mental retardation.

[c]"Low IQ" groups contained persons with moderate or severe mental retardation.

resulted in only $0.14 of program costs. Further, Wehman, Kregel et al. found that the cost per hour worked in Wehman et al. (1985) was $0.54. This ratio was much lower than the ratio reported by Lam (i.e., $3.36 of costs per hour worked by supported employees).

Nevertheless, there are some other major differences between Lam (1986) and Wehman et al. (1985). For example, it is unclear why Lam's sample of supported employees earned an average of 187% less than the minimum wage at the time (e.g., $3.35). According to Wehman and Kregel (1984) and Rusch (1986), supported employees must make at, or above, minimum wage in order to be considered competitively employed. Further, federal guidelines at the time required that supported employees work at least 20 hours per week (Rusch & Hughes, 1990). Lam's supported employment sample averaged only 16.17 h per week while other studies, such as Kiernan, McGaughey, and Schalock (1986) found that supported employees across the nation worked an average of 27.45 h a week. It is not known why Lam's sample of supported employees was underemployed compared to individuals presented in other studies. Because Lam's samples may be unrepresentative of supported and sheltered employees, his results should be viewed with caution.

It is also unclear how "work" was defined by Lam (1986) when applied to sheltered workshops. Workshops often provide supported employees with training activities that are distinctly different from paid tasks performed by individuals employed in the community (Wehman, 1986). Further, the duration over which data were collected presents some deficits. More recent studies (cf. McCaughrin et al., 1991; Rusch et al., 1993; Tines et al., 1990) conceded that supported employment costs more than sheltered workshops initially, but that benefits surpass costs. Because Lam only examined the relationships between supported employment and sheltered workshops for a 3-month period, little information was gained on the longitudinal costs and benefits of these programs.

D. Schloss, Wolf, and Schloss (1987)

Schloss, Wolf, and Schloss (1987) examined the financial implications of being employed full-time and part-time from the perspective of an individual with disabilities. The authors used a balance-sheet approach to determine the net financial gain to individuals in three hypothetical situations: (a) unemployed, (b) employed part-time (i.e., 20 hours a week) at $4.80 an hour, and (c) employed full-time (i.e., 40 hours a week) at $4.80 an hour.

Income included revenue from SSI, Medicaid, food stamps, and salary, whereas expenses consisted of cost associated with housing, food, transportation, taxes, and medical insurance. As income from salaries increased, subsidies from SSI, food stamps, and Medicaid decreased. Schloss et al. (1987) hypothesized that after accounting for expenses, the yearly net disposable income for unemployed individuals would have been $392. Finally, individuals employed part-time would have earned $4,992 in salary and sustained a net disposable income of $2,692. Individuals employed full-time would have earned $9,984 with a net disposable income of $2,667. The authors noted that, from the perspective of the individual, it was more beneficial monetarily to work part-time than full-time or remain unemployed.

Although these results resemble those obtained by Brickey and Campbell (1981), who found that individuals with disabilities profited more monetarily from working in workshops than in the community, Schloss and colleagues (1987) were sharply criticized by Knapp (1988). Specifically, Knapp (1988) pointed out that Schloss et al.'s (1987) assumption that Medicaid would no longer be available to individuals working full-time was incorrect. Amendments to the Social Security Act (PL 99-643), according to Knapp, would make Medicaid benefits available to individuals earning less than $14,000 a year. As a result, individuals in all Schloss et al.'s hypothetical situations would retain their benefits, thus increasing their net disposable incomes.

Further, Knapp noted that the federal income taxes included in Schloss et al. (1987) were miscalculated. Rather than being $83 for a part-time employee and $832 for a full-time employee, Knapp determined that federal income taxes withheld would have been $674 and $1,424, respectively. With these corrections, Knapp found that full-time employment provided greater net disposable income than part-time employment and unemployment (see Table XII).

Schloss, Schloss and Wolf (1988) responded to Knapp's (1988) criticisms. While conceding that the Amendments to the Social Security Act (PL 99-643) would protect an individual's Medicaid benefits, they maintained that employees earning over $300 a month were "routinely investigated for potential disability cessation" (Schloss et al., 1988, p. 182). As a result, many of these individuals would lose their Medicaid for reasons other than excess income; the authors gave no source to substantiate this claim, however. Finally, Schloss et al. noted that Knapp failed to consider standard deductions and exceptions when he calculated his revised taxes withheld figure.

In the end, the conclusions arrived at by Schloss et al. (1987) are influenced by two primary variables. The first variable is the amount of taxes individuals in each

TABLE XII
NET DISPOSABLE INCOME FOR PART-TIME AND FULL-TIME EMPLOYEES

Employed	Knapp (1988)	Schloss, Wolf, & Schloss (1987)
Part-time	$2,101	$2,692
Full-time	$3,275	$2,667

scenario would actually pay. It is interesting to note that neither Schloss et al. (1987, 1988) nor Knapp (1988) considered that most of the taxes withheld would eventually be refunded by the Internal Revenue Service at the end of the fiscal year (McCaughrin et al., 1993). As a result, working full-time would most likely generate a greater net income than working part-time.

The second variable involves whether Medicaid benefits would remain intact once individuals obtained full-time employment. It is unclear how likely this is to occur, although it is a concern to individuals leaving workshops to enter competitive employment (Walls, Dowler, & Fullmer, 1989). Regardless of these variables, Schloss et al. (1987) presented much-needed information about the impact that variation in hours worked has upon disposable income. Further, they are the only authors who have considered housing, food, and other ordinary expenses in their analyses.

E. Kregel, Wehman, and Banks (1989)

Kregel et al. (1989) examined the impact of placement approach and supported employee demographics on key employment outcomes for 1,550 supported employees receiving services through 96 programs across eight states. Employee demographics investigated included primary disability and functional characteristics. Employment outcomes included hourly wages, hours worked per week, increase in earnings from prior placement, and degree of integration at work sites.

All individuals, regardless of disability, were found to benefit from community employment with substantial increases of earning over those made in sheltered workshops. Further, persons with long-term mental illness and physical or sensory disabilities earned significantly higher wages than individuals with all levels of mental retardation. Individuals with physical or sensory disabilities also worked significantly more hours than individuals with severe or profound mental retardation (see Table XIII).

In relation to the models of support employment, individual placements yielded higher hourly wages and monthly earnings than all other approaches. No statistically significant differences were found among models based upon hours worked per week and monthly earnings prior to placement in supported employment (see Table XIV). However, group placement approaches (e.g., enclaves and mobile work crews) were reported to provide significantly fewer opportunities for both physical and social integration.

Mobile work crews, in particular, produced significantly inferior employment outcomes than other models. Additionally, as Table XIII illustrates, mobile work crews were found to be composed of mainly individuals with mild mental retardation, though this approach was traditionally designed for persons with more severe disabilities (Bourbeau, 1989). Finally, individuals with severe and profound mental retardation were more likely to be placed in enclaves than any other approach.

TABLE XIII
EMPLOYMENT OUTCOMES BY PRIMARY DISABILITY ACCORDING TO KREGEL, WEHMAN, AND BANKS (1989)[a]

Disability	Hourly wage ($)	Hours per week	Monthly earnings in supported employent ($)	Percent change[b]
Severe/profound mental retardation	$3.09*	22.7**	286***	536
Moderate mental retardation	3.30	26.8	372	576
Mild mental retardation	3.15	26.5	361	280
Borderline mental retardation	3.27	27.6	392	390
Mental illness	3.74	28.0	454	345
Physical/sensory disabilities	4.28	29.6	556	539

[a]Based upon a sample of 1,550.

[b]"Percent change" indicates the percentage of change in monthly income resulting from supported employment.

*$F(5, 1549) = 30.75, p < .0001$.

**$F(5, 1549) = 29.80, p < .0001$.

***$F(5, 1549) = 8.50, p < .0001$.

F. Thompson, Powers, and Houchard (1992)

Thompson et al. (1992) investigated the effects of placement approaches and employee demographics on employment outcomes in Michigan. Using a quasi-experimental design (cf. Cook & Campbell, 1979), the authors compared supported

TABLE XIV
EMPLOYMENT OUTCOMES BY PLACEMENT APPROACH ACCORDING TO KREGEL, WEHMAN, AND BANKS (1989)[a]

Disability	Hourly wage ($)	Hours per week	Monthly earnings in supported employent ($)	Percent change[b]
Individual placement	$3.68*	26.5	$424**	430
Enclaves	3.25	28.7	301	349
Mobile crews	2.32	27.6	253	164
Small business	1.30	25.4	149	224

[a]Based upon a sample of 1,550.

[b]"Percent change" indicates the percentage of change in monthly income resulting from supported employment.

*$F(3, 2549) = 243.27, p < .0001$.

**$F(5, 1549) = 69.16, p < .0001$.

***$F(5, 1549) = 8.50, p < .0001$.

employment programs to a sample of sheltered workshops. They found that males represented a higher proportion of supported and sheltered employees than females. Further, individuals in supported employment tended to have higher IQs and were younger than their sheltered employee counterparts.

Thompson et al. (1992) also found that the IQ of supported employees affected wages earned in 7 of the 11 fiscal quarters investigated. Wages increased with reported IQ levels. Specifically, individuals with profound mental retardation averaged earning $412.39 per quarter, whereas individuals with mild mental retardation averaged $546.73 per quarter.

Living arrangements also impacted wages during 5 of the 11 fiscal quarters. Specifically, independent and semi-independent living arrangements (i.e., family homes) were related to higher wages. Finally, gender and race were only significant in two and one quarters, respectively. The authors did not indicate in what manner these variables affected wages, however.

After controlling for IQ, ethnicity, gender, and number of disabilities, Thompson et al. (1992) found that, compared to workshops, supported employment led to a significant increase in number of hours worked in 6 out of 11 quarters. This increase averaged 58.77 hours per quarter, or 4.52 hours per week. Supported employment also led to significantly higher wages than workshops in 9 of 11 quarters, with an average hourly wage increase of $1.85.

Persons placed individually within the community earned more than individuals in any other approach, concurring with Lewis et al.'s (1992) findings. Further, persons in individual placements averaged $291.20 more a quarter than individuals in sheltered workshop. These findings were not affected by IQ or other demographics.

IX. SUMMARY OF THE WORKER'S PERSPECTIVE

A. Net Benefits

The benefits and costs of working in the community are well documented from the perspective of the supported employee. All 20 studies reviewed in this chapter discussed the benefits and costs of being employed. With the exception of Brickey and Campbell (1981), nearly each of these studies came to the same conclusion. That is, *generally* individuals with disabilities benefit monetarily from working within the community.

Brickey and Campbell (1981), on the other hand, determined that after losing their SS and SSI, individuals with disabilities would have a greater net income if they were unemployed than if working 20 hours a week within the community. Further, the authors found that supported employees without SS/SSI experienced a net loss of over $1,000 a year compared to what they could have earned in sheltered workshops. However, the authors failed to consider fringe benefits (e.g., vacation time) that would have increased the net benefits of being employed within the community. Had these employment outcomes been included in their analyses, Brickey and Campbell might have drawn different conclusions.

Contrary to Brickey and Campbell (1981), Kregel et al. (1989) found that all approaches to supported employment (i.e., enclaves, mobile work crews, and individual placements) offered supported employees greater monthly earnings than sheltered employees. Similarly, Conley et al. (1989) and Tines et al. (1990) found that supported employees increased their earning 37% over their previous placements. This figure increased to 67% during the second year that individuals were employed within the community (McCaughrin et al., 1991). Finally, Hill et al. (1987) determined that for every $1.00 of costs, such as forgone wages, supported employees earned $1.97 in benefits; the average net benefit per supported employee was $6,815.

Supported employment has also been found to produce other nonmonetary benefits for workers with disabilities. For instance, McCaughrin et al. (1993) determined that supported employment led to greater increases on most quality-of-life indicators than sheltered workshops. Specifically, supported employees with mild mental retardation were more integrated at work, were more involved with their nondisabled co-workers, and reported a higher quality of life than sheltered employees with mild mental retardation. In addition to the findings for individuals with mild mental retardation, supported employees with moderate and severe mental retardation were also less lonely than sheltered employees with moderate or severe mental retardation.

B. Impact of Mental Retardation

Despite the overwhelming agreement in the literature that, overall, supported employees benefit more from working in the community than in segregated settings, two areas of contention exist within the supported employment literature. The first of these involves the relationship between degree of mental retardation and the monetary gains achieved by supported employees. Specifically, there is still some question as to whether individuals with severe mental retardation benefit more monetarily from working in the community than working in workshops.

Six studies reviewed in this chapter examined the impact of mental retardation upon the benefits and costs from the worker's perspective (i.e., Cimera, 1997; Hill, Wehman, et al. 1987; Kregel et al., 1989; Lam, 1986; McCaughrin et al., 1993; Thompson et al., 1992). Of these, only Lam and Thompson et al. found that some individuals earned more in sheltered workshops than in the community. Specifically, Lam (1986) examined the effects of mental retardation on the costs per dollar earned by employees in supported employment and sheltered workshops. Lam observed that sheltered workshops were more cost-effective in providing individuals with severe mental retardation higher hourly wages and more hours worked than supported employment. Supported employees with high IQs worked fewer hours than sheltered employees with high IQs, but earned more per hour.

However, as noted earlier, weaknesses in Lam's (1986) study raise concerns about these findings. First, Lam examined only 3 months of data. This duration might not have taken into consideration the long-term employment trends experienced by supported employees. For example, supported employees commonly increase their hourly wages after a year of satisfactory service, as noted by Brickey and Campbell (1981).

Also, the concept of "work" was never defined by Lam (1986). This is important because workshops have been criticized for providing services that would not be considered work within the community (Rusch, Mithaug, & Flexer, 1986). For example, sheltered workshop clients may be asked to sort and then unsort items as part of their habilitation training.

Further, individuals without mental retardation were included in the high IQ subsample. Consequently, the ability level of individuals in this subsample may have been inflated. As a result, the validity of these findings may be drawn into question.

Thompson et al. (1992) also examined the employment outcomes achieved by 165 supported employees during 11 fiscal quarters, finding that sheltered employees averaged more earnings than supported employees in 4 of 11 fiscal quarters. Further, after adjusting for variables such as IQ and number of disabilities, supported employment increased wages over sheltered workshops in 10 of 11 fiscal quarters. The authors concluded that, for some individuals with severe mental retardation, sheltered employment presented greater monetary gains than supported employment.

The conclusions of Lam (1986) and Thompson et al. (1992) that individuals with severe mental retardation can earn more money in sheltered workshops than in the community are contradicted by Cimera (1997), Kregel et al. (1989), McCaughrin et al. (1993), and Hill, Wehman, et al. (1987). Each of these studies found that supported employees, regardless of disability, earned more than sheltered employees. However, these four studies obtained different results on the influence of mental retardation on earnings within the community.

For instance, Cimera (1997), Kregel et al. (1989), and McCaughrin et al. (1993) found that IQ was *positively* correlated to earnings. That is, as IQ increased, the amount of earnings also increased. Yet, supported employees with severe mental retardation still elevated their earnings over what they would have received in workshops. Specifically, Kregel et al. determined that supported employees with severe or profound mental retardation earned $3,432 a year more in the community than they would have in sheltered workshops. McCaughrin et al. reported this figure as $1,027 for supported employees with moderate or severe mental retardation. Additionally, Cimera found that the effect of mental retardation decreases over time.

Contrary to Kregel et al. (1989) and McCaughrin et al. (1993), Hill, Wehman, et al. (1987) found that IQ was *negatively* correlated to earnings. That is, individuals with moderate or severe mental retardation averaged more annual earnings per person than supported employees with mild mental retardation (i.e., $12,853 versus $10,833, respectively). Further, the authors found that supported employees with moderate or severe mental retardation were employed longer per person than supported employees with milder disabilities (i.e., 24.6 months vs. 17.0 months, respectively).

In summary, the six studies that examined the impact of IQ on employment outcomes all agreed that mental retardation affected earnings. However, different conclusions were reached on this issue. Specifically, Cimera (1997), Lam (1986), McCaughrin et al. (1993), and Kregel et al. (1989) found that degree of mental retardation was positively correlated with the wages earned by supported employees. But Cimera, McCaughrin et al., and Kregel et al. found that all individuals with mental retardation earned more in the community than in workshops, whereas Lam, and to some extent Thompson et al. (1992), found that individuals with moderate or severe mental retardation earned the most amount of money in workshops. Conversely, Hill, Wehman, et al. (1987) found that individuals with moderate or severe mental retardation earned more money in the community than individuals with mild mental retardation.

B. Impact of Governmental Subsidies

The second area of contention in the literature involves the reduction of governmental subsidies that often occurs as a result of working competitively. Specifically, Brickey and Campbell (1981) found that McDonald's employees who worked an average of 20 hours a week lost all of their SS and SSI after the first year of employment. Additionally, Schloss et al. (1987) theorized that it was more cost-efficient for individuals with disabilities to work part-time than full-time. According to these authors, the loss of income from governmental subsidies resulting from working full-time was not offset by a comparative increase in earned wages if individuals earned $4.25 per hour. However, these conclusions were disputed by Knapp (1988), who pointed out that reduction in subsidies as a result of working was not automatic due to changes in federal regulations (i.e., the Social Security Act Amendments of 1987).

Knapp's (1988) claim that governmental subsidies are not necessarily reduced due to competitive employment in the community was supported by Rusch et al. (1993), who found that the amount of governmental subsidies received by supported employees actually increased during the third year of their study. This increase in income would be considered a benefit to supported employees, rather than a cost.

However, with the exception of Rusch et al. (1993), nearly every examination of supported employment from the worker's perspective identified a reduction in governmental subsidies as a cost to the supported employee. For example, Hill et al. (1987) found that supported employees averaged a $2,350 reduction in governmental subsidies over a 21-month period. Further, Conley et al. (1989) found that 394 supported employees lost a combined total of over $26,000 in government subsidies in 1 year.

Similar to the impact of mental retardation on monetary outcomes, the issue of reduction in governmental subsidies as a result of being employed has not been completely settled. From the literature reviewed in this chapter, it is unclear whether or not reductions in subsidies occur once individuals become employed within the community. Moreover, the extent to which reductions take place is still being debated.

The importance of reduction in governmental subsidies and the impact of mental retardation on net benefits of being employed cannot be overstated. One of the primary obstacles to competitive employment for people with disabilities is the fear of losing eligibility for governmental programs, such as public assistance (Rusch et al., 1986). Further, many service providers feel that individuals with severe disabilities are better served in sheltered settings (Clark & Kolstoe, 1995). By gaining a greater understanding of the impact that the degree of mental retardation has upon net monetary benefits within the community, which includes the extent to which governmental subsidies are affected, service providers can better educate individuals with disabilities as to their employment options. Further, by understanding potential obstacles to competitive employment from the perspective of the worker, strategies for overcoming these obstacles may be developed.

X. CONCLUSIONS

From the 20 studies reviewed in this chapter, several common findings were identified (see Table XV). Specifically, the literature has found that, over time, supported employment is generally a better investment than sheltered workshops. That is, for every dollar society and taxpayers invest in supported employment, more than a dollar is returned. The primary reason for this appears to be that while monetary benefits and costs associated with sheltered workshops remain stationary, supported employment programs increase in cost-efficiency from year to year.

Within the benefit–cost literature, however, it remains unclear whether supported employment is cost-efficient for all purposes. For example, some studies found that individuals with severe mental retardation were more cost-efficient in sheltered workshops than supported employment, while other studies found that all individuals, regardless of disability, were cost-efficient to serve via supported employment. In short, there is little agreement whether individuals with severe or multiple disabilities should be served via supported employment or alternative placements.

TABLE XV
FINDINGS OF SUPPORTED EMPLOYMENT BENEFIT–COST LITERATURE[a]

Citation	Scope Region Length of data (Sample size)	Supported employment cost-efficiency perspectives			Level of mental retardation and cost-efficiency perspectives			Supported employment models perspectives		
		Worker	Taxpayer	Society	Worker	Taxpayer	Society	Worker	Taxpayer	Society
Cho & Schermann (1980)	Unknown 39 months (n = 34)	⇑								
Brickey & Campbell (1981)	None None (None)	⇔								
Schneider et al. (1981)	Illinois 2 years[b] (n = 22)			⇑						
Hill & Wehman (1983)	Virginia 47 months (n = 90)		⇑							
Wehman et al. (1985)	Virginia 75 months (n = 167)	⇑	⇑							
Lam (1986)[c]	Unknown 3 months (n = 100)	⇓ ⇔			⬆					
Schloss et al. (1987)[d]	None None	⇑								

	(None)								
Hill et al. (1987) Hill, Wehman et al. (1987)	Virginia 94 months (n = 214 & 117)	⇑	⇑		↑	↓			
McCaughrin (1988)[e]	Illinois 8 years (n = 22)		⇔						
Kregel et al. (1989)	Eight states 1 month (n = 1,550)	⇑			≈		I > G		
Conley et al. (1989) Tines et al. (1990)	Illinois 1 year (n = 394)	⇑	⇓	⇓					
Noble et al. (1991)	New York 21 months (n = 1,100+)	⇑	⇓	⇓	↑	↑			
McCaughrin et al. (1991)	Illinois 2 years (n = 588)	⇑	⇓	⇓					
Lewis et al. (1992)[f,g]	Minnesota 1 year (n = 856)		⇔	⇑			I > G	I > G	I > G
Thompson et al. (1992)[h]	Michigan 44 months (n = 2,400+)	⇔		↑					
McCaughrin et al. (1993)	Illinois 1 & 5 years	⇑	⇑	⇑	↑	↑	↑		

continues

TABLE XV *Continued*

Findings of Supported Employment Benefit–Cost Literature[a]

Citation	Scope Region Length of data (Sample size)	Supported employment cost-efficiency perspectives			Level of mental retardation and cost-efficiency perspectives			Supported employment models perspectives		
		Worker	Taxpayer	Society	Worker	Taxpayer	Society	Worker	Taxpayer	Society
	(n = 20)									
Rusch et al. (1993)	Illinois 3 years (n = 729)	⇑	⇓	⇓						
Cimera (1997)	Illinois 1990 &1994 (n = 111 & 57)	⬆	⇑	⇑	⬆	≋	≋			

⇑ indicates that supported employment was found to be cost-efficient (i.e., benefit-cost ratio exceeding 1.0); ⇓ indicated that supported employment was found to be cost-inefficient (i.e., benefit-cost ratio less than 1.0); ⇔ indicates that supported employment was sometimes found to be cost-efficient and sometimes cost-inefficient; ⬆ indicates that there was a positive relationship between supported employee intelligence and cost-efficiency (e.g., supported employees with mild mental retardation were more cost-efficient than supported employees with moderate or severe mental retardation); ⬇ indicates that there was a negative relationship between suppported employee intelligence and cost-efficiency (e.g., supported employees with severe mental retardation were more cost-efficient than supported employees with mental retardation); ≋ indicates that there was no relationship between supported employee intelligence and cost-efficiency; I > G indicates that "individual placements" were more cost-efficeint than "group placements;" G > I indicates that "group placements" were more cost-efficient than "individual placements."

[a]Supported employment models are categorized as "individual" versus "group" (i.e., enclaves, mobile work crews, small business).

[b]Schneider et al. (1981) gathered data during the first 2 years of program operation; they then projected cost-efficiency for 20 years into the future.

[c]Lam (1986) found that, in general, supported employment was less cost-efficient than sheltered employment in terms of generating annual wages for individuals with disabilities; cost-effectiveness, however, was determined by level of mental retardation.

[d]Schloss et al. (1987) found that being employed part-time was more beneficial than working full-time or not at all.

[e]McCaughrin (1988) found that the cost-efficiency of supported employment depended upon how costs were calculated.

[f]Lewis et al. (1992) found that supported employment programs were more cost-efficient from the taxpayer and societal perspectives than on-site programs (e.g., sheltered workshops) in 64% of the cases examined.

[g]Lewis et al. (1992) found that individual placements were more cost-efficient than group placements in 82% of the cases.

[h]Thompson et al. (1992) found that, when compared to sheltered workshops, supported employment offered more wages per quarter in 9 out of 11 quarters.

TABLE XVI
SUMMARY OF FINDINGS AND NEEDED RESEARCH

Agreements	Conflicting findings and needed research
• Over time, supported employment is a good investment for taxpayers and society.	• The affect of severity and number of disabilities on cost-efficiency (i.e., all perspectives) is unclear
• Generally, workers earn more in supported employment than sheltered workshops.	• Little is known about the cost-efficiency of various supported employment models (e.g., individual vs. group placements)
• The cost efficiency of supported employment programs varies among regions of the countries.	• A nationwide sample of supported employment and sheltered workshops programs are needed to better estimate cost-efficiency.
	• The monetary benefits and cost accrued during the entire working life of supported employees needs to be explored.
	• Future research needs to explore the effect of various training strategies on cost-efficiency.

In addition to the impact that severity of disability has upon cost-efficiency, many areas of research have yet to be fully explored within the literature (see Table XVI). For example, only two studies have investigated the cost-efficiency of various supported employment models (e.g., individual placements, enclaves, mobile work crews, small business approach). One study has examined the cost-efficiency of hiring workers with disabilities from the perspective of the employer, but it was methodologically flawed. Finally, only one study investigated the impact that various training strategies (e.g., natural supports) on cost-efficiency. Additional light needs to be shone upon these areas, for without employers willing to hire workers with disabilities or training strategies that effectively and efficiently teach individuals skills, supported employment could cease to be a viable program for legislators to fund.

REFERENCES

Arrow, K. J., & Lind, R. C. (1994). Risk and uncertainty: Uncertainty and the evaluation of public investment decisions. In R. Layard & S. Glaister (Eds.), *Cost-benefit analysis* (2nd ed., pp. 160).

Boorbeau, P. E. (1989). Mobile work crews: An approach to achieve long-term supported employment. In P. Wehman & J. Kregel (Eds.) *Supported employment for persons with disabilities: Focus on excellence* (pp. 53–68). New York: Human Sciences.

Brickey, M., & Campbell, K. (1981). Fast food employment for moderately and mildly retarded adults: The McDonald's project. *Mental Retardation, 19*(3), 113–116.

Buchanan, R. D. (1978, June). How to control turnover. *Food Service Marketing, 40*, 49–50; 55.

Burkhauser, R. V., & Haveman, R. H. (1982). *Disability and work: The economics of American policy.* Baltimore: Johns Hopkins Press.

Chadsey-Rusch, J. (1992). Toward defining and measuring social skills in employment settings. *American Journal on Mental Retardation, 96*, 405–418.

Cho, D. W., & Schuermann, A. C. (1980). Economic costs and benefits of private gainful employment of the severely handicapped. *Journal of Rehabilitation, 46*(4), 28–32.

Cimera, R. E. (1997). *The effects of supported employee demographics on individual benefit-cost ratios.* Unpublished doctoral dissertation, University of Illinois, Urbana-Champaign.

Cimera, R. E., Rusch, F. R., & Heal, L. W. (1997). *Supported employee independence from job coach involvement over a four-year period.* Manuscript submitted for publication.

Clark, G. M., & Kolstoe, O. P. (1995). *Career development and transition education for adolescents with disabilities.* Boston: Allyn and Bacon.

Conley, R. (1973). *The economics of mental retardation.* Baltimore: Johns Hopkins.

Conley, R. W., & Noble, J. H., Jr. (1990). Benefit-cost analysis of supported employment. In F. R. Rusch (Ed.), *Supported employment: Models, methods, and issues* (pp. 271–287). Sycamore, IL: Sycamore.

Conley, R. W., Rusch, F. R., McCaughrin, W. B., & Tines, J. (1989). Benefits and costs of supported employment: An analysis of the Illinois supported employment project. *Journal of Applied Behavior Analysis, 22*, 441–447.

Cook, T. D., & Cambell, D. T. (1979). *Quasi-experimentation: Design and analysis issues for field settings.* Chicago: Rand McNally.

Feldstein, M. S. (1972). The social time preference rate. In R. Layard (Ed.), *Cost-benefit analysis* (pp. 245–269). Baltimore: Penguin.

Hayden, M. F., & Depaepe, P. (1994). Waiting for community services: The impact on persons with mental retardation and other developmental disabilities. In M. F. Hayden & B. H. Avery (Eds.), *Challenges for a service system in transition: Ensuring quality community experiences for persons with developmental disabilities* (pp. 178–185). Baltimore: Brookes.

Heal, L. W., McCaughrin, W. B., & Tines, J. J. (1989). Methodological nuances and pitfalls of benefit-cost analysis: A critique. *Research in Developmental Disabilities, 10*, 201–212.

Hill, M. L., Banks, P. D., Handrich, R. R., Wehman, P. H., Hill, J. W., & Shafer, M. S. (1987). Benefit-cost analysis of supported competitive employment for persons with mental retardation. *Research in Developmental Disabilities, 8*, 71–89.

Hill, M., & Wehman, P. (1983). Cost benefit analysis of placing moderately and severely handicapped individuals in competitive employment. *Journal of the Association for the Severely Handicapped, 8*, 30–38.

Hill, M. L., Wehman, P. H., Kregel, J., Banks, P. D., & Metzler, H. M. D. (1987). Employment outcomes for people with moderate and severe disabilities: An eight-year longitudinal analysis of supported competitive employment. *Journal of the Association for the Severely Handicapped, 12*, 182–189.

Intagliata, J. C., White, B. S., & Cooley, F. B. (1979). Cost comparison of institutional community based alternatives for mental retarded persons. *Mental Retardation, 12*(3), 154–157.

Johnson, J. R., & Rusch, F. R. (1990). Analysis of hours of training provided by employment training specialists to supported employees. *American Journal on Mental Retardation, 94*, 674–682.

Johnston, M. V. (1987). Cost-benefit methodologies in rehabilitation. In M. J. Fuhrer (Ed.), *Rehabilitation outcomes: Analysis and measurement* (pp. 99–113). Baltimore: Brookes.

Joint Committee on Standards for Educational Evaluation. (1994). *The program evaluation standards* (2nd ed.). Thousand Oaks, CA: Sage.

Kee, J. E. (1994). Benefit-cost analysis in program evaluation. In J. S. Wholey, H. P. Hatry, & K. E. Newcomer (Eds.), *Handbook of practical program evaluation* (pp. 456–488). San Francisco: Jossey-Bass.

Kiernan, W. E., McGaughey, M., & Schalock, R. L. (1986). *National employment survey for adults with developmental disabilities.* Boston: Children's Hospital.

Knapp, S. F. (1988). Financial implications of half- and full-time employment for persons with disabilities: A response to Schloss, Wolf, and Schloss. *Exceptional Children, 55,* 181.

Kregel, J., Wehman, P., & Banks, P. D. (1989). The effects of consumer characteristics and type of employment model on individual outcomes in supported employment. *Journal of Applied Behavior Analysis, 22,* 407–415.

Lam, C. S. (1986). Comparison of sheltered and supported work programs: A pilot study. *Rehabilitation Counseling Bulletin, 30*(2), 66–82.

Layard, R. (1972). *Cost-benefit analysis.* Baltimore: Penguin.

Layard, R., & Glaister, S. (1994). *Cost-benefit analysis* (2nd ed.). Cambridge: Cambridge University Press.

Levin, H. M. (1983). *Cost-effectiveness: A primer.* Beverly Hills: Sage.

Lewis, D. R., Johnson, D. R., Bruininks, R. H., Kallsen, L. A., & Guillery, R. P. (1992). Is supported employment cost-effective in Minnesota? *Journal of Disability Policy Studies, 3,* 67–92.

McCaughrin, W. B. (1988). *Longitudinal trends of competitive employment for developmentally disabled adults: A benefit-cost analysis.* Unpublished doctoral dissertation, University of Illinois, Urbana-Champaign.

McCaughrin, W. B., Ellis, W. K., Rusch, F. R., & Heal, L. W. (1993). Cost-effectiveness of supported employment. *Mental Retardation, 31,* 41–48.

McCaughrin, W. B., Rusch, F. R., Conley, R. W., & Tines, J. (1991). A benefit-cost analysis of supported employment in Illinois: The first 2 years. *Journal of Developmental and Physical Disabilities, 3,* 129–145.

Moss, J. W., Dineen, J. P., & Ford, L. H. (1986). University of Washington employment training program. In F. R. Rusch (Ed.), *Competitive employment: Issues and strategies* (pp. 77–85). Baltimore: Brookes.

National Hotel and Restaurant Association (1983). Personal communication with Dr. Philip Nelan, Washington, DC.

Noble, J. H., Conley, R. W., Banjerjee, S., & Goodman, S. (1991). Supported employment in New York state: A comparison of benefits and costs. *Journal of Disability Policy Studies, 2*(1), 39–74.

Prest, A. R., & Turvey, R. (1965). Cost-benefit analysis: A survey. *Economic Journal, 75,* 685–705.

Revell, W. G., Wehman, P., Kregel, J., West, M., & Rayfield, R. (1994). Supported employment for persons with severe disabilities: Positive trends in wages, models, and funding. In P. Wehman & J. Kregel (Eds.), *New directions in supported employment: Volume 1* (pp. 30–39). Richmond, VA: Rehabilitation Research and Training Center on Supported Employment.

Rubin, S. E., & Roessler, R. T. (1995). *Foundations of the vocational rehabilitation process* (5th ed.). Austin, TX: PRO-ED.

Rusch, F. R. (1986). *Competitive employment issues and strategies.* Baltimore: Brookes.

Rusch, F. R. (1990). Preface. In F. R. Rusch (Ed.), *Supported employment: Models, methods, and issues* (pp. xv–xvi). Sycamore, IL: Sycamore.

Rusch, F. R., Conley, R. W., & McCaughrin, W. B. (1993). Benefit-cost analysis of supported employment in Illinois. *Journal of Rehabilitation, 59,* 31–36.

Rusch, F. R., & Hughes, C. (1990). Historical overviews of supported employment. In F. R. Rusch (Ed.), *Supported employment: Models, methods, and issues* (pp. 5–14). Sycamore, IL: Sycamore.

Rusch, F. R., Mithaug, D. E., & Flexer, R. W. (1986). Obstacles to competitive employment and transitional program options for overcoming them. In F. R. Rusch (Ed.), *Competitive employment: Issues and strategies* (pp. 7–22). Baltimore: Brookes.

Schalock, R. (1983). *Services for developmentally disabled adults: Development, implementation and evaluation.* Austin, TX: PRO-ED.

Schloss, P. J., Schloss, C. N., & Wolf, C. W. (1988). Continuing views of the financial implications of employment for persons with disabilities. *Exceptional Children, 55,* 182–183.

Schloss, P. J., Wolf, C. W., & Schloss, C. N. (1987). Financial implications of half- and full-time employment for persons with disabilities. *Exceptional Children, 54,* 272–276.

Schneider, K., Rusch, F. R., Henderson, R., & Geske, T. (1981). Competitive employment for mentally retarded persons: Costs vs. benefits. In W. Halloran (Ed.), *Funding and cost analysis* (pp. 63–82). Urbana: University of Illinois, Leadership Training Institute.

Stiglitz, J. E. (1994). Discount rates: The rate of discount for benefit-cost analysis and the theory of the second best. In R. Layard & S. Glaister (Eds.), *Cost-benefit analysis* (2nd ed., pp. 116–159). Cambridge: Cambridge University Press.

Thompson, L., Powers, G., & Houchard, B. (1992). The wage effects of supported employment. *The Journal of the Association for Persons with Severe Handicaps, 17,* 87–94.

Thompson, M. S. (1980). *Benefit-cost analysis for program evaluation.* Beverly Hills, CA: Sage.

Thornton, C. (1984). Benefit-cost analysis of social programs. In R. H. Bruinks & K. C. Lakin (Eds.), *Living and learning in the least restrictive environment* (pp. 225–244). Baltimore: Brookes.

Thornton, C. (1992). Uncertainty in benefit-cost analysis of supported employment. *Journal of Vocational Rehabilitation, 2*(2), 62–72.

Thornton, C., & Will, J. (1988). Benefit-cost analysis and special education programs. In R. H. Bruininks, D. R. Lewis, & M. L. Thurlow (Eds.), *Assessing outcomes, costs and benefits of special education programs* (pp. 158–189). Minneapolis: University of Minnesota, Department of Educational Psychology. University Affiliated Program on Developmental Disabilities.

Tines, J., Rusch, F. R., McCaughrin, W., & Conley, R. W. (1990). Benefit-cost analysis of supported employment in Illinois: A statewide evaluation. *American Journal on Mental Retardation, 95,* 44–54.

Vogelsberg, R. T. (1986). Competitive employment in Vermont. In F. R. Rusch (Ed.), *Competitive employment: Issues and strategies* (pp. 35–49). Baltimore: Brookes.

Walls, R. T., Dowler, D. L., & Fullmer, S. L. (1989). Cash and in-kind benefits: Incentives rather than disincentives for vocational rehabilitation. *Rehabilitation Counseling Bulletin, 33,* 118–126.

Wehman, P. (1981). *Competitive employment: New horizons for severely disabled individuals.* Baltimore: Brookes.

Wehman, P. (1986). Competitive employment in Virginia. In F. R. Rusch (Ed.), *Competitive employment issues and strategies* (pp. 23–34). Baltimore: Brookes.

Wehman, P. (1996a, April). Supported employment saves dollars and makes good sense. *The Advance, 7*(1), pp. 1, 7.

Wehman, P. (1996b). *Life beyond the classroom: Transition strategies for young people with disabilities* (2nd ed.). Baltimore: Brookes.

Wehman, P., Hill, M., Hill, J., Brooke, V., Pendleton, P., & Britt, C. (1985). Competitive employment for persons with mental retardation: A follow-up six years later. *Mental Retardation, 23,* 274–281.

Wehman, P., & Kregel, J. (1984). *A supported work approach to competitive employment for individuals with moderate and severe handicaps.* Richmond: Virginia Commonwealth University, Rehabilitation Research and Training Center.

Wehman, P., Kregel, J., Banks, P. D., Hill, M., & Moon, M. S. (1987). Sheltered versus supported work programs: A second look. *Rehabilitation Counseling Bulletin, 31,* 42–53.

Whitehead, C. W. (1979). Sheltered workshops in the decade ahead: Work and wages or welfare? In G. T. Bellamy, G. O'Connor, & O. C. Karan (Eds.), *Vocational rehabilitation of severely handicapped persons: Contemporary service strategies* (pp. 71–84). Baltimore: University Park.

Will, M. (1984). *Supported employment for adults with severe disabilities: An OSERS program initiative.* Unpublished paper. Office of Special Education and Rehabilitation Services, U.S. Department of Education, Washington, DC.

Worthen, B. R., & Sanders, J. R. (1987). *Educational evaluation: Alternative approaches and practical guidelines.* White Plains, NY: Longman.

Decision Making and Mental Retardation

LINDA HICKSON AND ISHITA KHEMKA

CENTER FOR OPPORTUNITIES AND OUTCOMES FOR PEOPLE WITH DISABILITIES
TEACHERS COLLEGE
COLUMBIA UNIVERSITY
NEW YORK, NEW YORK

I. INTRODUCTION

Major shifts in the guiding philosophies and realities of the systems that serve people with mental retardation have presented them with an array of new opportunities and challenges. Recent policies and laws emphasize concepts such as inclusion, independence, empowerment, and self-determination, or peoples' right to control their own lives (Ward, 1988; Wehmeyer, 1992, 1998). In keeping with these trends, educational and habilitative services for people with mental retardation have been moving away from sheltered, protective services toward programs that foster full community participation. Individuals with mental retardation are finding themselves in an increasing range of community settings where they are being challenged to make more decisions on their own. For example, Jiranek and Kirby (1990) reported a higher level of decision making among individuals with intellectual disability in less restrictive employment settings than in more sheltered employment settings. According to Morris, Niederbuhl, and Mahr (1993), service providers are increasingly being encouraged to allow "capable" adults with mental retardation to make their own decisions about medications, restrictive behavioral interventions, and invasive medical procedures. Brown, Belz, Corsi, and Wenig (1993) have offered their Choice Diversity Model to guide and encourage increased choice and decision-making opportunities across environments for all individuals, even those with severe cognitive disabilities.

All too often, however, increased opportunities for choice and decision making for individuals with mental retardation and developmental disabilities have been associated with increased vulnerability to exploitation and abuse, especially in social interpersonal situations. Dramatic examples are provided by two widely publicized court cases previously cited by Hickson, Golden, Khemka, Urv, and

INTERNATIONAL REVIEW OF RESEARCH IN
MENTAL RETARDATION, Vol. 22
0074-7750/99 $30.00

Yamusah (1998) and Greenspan (in press). In the Glen Ridge, New Jersey, case, cited by Hickson et al., a young woman with mental retardation was lured to a basement and sexually assaulted by a group of young men from her home community, who took advantage of her mental retardation to manipulate and coerce her into compliance. In the case of Richard LaPointe, discussed by Greenspan, a man with Dandy-Walker syndrome was sentenced to life in prison after being tricked into confessing to a murder that most believe he did not commit. It is easy to point to numerous examples that illustrate the vulnerability of people with mental retardation in a variety of community situations ranging from victimization in financial scams to extremely high rates of sexual coercion and abuse (Khemka & Hickson, in press; Sobsey, 1994; Sobsey & Doe, 1991).

The vulnerability of people with mental retardation in interpersonal choice and decision-making situations has been attributed to a number of factors, including generally impaired cognitive functioning. More specifically, there is evidence that individuals with mental retardation typically experience particular difficulty relative to their mental age (MA) levels with several cognitive components of decision making, including reasoning (Spitz, Webster, & Borys, 1982; Ross & Ross, 1978), working memory (Ferretti & Cavalier, 1991), and language comprehension (Bilsky, 1985; Abbeduto, Furman, & Davies, 1989). Others have attributed the interpersonal vulnerabilities of people with mental retardation to limited social competence (Greenspan & Driscoll, 1997; Gumpel, 1994). In Gumpel's model, decision skills constitute a stage in the attainment of social competence, whereas in Greenspan and Driscoll's model, social competence is composed of temperament, character, and social intelligence. Greenspan (1997) has identified social intelligence as a central, defining characteristic of mental retardation and has highlighted credulity and gullibility as key aspects of social intelligence that contribute to the vulnerability of people with mental retardation to exploitation and coercion. Motivational factors, including perceptions of control or personal agency beliefs and goal selection, have been suggested as possible additional sources of the difficulties experienced by people with mental retardation in interpersonal situations (Bandura, 1982; Ford, 1995; Greenspan, in press; Hickson et al., 1998; Short & Evans, 1990).

To date research on choice and decision making in individuals with mental retardation has focused largely on identifying the level of available opportunities to make choices and express preferences (Houghton, Bronicki, & Guess, 1987; Kishi, Teelucksingh, Zollers, Park-Lee, & Meyer, 1988) and assessing the capabilities of individuals with mental retardation to give consent and generate alternatives (Morris et al., 1993; Smith, 1986; Tustin & Bond, 1991). Choice and decision-making skills of individuals with mental retardation have been studied in the context of everyday situations, such as choosing leisure activities (Dattilo & Rusch, 1985; Koegel, Dyer, & Bell, 1987), expressing food preferences (Parsons & Reid, 1990), and handling major and minor personal and interpersonal situations (Jenkinson & Nelms, 1994), as well as in the context of life activities such as parenting (Tymchuk, Yokota, & Rahbar, 1990), health-care decisions (Morris et al., 1993), and sexual consent (Sundram & Stavis, 1994).

Although the terms *choice* and *decision making* are sometimes used interchangeably, our use of the terms in this chapter is generally consistent with Etzioni's (1988) distinction between *choice* as "all selections among options, however limited the scope of information process" (p. 92) and *decision making* as "deliberative" choices. Gumpel (1994) described decision making as encompassing the interpretation of a stimulus, generation of response options, analysis of the feasibility of those options, and execution of an "appropriate and executable" response choice (p. 195). With the exception of a few studies (Hickson et al., 1998; Jenkinson & Nelms, 1994; Tymchuk, Andron, & Rahbar, 1988), the use of the component steps of the decision-making process has not been closely examined in individuals with mental retardation.

The remainder of this chapter focuses on the current status of research and theory pertaining to the interpersonal decision-making capabilities of individuals with mental retardation. In the next section, the relatively sparse body of research and theory on interpersonal decision making and problem solving in individuals with mental retardation is reviewed. Because of the limited theoretical work on decision-making processes in individuals with mental retardation, in the third section, the focus shifts to relevant theory pertaining to decision making in individuals without mental retardation. In the fourth section, a framework for interpersonal decision-making research in mental retardation is proposed and discussed. The fifth and final section focuses upon conclusions and promising directions for future research.

II. RESEARCH AND THEORY IN MENTAL RETARDATION

Most previous studies of decision making in individuals with mental retardation have been conducted within a problem-solving framework. Within this broad framework, it is possible to view the interpersonal decision-making dilemma as a type of ill-defined problem and to view the more typical interpersonal problem-solving task as a more well-defined problem. Ill-defined problems may lack either clearly specified initial states, goal states, and/or rules to minimize the distance between the two states, whereas well-defined problems include clear specifications of each of these three components (Matlin, 1989; Short & Evans, 1990; Simon, 1974). Interpersonal decision-making dilemmas typically lack both a clearly defined goal state and clear rules on how to proceed. Problem-solving situations include at the least a clearly specified initial state and a clearly specified goal state and sometimes include rules on the generation of possible solutions. Illustrative examples of interpersonal decision-making and problem-solving vignettes from recent studies by Khemka (1997) and Edeh (1998) are presented in Table I.

TABLE I
EXAMPLES OF INTERPERSONAL DECISION-MAKING VIGNETTES[a] AND INTERPERSONAL PROBLEM-SOLVING VIGNETTES[b] WITH SELF AS THE KEY DECISION MAKER

Decision-making vignettes

1. During lunchtime, your best friend asks you to go eat in a park that is far away from work. You are afraid that you will get back to work late.
2. You are doing your best at work. However, your supervisor at work has been yelling at you for not working fast and calls you slow. Your supervisor tells you that you don't deserve any credit for your work.
3. One day on your way to work, a man from your neighborhood stops you. You have seen the man hanging out in the neighborhood before but you do not know him very well. The man offers you some money and asks you to deliver a packet for him.

Problem-solving vignettes

1. You are listening to your favorite music on your headphones during lunchtime. Your friend wants to borrow your headphones. You still want to use your headphones.
2. Your friends make fun of another child. Your friends want you to join them. You do not like to make fun of anybody.
3. Your friends want to skip classes. Your friends want you to skip classes with them. You do not want to skip classes.

[a]From Khemka, 1997.
[b]From Edeh, 1998.

A. Decision-Making Processes

The relatively few previous studies on personal and interpersonal decision making and problem-solving processes in individuals with mental retardation fail to provide a comprehensive picture of the capabilities of these individuals. Although most models of problem solving and decision making underscore the importance of at least four component processes, (1) framing the problem, (2) generating alternatives, (3) evaluating consequences, and (4) choosing a course of action, previous research in this area involving individuals with mental retardation has emphasized primarily the generation of alternatives. However, in a review of research in other domains of problem solving (i.e., academic, experimental, and scientific problem solving) where there is a larger body of available research involving individuals with mental retardation, Short and Evans (1990) presented evidence implicating several of these components, especially framing the problem, as possibly important loci of difficulty for individuals with mental retardation.

Among the studies that have examined the ability of individuals with mental retardation to generate alternatives, a study by Smith (1986) compared 11–13-year-old children with mild mental retardation with intellectually average children with comparable MAs and chronological ages (CAs) on an interpersonal problem-solving task. Pictures showing an interpersonal problem-solving situation were presented, and children were asked how many different ways they could solve the problems. Although the overall performance of the children with mental retardation was generally comparable to that of their equal-MA counterparts, it was markedly inferior to that of equal-CA children without mental retardation. The children with mental retardation exhibited fewer types of problem-solving strategies and less use of strategies that reflected higher levels of social understanding.

Wehmeyer and Kelchner (1994) examined the interpersonal problem-solving skills of adults with mental retardation using the Means–Ends Problem Solving (MEPS) procedure developed by Platt and Spivack (1989). The participants were presented with four problem situations in the form of stories. For each story, a statement of the problem to be solved and the final solution to the problem were provided. Participants were asked to generate strategies or steps to complete the middle of the story between the problem statement and the problem solution. Performance on two measures, total relevant means (total number of relevant solutions) and total relevancy ratio (proportion of relevant solutions relative to total solutions), was determined and the adults with mental retardation were compared with college students and noncollege adults from the MEPS assessment norms. Results indicated that adults with mental retardation generated both fewer relevant solutions and a lower proportion of relevant solutions than college students and noncollege adults without mental retardation. Of the total number of solutions proposed by individuals with mental retardation, 40% of the solutions were irrelevant to the problem as compared to 4 and 18% irrelevant solutions proposed by the college students and noncollege adults, respectively. Wehmeyer and Kelchner (1994) concluded by agreeing with Short and Evans (1990) that the problem solving of people with mental retardation is characterized by “cognitive rigidity” as reflected in their overreliance on a limited number of solutions drawn from past experience without flexibly adapting them to the demands of each new situation.

Tymchuk et al. (1990) came to a similar conclusion after conducting a study in which the decision-making performance of a group of mothers with mental retardation was compared to that of a group of mothers without mental retardation of the same socioeconomic level. Participants were presented with eight vignettes that included equal numbers of high-risk (e.g., baby is choking) and low-risk (e.g., baby continues crying after being fed and changed) child-care situations. Half of the vignettes were presented in a partial format, consisting of only a description of the situation, and half of the vignettes were presented in a full format, containing a description of the situation as well as several possible courses of action and their potential consequences. After exposure to each vignette, participants were asked what they would do and why. In addition, for full-format vignettes, participants were asked several questions about the alternatives and their consequences. The mothers with and without mental retardation did not differ in overall decision-making performance, but the mothers without mental retardation were more successful than the mothers with mental retardation at answering the questions on alternatives and their consequences. Both groups made more appropriate decisions for low-risk than for high-risk situations and for partial-format vignettes than for full-format vignettes. The authors suggested that the participants, especially those with mental retardation, may have been unable to take advantage of the additional information provided in the full-format vignettes because they were not following a deliberative, stepwise decision-making process involving the consideration of alternatives and their possible consequences. They suggested that, instead, they may have been drawing upon their past experience to produce automatic decision responses, some of which happened to be appropriate for the familiar situations used in the study. The authors went on to suggest that the lack of a systematic decision-making process was likely to impair participants' ability to make appropriate decisions in new and unfamiliar, especially high-risk, situations. Although the authors attributed their finding of superior performance with partial-format, rather than full-format, vignettes to the participants' apparent inability to utilize the additional information about alternatives and consequences provided in the full-format vignettes, an alternative interpretation seems possible. In the sample vignettes provided in the Tymchuk et al. article, the partial-format vignette consisted of an eight-sentence description of the decision situation, while the full-format vignette included only a two-sentence description of the situation, followed by a nine-sentence presentation of alternative solutions and their possible consequences. It is possible that the longer, more detailed descriptions of the situations in the partial-format vignettes fostered comprehension and framing of the decision situations in ways that facilitated making connections with relevant past experience to produce appropriate responses.

In another study, Jenkinson and Nelms (1994) compared the extent to which adults with and without mental retardation made vigilant decisions in response to vignettes depicting major or minor personal/interpersonal situations. Based on the decision-making theory of Janis and Mann (1977), vigilant responses were defined as responses reflecting a systematic search for all relevant information and the careful evaluation of alternatives to maximize possible benefits. Major decisions were those involving relatively long-term consequences or large sums of money and minor decisions were those not involving any long-term consequences. Jenkinson and Nelms reported that the adults without mental retardation made more vigilant decisions than the adults with mental retardation. In addition, both groups, but especially the group with mental retardation, were more likely to make vigilant responses for minor as opposed to major decisions. In interpreting this finding, Jenkinson and Nelms noted that participants with mental retardation made significantly more hypervigilant responses than participants without mental retardation for major decisions. Hypervigilant responses were maladaptive responses that suggested an impulsive, hasty action, or an overreaction. Jenkinson and Nelms's conclusion that limited decision-making experience may have contributed to the difficulties of the participants with mental retardation suggests that the participants may have had less relevant past experience with the major decision situations than with the minor decision situations.

Overall, the available research in mental retardation can be characterized by its emphasis on the cognitive aspects of interpersonal problem solving and decision making, to the exclusion of motivational and emotional factors. In some studies, the task has even been labeled interpersonal *cognitive* problem solving (e.g., Healey & Masterpasqua, 1992). In an effort to apply a broader perspective to the study of interpersonal decision making, Hickson et al. (1998) conducted two studies that considered motivational and emotional, as well as cognitive, factors as possible sources of the decision-making difficulties of individuals with mental retardation. In the first study, female and male adults with mental retardation listened to vignettes depicting situations in which a protagonist was faced with a decision involving the possibility of interpersonal conflict, physical danger, or sexual assault. In the second study, adults without mental retardation were presented with a paper-and-pencil version of the task. The vignettes each portrayed a situation in which a protagonist was faced with a potential conflict between a goal involving social or material gain (e.g., money) versus a goal involving a self-protective or socially responsible action to avoid a negative consequence (e.g., injury). Study participants were asked what the protagonist should do and why and responses were scored using criteria similar to those employed by Jenkinson and Nelms (1994) to determine the number of vigilant responses. Content analyses were subsequently performed on vigilant responses to describe the type of action recommended and the types of consequences specified. In addition, the participants in the second study were asked to rate each vignette as high-risk or low-risk.

Hickson et al. (1998) reported that the results of the two studies supported the broad-based conception of interpersonal decision making as tapping cognitive, motivational, and emotional processes. As expected, a major cognitive component was reflected in large performance differences between the adults with mental retardation, who made vigilant decisions only 50% of the time, and the adults without mental retardation, who made vigilant decisions about 92% of the time. The content analyses indicated that the groups also exhibited somewhat different goal-selection patterns, possibly reflecting motivational differences. In keeping with the risks inherent in the vignettes, more than 75% of the vigilant decisions for both groups involved recommending that the protagonist take actions aimed at minimizing risks and/or acting in a socially responsible way. Of the remaining vigilant responses, the adults without mental retardation were somewhat more likely to recommend a negotiation approach that blended gain-oriented and safety/responsibility-oriented goals and the adults with mental retardation were slightly more likely to recommend actions that involved seeking assistance.

A comparison of the patterns of performance for the women and men who participated in the two studies reported by Hickson et al. provided further indications of the potential importance of motivational and emotional factors. The women, both with and without mental retardation, produced more vigilant responses than the men and were more likely to state possible negative consequences of failing to take vigilant action. These differences may have reflected higher levels of relevant past experience on the part of the women with some of the situations depicted in the vignettes, especially those involving a threat of sexual or physical assault. Hickson et al. suggested that the women may have been more sensitive to the risks inherent in the vignettes, an interpretation that was supported by their finding in the second study that women were more likely than men to rate vignettes as high-risk. It was suggested that the sensitivity of the women to the risks implicit in the vignettes could have both enhanced the emotional significance of the task, inducing deeper processing of the information, and also increased motivation to recommend self-protective and socially responsible actions.

B. Decision-Making Training

To date most training studies have distinguished between social skills training aimed at adding specific behaviors to a person's repertoire and social problem-solving/decision-making training that emphasizes strategies. In keeping with the focus of the present review, studies dealing exclusively with social skills training are not discussed. However, it is worth noting that a few studies (e.g., Park & Gaylord-Ross, 1989) have reported increased generalization when a stepwise problem-solving approach is used to teach social skills. Like the research on decision-making processes, most previous research aimed at developing training approaches to improve problem solving and decision making has emphasized cognitive strategies. In a review of research on interpersonal problem-solving training, Coleman, Wheeler, and Webber (1993) noted that social incompetence is typically viewed as a cognitive deficit, and most interpersonal problem-solving training studies have focused on teaching a series of problem-solving steps. Although their review indicated that students with a variety of learning and behavior problems can acquire a sequence of social problem-solving steps, results of the studies often revealed that gains were limited to cognitive measures and did not extend to observations of actual behavior. Drawing upon a construct introduced by Strain, Cooke, and Appolloni (1976), Coleman et al. proposed that most of the training studies may have been addressing repertoire deficits, but not performance deficits. Repertoire deficits reflect a lack of problem-solving knowledge or skills, whereas performance deficits occur when individuals possess the needed knowledge and skills but fail to exhibit the behavior for "another reason such as emotional interference or situational parameters" (p. 33). Although Coleman et al. (1993) reviewed studies involving students with learning disabilities and behavior problems as well as students with mental retardation, their observations appear equally applicable to most available training studies involving individuals with mental retardation.

The approaches used to train individuals with mental retardation to handle interpersonal problems and decisions have been heavily influenced by the work of D'Zurilla and Goldfried (1971) and Spivack, Platt, and Shure (1976), who applied models highlighting the stepwise components of problem solving and decision making to improve the performance of children and adolescents without disabilities. Despite this influence, most training studies involving individuals with mental retardation have not comprehensively addressed the complete constellation of components. Some studies have monitored the number of steps identified and/or applied, but more typically the studies have focused on a single step in the process, usually the generation of alternatives. This is not surprising, however, as most of the training studies have focused on problem solving with a defined goal rather than decision making, where a goal must be specified as part of the solution. With the exception of two studies, the training studies in the mental retardation literature have addressed problem solving rather than decision making. In one of the two studies, Ross and Ross (1978) trained children with mental retardation to select the best of several alternative solutions to social or environmental problems and decision-making situations. In the other study, Tymchuk et al. (1988) used a multiple-baseline design to train nine mothers with mental retardation to identify and apply the following decision-making components to a set of child-care vignettes: (a) decision identification, (b) goal definition, (c) who should make the decision, (d) where to obtain help, (e) alternatives, and (f) selection of an optimal decision. The women improved from the base line to the training phase in identifying (i.e., naming) and applying (i.e., stating how a step would be applied to a particular vignette) the steps with both training and generalization vignettes. These gains were maintained in a 1-month follow-up. However, appropriateness of final decisions improved only for high-risk training vignettes, but not for low-risk training vignettes or generalization vignettes, indicating that aquisition of a stepwise decision-making procedure did not necessarily result in better decisions.

All of the remaining studies reviewed focused on the generation of solutions to problem situations where the goal was specified. Most of these studies used either a cognitive (Browning & Nave, 1993; Castles & Glass, 1986; Nezu, Nezu, & Arean, 1991; Ross & Ross, 1973, 1978) or behavioral (Martella, Marchand-Martella, & Agran, 1993; Park & Gaylord-Ross, 1989) approach to teach a stepwise process for generating alternative problem solutions. Even in a study by Vaughn, Ridley, and Cox (1983), which employed a broad-based social–cognitive training approach, the outcome focus was on number of alternative solutions generated. Although these training studies were generally successful at teaching the participants to apply the steps to training problems, some of the studies suffered from methodological flaws such as small *ns* and brief training periods. Generalization was limited and dependent variables generally failed to include measures of behavior in natural settings.

Perhaps the greatest shortcoming of this body of research is the absence of an emphasis on the *content* of the problem-solving and decision responses. If training in problem solving and decision making is to enable people with mental retardation to make better decisions in real-life community situations, many of which carry threats of danger, coercion, or abuse, then the content of each decision is of paramount importance. The literature on decision processes suggested that people with mental retardation may make appropriate decisions in some situations but that these decisions are often rote decisions based on past experience with similar situations. In other words, there is often no evidence that a deliberative, stepwise decision-making process is being followed. The training literature, on the other hand, indicates that although it is possible to teach people with mental retardation to apply a stepwise decision process, that does not necessarily improve the quality of their decisions.

Khemka (1997), in a recent study, did address decision quality by comparing the effectiveness of two training approaches aimed at improving the independent decision-making skills of women with mental retardation in response to videotaped situations portraying a key decision maker who was faced with a decision involving interpersonal conflict or abuse. The two training approaches include, (a) decision-making training: a training approach that provided instruction in the use of a cognitive decision-making strategy that included generating alternative solutions and considering possible consequences; and (b) self-directed decision-making training: an integrated cognitive and motivational training approach that provided instruction in the use of a cognitive decision-making strategy within a context designed to foster goal clarification and greater perceptions of control and responsibility in decision making. The features of the self-directed decision-making training model are highlighted in Figure 1. The decision-making training condition included the four cognitive steps shown at the right of the figure, but not the motivational activities portrayed in the panel at the left. Although both training methods were effective relative to a control condition, the self-directed decision-making training method was superior to the decision-making training method that included only instruction in the use of a cognitive strategy. The superiority of the self-directed training condition was reflected in posttest performance with the video vignette task, a version of which was used for training, as well as on a verbally presented generalization task that required the respondent to state what they would do if they were ever in that situation themselves. For both tasks, independent decision-making responses were defined as self-initiated actions by the decision maker that addressed the situation effectively in a timely manner. The findings of Khemka's study suggest that, in order to increase independent decision making, it may be necessary to augment training in the cognitive processes of decision making with training that addresses the motivational processes—including goal setting and perceptions of control—that affect the specific nature of decision responses.

• Setting Self-Directed Goals (examples)
•Safety
•Privacy and Respect
•Do things on your own/ speak up for yourself
•Act on time to stop the problem
• Reinforcing Internal Perceptions of Control
• Building Decision - Making Confidence and Motivating Self-Responsibilty in Decision-Making
1. Recognition of Problem
• Is ____ faced with a problem?
• What is the problem here?
• How do you think ____ is feeling in this situation?
• Does ____ need to do something about this situation?
• Does ____ need to make a decision?

2. Generate Alternatives and List Consequences
• What are some of the things that ____ can do to solve the problem in this situation?
• What will happen if? (for each choice generated)

3. Evaluate Consequences
• Will the person be safe?
• Will the problem be solved?
• Is this a real emergency/ do we need to call the cops?
• Does the choice meet all self-directed goals?

4. Eliminate Choices and Make Decision
•Eliminate ineffective choices
•Select among effective choices

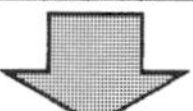

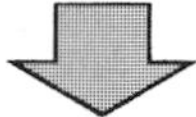

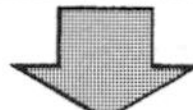

FIG. 1. Self-directed decision-making training model. (From Khemka, 1997.)

III. DECISION THEORY

This section of the chapter presents a broad overview of the theories of decision making and related factors that have formed a basis for the study of individual choice and decision-making behavior in people without mental retardation. The overview provides a theoretical context for understanding the complex issues involved in defining and studying human decision making and lays the groundwork for a framework for decision-making research in individuals with mental retardation.

A. Prescriptive Theories

A review of the literature on decision making reveal several theories that have been prescriptive in nature in the analysis of decision behavior, providing explanations of how decisions should be made (von Neumann & Morgenstern, 1944). One of the most important among them has been rational choice theory. *Rational choice theory* assumes that decision makers can estimate the value and the probability distributions of all variables relevant to a decision and can then use this information to make optimal decisions. It is assumed that decision makers are knowledgeable about their preferences; have stable rankings of their preferences; possess full information about the decision problem, the available alternatives, and the consequences (i.e., possess optimal cognitive understanding of the decision situation); and can rank all alternative choice options for maximizing self-interest (Fischhoff, 1982). This approach views human decisions and actions as fixed and predetermined and discounts the possibility of decision makers diverging from their capacity for rational decision making.

The human mind is however limited in its capacity for memory, attention, and information processing (Anderson, 1990; Baddeley, 1986; Miller, 1956; Newell & Simon, 1972). The effects of these limitations on decision making may be significant and result in nonrational decisions. Decision makers often have little insight into or control of their own decision-making behavior (Dawes, 1988; Hogarth, 1987; Kahneman, Slovic, & Tversky, 1982; Simon, 1985). Decision makers may not always know all available alternatives at the time of decision making or be aware of future alternatives not presently available. Furthermore, the outcomes of selected alternatives may be uncertain, and the knowledge base of the decision makers may be insufficient or irrelevant to the decision at hand. Due to these limitations, individuals tend to simplify decision-making situations and formulate decisions based on limited viewpoints that focus on some aspects of the decision-making situation while ignoring others (Carroll & Johnson, 1990). This has led decision-making researchers to redefine the concept of rationality and to acknowledge that decision makers in actuality engage in the decision-making process with less than optimal cognitive understanding of the domains relevant to their decisions (Zey, 1992).

Simon (1957) proposed the notion of *bounded rationality* to identify human limitations for highly complex and normative calculations of choice. According to him, human rationality is bounded or constricted by several factors including the limited cognitive or information-processing capacities of individuals, the ability to frame problems appropriately, etc. People handle complexity in decision making by selectively reducing problems to levels that are manageable in the real world, and therefore reducing the cognitive demands of decision making (Simon et al., 1986; Tversky & Kahneman, 1974). Simon proposed that the goal of decision making should be viewed in terms of searching and finding a satisfactory solution to a problem, a process he labeled "satisficing," rather than aiming to choose the best of all possible alternatives as expected under the rational choice theory. The primary mechanism through which individuals reduce their need to search for information and process all possible alternatives and outcomes is the adoption of aspiration levels (Simon, 1957). A decision maker sets an aspiration level—a level to which she or he aspires and which is acceptable, given her or his goals and needs. The aspiration level varies with different decision tasks and may be adjusted within the process of decision making itself. Given this aspiration level, she or he then searches for a reasonable solution within the limited scope of the decision problem. In this context, an individual's decision making reflects choices that are reasonable and purposeful given her or his goals and inherent limitations (Hogarth, 1987).

B. Reasoning Theories

Given that deviation from an optimal rationality criterion is only natural to human thinking, a number of theories—broadly classified as reasoning theories—have sought to identify alternative mental mechanisms that individuals could apply during decision making in order to maximize their decision-making competence. For example, the *mental-logic theory* (Braine, 1978; Inhelder & Piaget, 1958; Johnson-Laird, 1975) proposes the use of formal syntactic inference rules of the type "if p then q" for encoding and inference of a problem. Alternatively, the *mental-models theory* (Johnson-Laird & Byrne, 1991) focuses on the nature of the semantic encoding of an inference rule and subsequent manipulation of content for reasoning. Svenson (1979) described two major types of decision rules or strategies, *compensatory* and *noncompensatory* in nature, that individuals employ to reach decisions. Compensatory strategies allow an individual to confront the conflicts inherent in the choice situation by trading off one alternative option against another alternative option to effectively reach a balanced decision. On the other hand, noncompensatory strategies are conflict avoiding in nature where the decision maker avoids any trade-off between alternative options. Instead, decision makers may set a limiting point on the various dimensions of an alternative and eliminate alternatives that fall below that limit (e.g., *conjunctive models*) or they may set a low limit on one or a few dimensions and very high levels on another or other dimensions of an alternative, thereby eliminating alternatives that do not match the set limit (e.g., *disjunctive models*). In different circumstances decision makers have been found to use one or the other strategy, or a combination of both, depending on the complexity of the decision, the importance of choice, availability of information, and uncertainty associated with the decision (Klayman, 1985; Payne, 1976).

C. Descriptive Theories

The theories described above have held explanatory power in predicting the likelihood for optimal decision outcomes. However, the validity of these theories is restricted to controlled, laboratory task situations and strategies that are not necessarily applicable to real-life decisions and everyday circumstances (Oaksford & Chater, 1993). Furthermore, these theories are restricted in their ability to provide an adequate description of the decision-making process or explain why individuals under similar circumstances make different choices. Many decision researchers prefer more ecologically valid, context-free explanations of human reasoning that reflect everyday preferences, strategies, and processes used by decision makers. Descriptive theories of decision making, such as the *reasoned choice models*, that view decision making as a process and examine how people rationalize as they undertake the process of decision making, have become popular in decision-making research. Reasoned choice models identify decision-making components that describe the process used by decision makers to arrive at reasoned choices. The emphasis is on the process of decision making and not on finding means to achieve predicted ends or apply specific inference rules (Zey, 1992).

Stage-based or process models of decision making conceptualize the decision-making process as a series of fairly well-defined sequential or temporal stages, with some overlap or backtracking between the stages during complex decision making. Janis and Mann's (1977) *conflict model* of decision making provides an example of this approach. The model was developed to describe decision making in the context of emergency decisions and is applicable to all situations involving consequential personal decisions. The model is based on the assumption that during decision making an individual faces some level of decisional conflict in the form of simultaneous opposing tendencies to accept or reject a given course of action, expressed as psychological stress, anxiety, or feelings of uncertainty. A decision-maker's attempt to reduce decisional conflict is influenced by specific psychological conditions relating to decisional self-esteem and the ability to handle stress. These conditions in turn determine distinctive coping styles that individuals adopt in their approach to a decision-making situation.

The most adaptive or efficient coping style that leads to successful and informed resolution of decisional conflict is referred to as a vigilant style. Janis and Mann

(1977) highlighted seven procedural criteria that result in vigilant information processing: (a) canvassing a wide range of alternative courses of action; (b) surveying the full range of objectives to be fulfilled; (c) weighing the costs and benefits of negative and positive consequences of each alternative; (d) intensive information search for evaluation of alternatives; (e) adequately assimilating and taking into account new information or expert judgment; (f) reexamining the positive and negative consequences of all known alternatives before making a choice; and (g) thorough planning for implementing or executing the chosen course of action and handling contingencies. In contrast, coping styles such as unconflicted adherence (ignoring the need to make a decision); defensive avoidance (devaluing the importance of the decision and the search for alternatives or procrastinating); and hypervigilance (making a hasty or panicky decision) interfere with the cognitive processes specified by the model. These coping styles are considered maladaptive as they usually lead to low-quality decisions and inefficient action (Janis & Mann, 1977; Radford, Mann, Ohta, & Nakane, 1993).

D. Normative and Affective Factors in Decision Making

The decision-making theories described above posit that individuals follow some decision rules to sort through and evaluate alternatives when making decisions. The decision rules vary in their formality and complexity from being exact and prescriptive in nature as under the rational choice theory or reasoning models, to outlining specific processes of decision making, as under the descriptive models of decision making. However, several researchers (Einhorn & Hogarth, 1981; Evans, 1983; Kahneman & Tversky, 1979) have suggested that individuals may not always apply formal or specific decision rules to reach a decision. Individuals might replace precise decision rules with less formal decision rules, commonly referred to as heuristics, in recognizing and structuring decision situations and in evaluating preferences. Heuristics are a mental shorthand that generates a basis for decisions without having to follow detailed decision rules. Under the heuristic approach, alternatives or attributes of alternatives are eliminated early in the search process and the decision maker operates within a much narrower decision-making context for the final solution. Heuristics frequently documented in the research on decision making are based on judgments, habits, past or stereotypic choice, and moral values (Camic, 1992). For example, individuals making stereotypic decisions may choose the most representative behavior of the group to which they belong, without engaging themselves in the decision-making process. Thus, an individual may buy a particular commodity brand not because it is the best choice available but because it is customary to buy that brand in his or her family. Based on past experience, a known element or quantity might serve as an anchor or a benchmark, against which other decisions are judged. For example, when shopping for clothes an individual might choose to exclude all synthetic materials and consider only clothes made from cotton. In this case, cotton serves as an anchor against which other decisions (e.g., price, color, style) are made. Similarly, decisions can be driven by normative factors that include moral values, superstitions, or long-held beliefs (Etzioni, 1988; Gilovich, Vallone, & Tversky, 1985).

Affective factors are also relevant in decision making. Affective states or individual emotions like passion, rage, fervor, and so on are known to play a role in decision making. The effectiveness of decision making may decline in situations of high stress, anxiety, or emotion (Holsti, 1979 [cited in Zey, 1992]); Janis & Mann, 1977). According to Elster (1985), emotions play a negative role by overwhelming or subverting the rational mental processes of an individual during decision making. Similarly, Toda (1980) labeled emotions as having "a noisome, irrational effect on decision-making" (p. 133). On the other hand, Maslow (1962) and Zajonc (1980) maintained that emotions serve a positive function in decision making. Other theorists have attributed a more neutral role to emotion, attributing to it the primary function of reordering processing priorities in order to adapt to changing situations (Clore, Schwarz, & Conway, 1994; Simon, 1967). Epstein (1994), in his cognitive-experiential self-theory, has described two separate processing systems, each of which can lead to positive decision outcomes under particular circumstances. The experiential system, intimately associated with emotion or affect, accounts for responses that are nonrational, impulsive, and tied to concrete representations of experience that may be intuitive, heuristic, and potentially rapid and efficient. The rational system, which typically operates in the absence of strong emotion, is abstract, sequential, analytical, and deliberative. Although the rational system would support stepwise, cognitive decision-making processes, individuals may be forced to rely on their experiential system under conditions of extreme stress or time pressure.

Etzioni (1988) has developed a normative–affective model of decision making that recognizes the constructive basis of normative values and affect in behavior and decision making. According to his model, normative commitment (values) or affective involvement (emotions) governs the majority of choices or decisions that individuals make by influencing which information is considered, how it is processed, and which options are considered and chosen. The degree to which normative–affective considerations as opposed to cognitive information processes drive decision making is represented by a continuum. At one extreme, decision-makers may choose a course of action without exploring any alternatives (i.e., cognitive processing is completely excluded). In this case, choice is made exclusively on normative grounds. Alternatively, decision makers may engage in some sort of information search and evaluation of options, but their choices may be extensively "loaded" or "ranked" by normative-affective factors. At the other extreme, individuals may consciously regulate or control their decision making in order not to divert from a logical flow of information processing or reasoning, completely excluding normative–affective factors. The decision to remain indifferent to the influence of normative–affective factors, and to base a decision on a cognitive decision-making process, is itself determined by normative–affective considerations. Factors such as stress, lack of concentration, and level of stamina may also play a significant role in decision making.

E. Motivational Factors and Self-Perceptions

Motivational factors are also important determinants of decision-making performance. Motivation pertains to the purpose of behavior, or to goal-related processes (Kuhl, 1986; Spaulding, 1994). In the context of decision making, motivation can affect whether a person chooses to engage in a decision-making process at all as well as their selection of a goal and of a means for attaining that goal. Traditional models of decision making have highlighted the motivational relevance of a person's self-perceptions of their ability to attain a particular goal and the extent to which they value that goal.

An individual's self-awareness of her or his own decision-making capabilities and level of confidence are critical to decision-making performance (Cacioppo & Petty, 1982; Fischhoff, 1975; Verplanken, 1993). Elms (1976), Janis (1974), Janis and Mann (1977), Lefcourt (1982), Mann, Harmoni, and Power (1989), and Radford et al. (1993) have emphasized the role of self-esteem, locus of control, self-efficacy, and other predispositional characteristics of the decision maker in influencing decision-making competence. The self-esteem of a decision maker as reflected in an increased sense of confidence and self-perception of ability to make competent decisions has been linked to the use of adaptive decision response styles (Burnett, Mann, & Beswick, 1989; Radford et al., 1993). Ollendick, Greene, Francis, and Baum (1991) have found external locus of control to be related to impulsive decision making and distractibility. Studies by Deci and Ryan (1987) and Lent and Hackett (1987) have shown that perceived control, of which locus of control is a dimension, can influence the type of choices an individual makes.

According to Ford's (1992, 1995) motivational systems theory, goals, emotions, and personal agency beliefs all work together in the process of decision making. Goals are viewed as thoughts about desired (and undesired) future outcomes and are closely tied to emotional priorities. Personal agency beliefs, similar to the concept of perceptions of control discussed by other theorists, pertain to a person's belief about the extent to which a goal is attainable. Ford described two types of personal agency beliefs, capability beliefs relating to self-perceived skill levels, and context beliefs, relating to expectancies about the extent to which the environment will support goal attainment. Personal agency beliefs affect peoples' decisions about how much time and effort to invest in attempting to attain a particular goal.

Cacioppo and Petty (1982) linked an individual's readiness to engage in information search for decision making to his or her motivation to process information, an attribute they termed as "need for cognition." Similarly, Kruglanski (1996) has advanced the concept of "the need for cognitive closure" as determining primary motivational tendencies that influence the way an individual comprehends a decision-making situation and then approaches a decision solution. The need for cognitive closure refers to "an individual's desire for a firm answer to a question and an aversion to ambiguity" (p. 467), and occurs on a continuum from a strong need for closure to a strong need to avoid closure. Individuals with a high need for closure are motivated to act quickly in reaching a decision and may engage in only a partial or cursory information search prior to decision making. Conversely, individuals with a low need for closure are not motivated to commit quickly to a course of action and may engage in a more detailed and careful processing of relevant information prior to decision making. The need for closure, independent of individual differences, may change depending on the conditions under which decisions have to be made. The need for closure is heightened in situations of time pressure where a quick solution is desired and lessened in situations where a decision involving either long-term commitment or significant magnitude is sought. The effects of time pressure on the decision-making processing of individuals have been noted elsewhere in the literature (Svenson & Maule, 1993). In response to time pressure in decision tasks, individuals may either accelerate information processing; show greater selectivity for predecisional choices or information; or shift to less complex decision strategies and the use of heuristics (Maule & Mackie, 1990; Verplanken, 1993). Verplanken (1993) also found individuals to report less confidence in their decision-making ability under time pressure.

Decision makers are sometimes not motivated to enter a decision-making process. For instance, individuals with low decisional confidence experience very little motivation to engage in choice selection (Janis & Mann, 1977). Corbin (1980) has identified three possible types of no-action choices that individuals can adopt. These actions include refusal, delay, and inattention, and are similar to the unconflicted adherence choice option suggested by Janis and Mann (1977). In a no-action response, the individual chooses to maintain the status quo which then functions as her or his aspiration level. A no-action response may be chosen when the individual perceives less uncertainty in doing nothing than in finding or choosing among other alternatives. Corbin argues that a person's subjectively perceived state of uncertainty must fall below a certain threshold before she or he can be motivated to precipitate an action and make a decision negating the status quo. Individual motivation may therefore be tied to the uncertainty of finding a satisfactory solution to a decisional problem.

Hogarth (1987) offered a broader view of how people decide whether to engage in active decision making. He proposed that the choice of whether to engage in action or not is determined by an individual's perception of the environment, general expectations, and the extent to which an individual engages in clarifying goals and preferences, seeking more information, and reformulating a problem to discover alternative solutions. According to Hogarth, conflict in the form of incompatibility between different alternative choice options is inherent in the process of decision making. Conflict is resolved through a dynamic process that is guided by an individual's needs and goals and the need to balance the costs and benefits of alternative choice actions. By adopting a sequential process of choice, an individual can engage in the following steps: problem representation, information search, and evaluation of different choice points. At various choice points, an individual decides to either engage in the mental effort of analyzing the decision problem leading to a potential solution or to opt out of the situation, or to preserve the status quo by making no choice and leaving needs unfulfilled.

The substantive content of a decision may also dictate whether an individual engages herself or himself in the decision-making process (Simon, 1985; McGuire & McGuire, 1991). Some decisions may be of little interest to the decision maker, whereas other decisions may engage the decision maker but later be considered unimportant or insignificant by the decision maker. McGuire and McGuire (1991) argued that the personal relevance of an event to an individual influences how much an individual may think about that event, thereby shaping the individual's behavioral actions or decisions in response to that event.

People's response to problems in decision-making situations depends, in part, on how they view the problem. Mithaug (1993) refers to problems as being "relative" (i.e., what may be a problem for one person may not be a problem for another person). An individual's need to engage in active problem solving or decision making arises when an individual wishes to achieve or move closer to unsatisfied goal conditions (Gilhooly, 1989; Mithaug, 1993). Tversky and Kahneman (1981) have talked about the effects of framing, the context within which problems are presented, as being important to decision making. Framing influences the way in which problems are represented for comprehension. A problem presented in different frames may lead to different interpretations of the importance of the situation and the extent to which it merits active decision making.

Motivation also plays a central role in determining which goal a person selects and how she or he evaluates the possible consequences of a decision. Higgins's (1997) regulatory-focus theory posits that individuals regulate themselves in decision-making situations, seeking either promotion-focused or prevention-focused outcomes. Promotion-focused regulation is aimed at seeking motivational goals relating to accomplishment, advancement, nurturance, and growth. On the other hand, prevention-focused regulation is motivated by goals of avoiding danger and loss, maintaining safety, responsibility, and protection. Higgins's theory also implies that fundamentally different motivations may result from the emotions (e.g., hope, optimism, terror, and depression) that arise as a function of the type of regulatory focus an individual chooses to adopt when seeking decision solutions. The type of regulatory focus an individual adopts produces different motivation incentives and different decision outcomes.

Goal selection in decision making is also influenced by a person's orientation toward risk. An individual's inclination to engage or not to engage in risky action is a factor in choice among alternative courses of action. Risk taking has been defined as engaging in an action or inaction that entails a chance of loss, the loss being defined in terms of the decision-maker's beliefs and values (Furby & Beyth-Marom, 1992). Decision theory has been used to estimate an individual's potential for risk taking by examining the components of her or his decision-making process and ability to anticipate the possible outcomes of behaviors (Beyth-Marom, Austin, Fischoff, Palmgren, & Jacobs-Quadrel, 1993; Yates, 1990). Furby and Beyth-Marom (1992) have identified the processes that individuals should follow to minimize risks in decision-making situations. These processes include (a) identifying all the possible response options, (b) identifying possible consequences that may result from each of the listed options, (c) evaluating the desirability of each of those consequences, (d) assessing the likelihood of those consequences, (e) combining all the above steps according to some decision rule to arrive at the best option, given the decision-maker's knowledge, personal values, and perceptions. Furby and Beyth-Marom also emphasized the importance of consequence perception ability by a decision maker in risky situations.

The growing appreciation of the interplay of cognitive, emotional, and motivational factors in decision making presents the need for developing decision-making models that address these factors in an integrated manner. Kuhl (1986) has presented a taxonomy that emphasizes the interdependency of cognition, motivation, and emotion elements in decision making. According to Kuhl, cognition, emotion, and motivation each operate as a separate information-processing subsystem performing unique functions in the process of decision making. The cognitive processes in decision making are involved in mediating the acquisition and representation of knowledge and information upon which decisions are made. The emotional processes are involved in evaluating the personal significance of information collected during decision making. The motivational processes are involved in the selection of goals relating to various alternative courses of action. At various stages of the decision-making process, the three components interact with each other in a variety of ways to determine final decision outcomes (see Kuhl, 1986).

The literature reviewed in this section of the chapter highlights the growing consensus on the interrelatedness among cognitive and noncognitive factors in decision making. This body of work suggests numerous possible explanatory mechanisms for the decision-making difficulties of people with mental retardation. For example, as a way of coping with the overwhelming amount of relevant information needed to fully apply a rational decision-making strategy, individuals with mental retardation may be even more likely than people without mental retardation to disregard some of the information in an effort to simplify the task. Or in light of their cognitive limitations, individuals with mental retardation may be overly reliant on normative–affective factors to guide their decision making. Alternatively, low self-perceptions or personal agency beliefs may undermine the motivation of individuals with mental retardation to choose ambitious goals or to actively engage in a stepwise decision-making process. In the next section, we propose a framework for interpersonal decision-making research with individuals with mental retardation in an effort to encourage systematic research aimed at increasing understanding of individual differences in decision making.

IV. A FRAMEWORK FOR DECISION-MAKING RESEARCH

Previous research on decision making with individuals with mental retardation has focused almost exclusively on the cognitive aspects of this process. The decision-making difficulties of individuals with mental retardation have been attributed primarily to cognitive limitations such as the inability to comprehend a decision-making situation, generate a sufficient range of alternative choice options, or effectively follow a stepwise decision-making process. To date, this body of research has not provided a clear and comprehensive picture of how cognitive factors interact with noncognitive factors to produce specific decision outcomes. However, a broader survey of related research and theory that includes individuals without mental retardation indicates that individual differences in decision making cannot be adequately accounted for in terms of cognition (e.g., Etzioni, 1988; Kuhl, 1986; Short & Evans, 1990). A series of recent studies (e.g., Hickson et al., 1998; Khemka, 1997; Khemka & Hickson, in press), conducted to examine the decision-making performance of individuals with mental retardation in social interpersonal situations, have highlighted several potentially important factors. In particular the study by Hickson et al. (1998) pointed to the relevance of motivational, emotional, and experiential factors, in addition to cognitive factors, in the interpersonal decision-making performance of individuals both with and without mental retardation.

The proposed framework presented in Figure 2 is intended to encourage researchers to adopt a broader focus as they continue the investigation of decision making in individuals with mental retardation. The framework is based on the notion that interpersonal decision making is a multidimensional phenomenon shaped by a number of factors (e.g., Kuhl, 1986), including the cognitive, motivational, and emotional basic process variables identified in the figure. Although the framework reflects the influence of a wide range of previous theoretical and empirical works, it flows most directly from several molar models of self-determination and personal/social competence that have emphasized the importance of decision-making skills for people with mental retardation. For example in their models of self-determination, both Abery (1994) and Wehmeyer (1996) acknowledged decision making as part of the skills base that is necessary for self-determination. In Abery's process model of self-determination, personal choice and decision making were specified, along with self-regulation, personal advocacy, and problem

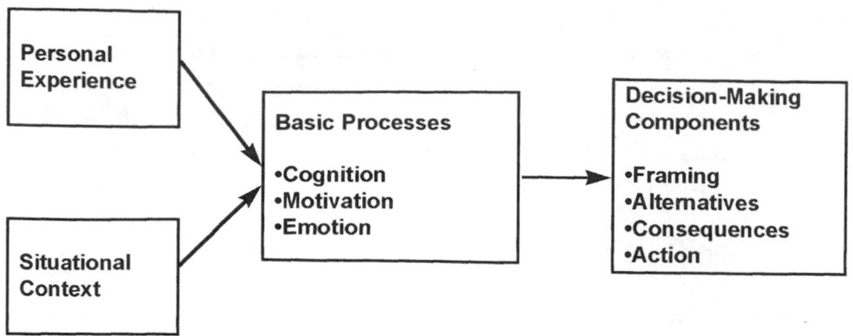

FIG. 2. Framework for interpersonal decision-making research.

solving, as social skills that are essential to the ability to exert personal control. In Wehmeyer's presentation of his model depicting autonomy, self-regulation, self-realization, and psychological empowerment as the four essential elements of self-determination, he listed nine component elements as integral to their development. Choice making, decision making, and problem solving were the first three component elements listed.

Similarly, recent models of personal and social competence have pointed to the centrality of decision-making skills. Decision skills constituted the second stage of Gumpel's (1994) six-stage model of social competence. Gumpel pointed out that by using decision skills to interpret stimuli and generate response options, individuals with mental retardation could develop the competence needed to deal independently with social situations. Decision-making skills are also integral components of two recently proposed models of personal competence (Greenspan & Driscoll, 1997) and social effectiveness (Greenspan, in press). In proposing their 1997 model, which builds upon earlier versions developed by Greenspan and his colleagues (Greenspan, 1979, 1981; Greenspan & Granfield, 1992), Greenspan and Driscoll defined personal competence as a construct comprising "all the skills that contribute to attaining (valued and/or desired) goals or solving challenges" (p. 131). Within the framework depicted in Greenspan and Driscoll's model, decision making can be viewed as an instance of everyday competence, which along with physical competence, affective competence, and academic competence, is one of the four major domains of personal competence. Everyday competence, the "ability to think about and understand problems" (p. 134) in a variety of real-world settings relies upon both practical intelligence and social intelligence. Greenspan's emphasis on social intelligence is maintained in his more recent (in press) dynamic action model aimed at predicting and explaining social effectiveness. In that model, social intelligence, along with context demands, biology, and motivation, is one of four predictors of ineffective social behavior. In that chapter, Greenspan advocates a contextualist strategy for the study of social intelligence, which involves looking at performance with actual problems that are critical to successful functioning in community settings, particularly complex problems involving social ambiguity with the potential for deception, manipulation, and exploitation. Our discussion of the decision-making framework proposed in Figure 2 is very much in keeping with this approach. Although the framework is potentially applicable to other types of decision-making situations, it was developed in the context of our interest in how people with mental retardation handle risky interpersonal situations involving a threat of coercion or abuse.

A. A Proposed Framework

As shown in Figure 2, the proposed framework is designed to assist in determining the relative contributions of three key BASIC PROCESSES in the prediction of decision-making performance and in identifying major loci of individual differences. Although the three processes, cognition, motivation, and emotion, were selected because of their importance in decision making, each of these basic processes has also been implicated as a possible contributor to the decision-making difficulties experienced by people with mental retardation. By including personal experience and situational context as factors that can influence the operation of the three basic processes, we emphasized that the relative contributions of cognition, motivation, and emotion can be expected to vary as a function of personal experience and the specific situational context of the decision. The four decision-making components appear at the right of Figure 2. The specification of the components of the decision-making process itself is intended to underscore the importance of designing future research to monitor the differential effects of key variables on each of the component processes.

The centrality of the role of COGNITION in decision making and as a source of individual differences in all four component processes of decision making is well established. In view of the present focus on decision making in interpersonal conflict situations, which often carry the risk of exploitation and abuse, the contributions of social cognition/social intelligence are of particular interest. Social intelligence, as defined by Greenspan and Driscoll (1997), is the "ability to think about and understand problems found in relationships with other people" (p. 134). People with mental retardation are often characterized by their difficulties in this domain (Greenspan, 1997). Limitations relating to social intelligence have been documented with tasks such as social perspective taking (Affleck, 1977; Bradley & Meredith, 1991), "theory of mind," or ability to reason about the mental states of others (Benson, Abbeduto, Short, Nuccio, & Maas, 1993), and credulity (inability to detect false assertions) and gullibility (vulnerability to being tricked) (Greenspan, in press).

There are many indications that MOTIVATION plays an important role in decision making, in terms of both goal setting and self-perceptions. With respect to goals, research findings have indicated that people with mental retardation are somewhat more likely than others to select goals relating to comfort and safety and less likely to seek goals involving challenge and mastery (Haywood, 1981; Haywood & Switzky, 1986; Koestner, Aube, Ruttner, & Breed, 1995) and that they tend to be more extrinsically than intrinsically motivated (Switzky, 1997). With respect to self-perceptions, or personal agency beliefs, research has indicated that people with mental retardation tend to perceive themselves as having less control over situations than individuals without disabilities, as reflected by an external locus of control and low feelings of self-efficacy (Abery, 1994; Wehmeyer, 1994; Wehmeyer & Palmer, 1997). Taken together, these characteristics may discourage a person with mental retardation from making an effort to actively engage in a stepwise decision-making process or they may limit her or his willingness to consider a wide range of alternative solutions as potentially attainable. The findings of a recent study by Wehmeyer and Kelchner (1994) support this possibility. When they investigated the role of individual perceptions of control, self-efficacy, outcome expectancy, self-esteem, and self-concept in the interpersonal problem-solving performance of individuals with mental retardation, a small (6 to 7%) but significant amount of variability in interpersonal problem-solving scores was accounted for by these factors. Problem solvers who were able to generate a greater number of relevant solutions to problems held significantly higher perceptions of control (measured as greater internality on a locus-of-control scale), self-esteem, and outcome expectancies. Similarly, the proportion of relevant to total solutions to a problem was linked to higher perceptions of control, self-efficacy, outcome expectancies, and self-esteem among the problem solvers. Wehmeyer and Kelchner concluded that the extent to which study participants believed in their ability to exercise control over their environment was predictive of their ability to be efficient as opposed to inefficient problem solvers. In a study exploring the motivational beliefs of individuals with mental retardation, Kreitler and Kreitler (1988) reported that the behavioral rigidity of participants could be reduced by modifying their motivational beliefs.

Emotion and related affective factors have also been identified as potentially important contributors to decision-making. As noted earlier, Etzioni (1988) has asserted that most decisions are made largely on the basis of affective–normative considerations. It is possible that, because of their cognitive limitations, people with mental retardation may be even more inclined than people without mental retardation to bypass a cognitive decision-making process in favor of basing decisions on their emotional involvements or normative commitments. According to Wicker, Wiehe, Hagen and Brown (1994), most decision makers are more likely to act on goals aimed at avoiding negative emotions (e.g., safety-related goals) than goals aimed at seeking positive emotions (e.g., wealth-related goals). The extent to which this is also the case for individuals with mental retardation will have important implications for how they will handle risky situations.

Personal experience was included in the framework to underscore its potential importance in predicting decision making. Personal experience is the avenue through which a decision maker's background knowledge and skills, values, cultural norms and commitments, aspirations, and sensitivities to risk enter the decision-making process. Individuals with mental retardation may lack important relevant experiences, especially with a wide range of independent choice and decision-making situations (e.g., Sands & Kozleski, 1994). Limited personal experience with relevant situations may have a particularly devastating impact on the decision-making capabilities of people with mental retardation because they appear to be even more likely than individuals without mental retardation to base their decisions on past experience rather than a stepwise decision-making process (e.g., Wehmeyer & Kelchner, 1994).

The inclusion of situational context in the framework reflects its essential role in predicting decision outcomes. The type and nature of the decision problem are known to present unique demands for the decision maker (Khemka, 1997), suggesting that it is essential to consider situational variables when studying the decision-making performance of individuals with mental retardation. In a recent study by Khemka and Hickson (in press), women and men with mental retardation made significantly more direct prevention-focused decision responses to video vignettes portraying situations of physical abuse than to situations of sexual or verbal abuse. They also reported significantly more direct prevention-focused responses for sexual abuse situations than for verbal abuse situations. Greenspan and Driscoll (1997) underscored the importance of considering the "full array of task demands, social expectations, and success routes operating in specific situations" (p. 144). It is anticipated that type of decision will function as a "situational moderator" (Humphreys & Revelle, 1984, p. 153) in efforts to predict the likelihood that individuals with mental retardation will make effective decisions and/or employ a stepwise process. As suggested by Greenspan (in press), individuals with mental retardation who may appear competent in routine situations may exhibit incompetence in novel situations. Specifically, Greenspan proposes that a "social intelligence deficit may manifest itself in relatively benign and minor forms in routine social situations, but may be quite disabling (i.e., risk-creating) in situations of deliberate deception and manipulation" (p. 21).

At the far right of the framework in Figure 2, the decision-making components are enumerated, based on various descriptions of the decision-making process found in the literature (e.g., Spivack et al., 1976; Tymchuk et al., 1988). These steps may vary from one situation to another or, as suggested earlier, they may be skipped entirely, especially by individuals with mental retardation who tend to base choices and decisions on past experience, thereby bypassing a stepwise process (e.g., Short & Evans, 1990; Tymchuk et al., 1988, 1990).

The framework proposed in Figure 2 is intended to suggest a systematic approach to identifying the mechanisms and causes of ineffective decision making in individuals with mental retardation. How do cognitive, motivational, emotional, and experiential variables combine to influence a particular decision? How do attributes of the situational context influence the demands imposed on a decision maker? Which personal experience factors are most central to the decision-making difficulties of people with mental retardation? Finally, given the complex, interactive nature of decision making, what kind of decision aids, tools, and intervention strategies will be most helpful in improving the decision-making strategies of people with mental retardation? By outlining some of the underlying dimensions of decision making, the framework offers a structure for understanding the processes of decision making in individuals with mental retardation across different life situations and for developing and empirically validating effective decision-making training methods.

B. Preliminary Application of the Framework

Preliminary empirical support for this framework is provided by the findings of a recent study in which Hickson and Khemka (1998) examined the potential of several variables suggested by the theoretical and empirical literature to predict decision-making performance of adults with mild mental retardation in video situations involving interpersonal conflict and abuse. Predictor variables included: IQ, fact comprehension, inference comprehension, and comprehension of emotions/feelings, self-efficacy, locus of control, degree of community independence (based on how often participants reported going out in the community on their own), and degree of residential independence. The three comprehension measures were based on responses to a series of brief, verbally presented interpersonal decision situations followed by multiple-choice questions pertaining to facts, inferences, or the feelings of the key decision maker in the passages.

A stepwise multiple regression analysis, with each of these variables entered as potential predictors, was conducted with effective decision-making scores as the criterion variable. Decision-making responses were scored as effective if the participants were able to suggest either an independent or other-dependent action to resolve the conflict presented in the vignette. Eighty-eight adults (44 women, 44 men) with mild mental retardation participated in this study. The multiple regression analysis was completed in four steps that accounted for 39% of the variance. The four factors that contributed to the proportion of the variance accounted for were IQ (16%), self-efficacy (10%), community independence (8%), and comprehension of emotions and feelings (5%). These four predictors spanned the three basic process factors at the center of the framework in Figure 2 (*cognition*: IQ; *motivation*: self-efficacy; *emotion*: comprehension of emotions and feelings) as well as *personal experience* (community independence).

C. Generality of the Framework

The decision-making framework presented in Figure 2 is not exhaustive in addressing all the issues that may be pertinent to the study of decision making among individuals with mental retardation. The framework was developed in the context of research studies that have focused primarily on the interpersonal decision making performance of adults with mild and moderate mental retardation. The framework is intended to be a model-in-progress that provides a comprehensive picture of the current understanding of the decision-making processes of individuals with mental retardation and that can serve as a guide for future research in this area.

Individual decision-making behavior develops in a social-cultural context. The role of culture in shaping individual decision-making styles and strategies may be significant (Radford et al., 1993; Wright, 1985). The study of cultural influences on decision-making performance of individuals with mental retardation is virtually absent. A recent study by Edeh (1998), although conducted within the domain of interpersonal problem solving rather than decision making, indicated that cultural factors play a critical role in determining the problem-solving styles of individuals with mental retardation, with children in Nigeria using more cooperative interpersonal problem-solving styles than either African-American or Euro-American children in the United States. Future examination of interpersonal decision making in individuals with mental retardation will need to address the potentially complex influences of cultural factors on performance.

The utility of the framework for application with younger age groups will also need to be assessed. In general, the study of developmental issues in decision making from childhood to adulthood has been modest (Byrnes & McClenny, 1994; Furby & Beyth-Marom, 1992). Byrnes and McClenny found adolescents and adults to differ in their decision-making strategies. In a study by Khemka, Chatzistyli, Hickson, Manhertz, Miano, and Yamusah (1996), the interpersonal decision-making strategies of adolescents and adults with developmental disabilities were compared. Significant differences in decision-making performance related to the age of the participants were found, with younger participants suggesting more risk-taking actions and showing lower consequence-perception ability.

D. Methodological Considerations

An underlying purpose of this chapter is to stimulate high-quality, systematic research on decision making in individuals with mental retardation. Although the literature review and proposed framework are offered with that end in mind, several methodological issues pose potential barriers to the production of a cohesive body of research and theory on this topic. In this section, the issues are discussed along with some suggestions on how they might be addressed.

First, the decision-making situational context determines the level and nature of decision-making task demands. The possible task variations in this domain are extensive. At the present time, no clear basis has been established in the literature for comparing studies that use widely varying versions of problem-solving or decision-making tasks. To address this issue, it is important for researchers to reach a consensus on operational definitions of problem solving and decision making and to use consistent terminology to identify the tasks used in their studies. As suggested earlier in this chapter, the term *problem solving* might best be reserved for tasks in which a goal state is specified and the problem solver is required only to provide strategies for reaching that goal. The term decision making could then be reserved for tasks in which the goal state is not specified and the decision maker must select a goal as well as strategies for attaining it. Comparisons among decision-making research studies would also be facilitated to the extent that studies could be classified according to one or more taxonomies of task variations across situational context domains. An example of one such taxonomy is presented in Figure 3, which identifies three domains of decision making. The shaded panel at the right of the figure highlights interpersonal decision-making situations, which have been the focus of this chapter. Examples of impersonal decision-making situations that focus on the decision-maker's activities in relation to abstract tasks or inanimate objects are shown in the panel at the left of the figure. Personal decision-making situations that focus on decisions concerning primarily the decision-maker herself or himself are included in the center panel. The top and bottom portions of the

	Impersonal	Personal	Interpersonal	
			Self orientation	Social orientation
Minor / minimal consequences	• Abstract problems • Games • Puzzles	• Food • Clothing • Exercise	• Peer relations • Family and supervisor relations • Dating	• Workplace conduct • Community responsibility • Social ethics
Major / significant consequences	• Work machinery • Computers • Home appliances	• Health / medical • Housing • Financial / employment	• Physical danger • Sexual, physical and verbal abuse • Manipulation / trickery	• Child care • Parenting • Stealing / crime related

FIG. 3. Domains of decision making.

figure are differentiated according to the seriousness of the decision in terms of its potential impact. The decision situations in the top section of the figure can generally be classified as having minor or minimal consequences (low risk), whereas the decision situations in the bottom section can be classified as having major or significant consequences (high risk). For impersonal and personal decisions, consequences would affect primarily the self. However, for interpersonal decisions, consequences may be viewed in terms of their impact on either the self (self-orientation) or others (social orientation).

A second methodological issue pertains to the wide range of measurement approaches and scoring criteria that have been used in the existing research studies on decision making. These variations and inconsistencies have posed major barriers to comparisons among studies. Measurement is complicated by the multiple modes of presentation used to present the decision-making situations, including verbally presented vignettes of various lengths, video scenarios, and role-play situations. Although most studies have employed self-report measures, some have utilized multiple-choice and short-answer formats. As pointed out by Heal and Sigelman (1995), all of these measures pose risks of response biases when used with respondents with mental retardation. There has been particular confusion surrounding the selection of criteria for scoring self-report responses. We believe that much of this confusion stems from lack of agreement on an operational definition of effective decision making. Although some investigators have focused on cognitive criteria, like number of steps enumerated, others have focused on the content of the decision response itself in terms of the type of goal selected (e.g., prevention-focused action to escape from threat of physical harm). We propose, as shown in Table II, that scoring methods be explicitly linked to the domain of the decision and the specific situational context. For example, in a routine situation of

TABLE II

GUIDE FOR SCORING DECISION-MAKING RESPONSES FOR SITUATIONS INVOLVING INTERPERSONAL CONFLICT AND ABUSE

Interpersonal conflict situations	Abuse situations
Effective or vigilant decision making	Prevention-focused decision making
• Independent action or negotiation	• Independent direct prevention-focused action
• Other dependent action/reporting/ seeking help or advice	• Other-dependent action/reporting/seeking help or assistance
Noneffective decison making	Nonprevention-focused decison making
• Maladaptive decision	• Ineffective prevention
Hypervigilant	Impulsive/hasty reaction
Avoidant	Avoiding/delaying action
Complacent	Complying with abuse
• No decision	• No decision

interpersonal conflict or disagreement with minor consequences, an effective decision may involve compromise or negotiation. However, in an abuse situation, an effective decision may require the decision maker to take immediate independent action to escape from the abuse.

A final and extremely important methodological issue is that ecological validity is a concern in almost all of the existing studies involving people with mental retardation, especially the training studies. Improved responses to interview questions, simulated video situations, or role-play activities do not guarantee improved performance in real-life community situations. The steps required for generalization from research tasks and settings to real-life decisions must be clearly specified and incorporated into future studies. We believe that research with hypothetical situations that are carefully designed to span a particular domain of decision making can provide a valuable starting point for gaining a better understanding of the decision-making processes of people with mental retardation. The findings of research with a wide range of hypothetical situations, which can be manipulated to include situational contexts where another person is portrayed as the decision maker and those where the self is the decision maker, can provide a conceptual base for the development of intervention approaches that are calibrated to the demands of specific situational contexts. Finally, research will need to focus on the generalization of acquired decision-making skills and strategies to the types of real-life situations that can make a meaningful difference in the lives of people with mental retardation.

V. CONCLUSIONS AND FUTURE DIRECTIONS

The final section of the chapter includes a brief synopsis of the current state of knowledge about decision making in people with mental retardation. The chapter ends with a discussion of some suggested directions for the kinds of future research that will be needed if we are to empower individuals with mental retardation to make effective, independent, and self-protective decisions in all aspects of their lives.

A. Conclusions

As part of a growing acknowledgment that people with disabilities have a right to be fully participating, self-determined members of the community, people with mental retardation are increasingly faced with making their own decisions, important ones as well as unimportant ones. Unfortunately, the limited decision-making competence of many individuals with mental retardation is well documented, especially in nonroutine, potentially manipulative and coercive interpersonal situations. In one study, Hickson et al. (1998) reported effective decision making in response to hypothetical interpersonal situations about 50% of the time for adults with mental retardation in contrast to about 92% of the time for adults without mental retardation. In a specific example from that study, one of the vignettes portrayed a situation which was similar to the initiating event in the Glen Ridge, New Jersey, case that involved the sexual assault of a young woman with mental retardation by a group of young men. In that vignette, Jeff, who has made fun of Emily in the past, attempts to entice Emily to accompany him to the house of two of his friends by promising her a date with his brother. All but one of the respondents without mental retardation said that Emily should not go with Jeff. However, only one-third of the respondents with mental retardation said that Emily should not go with Jeff. Even with the limited existing research, it is clear that community participation may involve significant risks of harm and victimization for individuals with mental retardation unless their decision-making competence can be enhanced.

To date, several specific shortcomings in the decision making of people with mental retardation have been reported. In many situations, people with mental retardation appear not to apply a stepwise decision-making process, but seem to rely on a limited number of solutions drawn from their past experience that they apply to new situations in a "rigid," inflexible manner. In other situations, people with mental retardation may attempt to apply a stepwise decision-making process, but with limited success at each stage of the process. Specifically, it has been reported that people with mental retardation tend to construct representations of situations that do not adequately frame the problem, generate fewer relevant alternative solutions and strategies, are less able to anticipate consequences of possible courses of action, and are less likely to select an appropriate course of action. Although there are indications that gender, age, culture, and level of intelligence, especially social intelligence, may play an important role in decision making, little is known about specifically how they operate.

The success of existing training studies has been limited. Many of these studies have focused upon problem-solving situations that emphasized the generation of alternative strategies rather than engagement in the entire decision-making process. Most studies, addressing "repertoire" deficits rather than "performance" deficits, have failed to assess the application of acquired strategies in natural settings. Although it has been demonstrated that it is possible to teach a stepwise decision-making process to individuals with mental retardation, application of that process has not necessarily led to higher quality decisions. The findings of a recent study (Khemka, 1997) suggest that it will be necessary to employ more broad-based training approaches that address motivational, as well as cognitive, issues in order to obtain meaningful improvements in decision quality.

B. Future Directions

Drawing upon theory and research involving individuals with and without mental retardation, we offer several suggestions for future research on decision making.

First, we have proposed a framework (see Figure 2) aimed at broadening the scope of decision-making research in mental retardation. We hope that the framework will stimulate research that will increase understanding of how cognitive, motivational, and emotional processes contribute to decision making in various situational contexts. It will be important to identify the types of situation in which effective decisions may be based on experiential or normative–affective considerations without undue risk to the decision maker as opposed to those situations where a deliberative decision-making process must be applied to achieve valued goals and avoid harm.

Second, it is essential to develop methods for assessing and profiling individual strengths and weaknesses across decision-making domains in a wide range of high- and low-risk situational contexts (see Figure 3). The relative merits of a variety of measurement strategies should be explored, including verbal interviews, video presentations, role-play situations, and observations in natural settings. Items on these measurement instruments should resemble as closely as possible real-life situations likely to be encountered by individuals with mental retardation in their everyday lives.

Third, research is needed to identify key sources of individual differences in decision-making competence. This research should be sensitive to the influences of gender, culture, age, and ability.

Fourth, building on the work of Khemka (1997), studies are needed to develop effective interventions for individuals representing a range of decision-making profiles. These interventions should teach participants how to identify situations where it is necessary to apply a stepwise, cognitive decision-making process and how to apply such a process. Training methods should also include components that address motivational issues, such as self-perceptions—or personal agency beliefs—and goals clarification as well as components that address emotional factors.

Finally, research is needed to explore the usefulness of structural supports for the maintenance and generalization of improved decision-making strategies. These structures might include various types of school-based or community-based support groups and self-advocacy groups that can provide expanded opportunities for decision making as well as a supportive environment that allows participants to examine pending decisions as well as obtain any necessary protections in the event of serious threat of harm. The long-term goal of these groups would be the empowerment of individuals with mental retardation as independent decision makers who can effectively handle the variety of challenges they encounter in their lives in the community.

ACKNOWLEDGMENTS

We would like to thank Harriet Golden and Michael L. Wehmeyer for their very helpful comments on this chapter.

REFERENCES

Abbeduto, L., Furman, L., & Davies, B. (1989). Relation between the receptive language and mental age of persons with mental retardation. *American Journal on Mental Retardation, 93*, 535–543.

Abery, B. (1994). A conceptual framework for enhancing self-determination. In M. Hayden & B. Abery (Eds.), *Challenges for a service system in transition* (pp. 345–380). Baltimore, MD: Brookes.

Affleck, G. G. (1977). Interpersonal competencies of the mentally retarded: A Piagetian perspective. In P. Mittler (Ed.), *Research to practice in mental retardation, education and training*, Vol. II. Baltimore, MD: University Park Press.

Anderson, J. R. (1990). *Cognitive psychology and its implications* (3rd ed.). New York: W. H. Freeman.

Baddeley, A. (1986). *Working memory*. Oxford: Oxford University Press.

Bandura, A. (1982). Self-efficacy mechanism in human agency. *American Psychologist, 37*, 122–147.

Benson, G., Abbeduto, L., Short, K., Nuccio, J. B., & Maas, F. (1993). Development of a theory of mind in individuals with mental retardation. *American Journal on Mental Retardation, 98*, 427–433.

Beyth-Marom, R., Austin, L., Fischoff, B., Palmgren, C., & Jacobs-Quadrel, M. J. (1993). Perceived consequences of risky behaviors: Adults and adolescents. *Developmental Psychology, 29*, 549–563.

Bilsky, L. H. (1985). Comprehension and mental retardation. In N. R. Ellis & N. Bray (Eds.), *International review of research in mental retardation, Vol 13* (pp. 215–246). Orlando, FL: Academic Press.

Bradley, L. J., & Meredith, R. C. (1991). Interpersonal development: A study with children classified as educable mentally retarded. *Education and Training in Mental Retardation, 26*, 130–141.

Braine, M.D.S. (1978). On the relation between the natural logic of reasoning and standard logic. *Psychological Review, 85*, 1–21.

Brown, F., Belz, P., Corsi, L., & Wenig, B. (1993). Choice diversity for people with severe disabilities. *Education and Training in Mental Retardation, 28*, 318–326.

Browning, P., & Nave, G. (1993). Teaching social problem-solving to learners with mild disabilities. *Education and Training in Mental Retardation and Developmental Disabilities, 28*, 309–317.

Burnett, P. C., Mann, L., & Beswick, G. (1989). Validation of the Flinders Decision Making Questionnaire in course decision-making. *Australian Psychologist, 24*, 285–292.

Byrnes, J. P., & McClenny, B. (1994). Decision-making in young adolescents and adults. *Journal of Experimental Child Psychology, 58*, 359–388.

Cacioppo, J. T., & Petty, R. E. (1982). The need for cognition. *Journal of Personality and Social Psychology, 42*, 116–131.

Camic, C. (1992). The matter of habit. In M. Zey (Ed.). *Decision making: Alternatives to rational choice theory* (pp. 185–232). Newbury Park, CA: Sage Publications.

Carroll, J. S., & Johnson, E. J. (1990). *Decision research: A field guide*. Newbury Park, CA: Sage Publications.

Castles, E. E., and Glass, C. R. (1986). Training in social and interpersonal problem-solving skills for mildly and moderately mentally retarded adults. *American Journal of Mental Deficiency, 91*, 35–42.

Clore, G. L., Schwarz, N., & Conway, M. (1994). Affective causes and consequences of social information processing. In R. S. Wyer & T. K. Srull (Eds.). *Handbook of social cognition*, Vol. 1. (pp. 323–417). Hillsdale, NJ: Erlbaum.

Coleman, M., Wheeler, L., & Webber, J. (1993). Research on interpersonal problem-solving training: A review. *Remedial and Special Education, 14*(2), 25–37.

Corbin, R. (1980). Decisions that might not get made. In T. S. Wallsten (Ed.) *Cognitive processes in choice and decision behavior* (pp. 47–68). Hillsdale, NJ: Erlbaum.

D'Zurilla, T. J., & Goldfried, M. R. (1971). Problem solving and behavior modification. *Journal of Abnormal Psychology, 78*, 107–126.

Dattilo, J., & Rusch, F. R. (1985). Effects of choice on leisure participation for persons with severe handicaps. *Journal of the Association for Persons with Severe Handicaps, 10*, 194–199.

Dawes, R. (1988). *Rational choice in an uncertain world*. New York: Harcourt Brace Jovanovich.

Deci, E. L., & Ryan, R. M. (1987). The dynamics of self-determination in personality and development. In R. Schwarzer (Ed.), *Self-regulated cognitions in anxiety and motivation* (pp. 171–194). Hillsdale, NJ: Erlbaum.

Edeh, O. (1998). *Social interpersonal problem-solving and culture: The effect of general cognitive strategy training among students with mild mental retardation*. Unpublished doctoral dissertation, Teachers College, Columbia University, New York, NY.

Einhorn, H. J., & Hogarth, R. M. (1981). Behavioral decision theory: Processes of judgement and choice. *Annual Review of Psychology, 32*, 53–88.

Elms, A. C. (1976). *Personality and politics*. New York: Harcourt Brace Jovanovich.

Elster, J. (1985). Sadder but wiser? Rationality and the emotions. *Social Science Information, Vol. 24* (pp. 375–406). London: Sage Publications.

Epstein, S. (1994). Integration of the cognitive and the psychodynamic unconscious. *American Psychologist, 49*, 709–724.

Etzioni, A. (1988). Normative-affective factors: Toward a new decision-making model. *Journal of Economic-Psychology, 9*, 125–150.

Evans, J.St.B.T. (Ed.). (1983). *Thinking and reasoning: Psychological approaches*. London: Routledge & Kegan Paul.

Ferretti, R. P., & Cavalier, A. R. (1991). Constraints on the problem solving of persons with mental retardation. In N. W. Bray (Ed.), *International review of research in mental retardation, Vol. 17*, (pp. 153–192). New York: Academic Press.

Fischhoff, B. (1975). Hindsight = foresight: The effect of outcome knowledge on judgement under uncertainty. *Journal of Experimental Psychology: Human Perception and Performance, 1*, 288–299.

Fischhoff, B. (1982). Debiasing. In D. Kahneman, P. Slovic, & A. Tversky (Eds.). *Judgement under uncertainty: Heuristics and Biases*. New York: Cambridge University Press.

Ford, M. E. (1992). *Motivating humans: Goals, emotions, and personal agency beliefs*. Newbury Park, CA: Sage Publications.

Ford, M. E. (1995). Motivation and competence development in special and remedial education. *Intervention in School and Clinic, 31*, 70–83.

Furby, L., & Beyth-Marom, R. (1992). Risk taking in adolescence: A decision-making perspective. *Developmental Review, 12*, 1–44.

Gilhooly, K. J. (1989). (Ed.). *Human and machine problem-solving*. New York: Plenum Press.

Gilovich, T., Vallone, R., & Tversky, A. (1985). The hot hand in basketball: On the misperception of random sequences. *Cognitive Psychology, 17*, 295–314.

Greenspan, S. (1979). Social intelligence in the retarded. In N. R. Ellis (Ed.), *Handbook of mental deficiency, psychological theory and research* (2nd ed., pp. 483–531). Hillsdale, NJ: Erlbaum.

Greenspan, S. (1981). Defining childhood social competence: A proposed working model. In B. K. Keogh (Ed.), *Advances in special education*, Vol. 3. (pp. 1–39). Greenwich, CT: JAI Press.

Greenspan, S. (1997). Dead manual walking? Why the 1992 definition needs redoing. *Education and Training in Mental Retardation and Developmental Disabilities, 32*, 179–190.

Greenspan, S. (in press). A contextualist perspective on adaptive behavior. In R. Schalock (Ed.), *Adaptive behavior: Conceptual basis, measurement, and use*. Washington, DC: AAMR.

Greenspan, S., & Driscoll, J. (1997). The role of intelligence in a broad model of personal competence. In P. P. Flanagan, J. L. Genshaft, & P. L. Harrison (Eds.), *Contemporary intellectual assessment: Theories, tests, and issues*. New York: Guilford.

Greenspan, S., & Granfield, J. M. (1992), Reconsidering the construct of mental retardation: Implications of a model of social competence. *American Journal on Mental Retardation, 96*, 442–453.

Gumpel, T. (1994). Social competence and social skills training for persons with mental retardation: An expansion of a behavioral paradigm. *Education and Training in Mental Retardation and Developmental Disabilities, 29*, 194–201.

Haywood, H. C. (1981). Reducing social vulnerability is the challenge of the eighties (AAMD Presidential Address). *Mental Retardation, 19*, 190–195.

Haywood, H. C., & Switzky, H. N. (1986). Intrinsic motivation and behavior effectiveness in retarded persons. In N. R. Ellis & N. W. Bray (Eds.), *International review of research in mental retardation, Vol. 14*. Orlando, FL: Academic Press.

Heal, L. W., & Sigelman, C. K. (1995). Response biases in interviews of individuals with limited mental ability. *Journal of Intellectual Disability Research, 39*, 331–340.

Healey, K. N., & Masterpasqua, F. (1992). Interpersonal cognitive problem-solving among children with mild mental retardation. *American Journal on Mental Retardation, 96*, 367–372.

Hickson, L., Golden, H., Khemka, I., Urv, T., & Yamusah, S. (1998). A closer look at interpersonal decision making in adults with and without mental retardation. *American Journal on Mental Retardation, 103*, 209–224.

Hickson, L., & Khemka, I. (1998). *Examining social interpersonal decision-making skills of adults with mental retardation: Implications for training*. Paper presented at the Gatlinburg Conference on Research and Theory in Mental Retardation and Developmental Disabilities, Charleston, SC.

Higgins, E. T. (1997). Beyond pleasure and pain. *American Psychologist, 52*, 1280–1300.

Hogarth, J. (1987). *Judgement and choice: The psychology of decision* (2nd ed). New York: John Wiley.

Houghton, J., Bronicki, B., & Guess, D. (1987). Opportunities to express preferences and make choices among students with severe disabilities in classroom settings. *Journal of the Association for Persons with Severe Handicaps, 12*, 18–27.

Humphreys, M. S., & Revelle, W. (1984). Personality, motivation, and performance: A theory of the relationship between individual differences and information processing. *Psychological Review, 91*, 153–184.

Inhelder, B., & Piaget, J. (1958). *The growth of logical thinking*. New York: Basic Books.

Janis, I. L. (1974). Vigilance and decision-making in personal crises. In D. A. Hamburg & C. V. Coelho (Eds.), *Coping and adaptation*. New York: Academic Press.

Janis, I. L., & Mann, L. (1977). *Decision making: A psychological analysis of conflict, choice and commitment*. New York: The Free Press.

Jenkinson, J., & Nelms, R. (1994). Patterns of decision-making behaviour by people with intellectual disability: An exploratory study. *Australia and New Zealand Journal of Developmental Disabilities, 19*, 99–109.

Jiranek, D., & Kirby, N. (1990). The job satisfaction and/or psychological well-being of young adults with an intellectual disability and nondisabled young adults in either sheltered employment, competitive employment or unemployment. *Australia and New Zealand Journal of Developmental Disabilities, 16*, 133–148.

Johnson-Laird, P. N. (1975). Models of deduction. In R. J. Falmagne (Ed.), *Reasoning: Representation and process*. Hillsdale, NJ: Erlbaum.

Johnson-Laird, P. N., & Byrne, R. (1991). *Deduction*. Hillsdale, NJ: Erlbaum.

Kahneman, D., Slovic, P., & Tversky, A. (Eds.). (1982). *Judgement under uncertainty: Heuristics and biases*. New York: Cambridge University Press.

Kahneman, D., & Tversky, A. (1979). Prospect theory: An analysis of decision under risk. *Econometrica, 47*, 263–291.

Khemka, I. (1997). *Increasing independent decision-making skills of women with mental retardation in response to social interpersonal situations of abuse*. Unpublished doctoral dissertation, Teachers College, Columbia University, New York, NY.

Khemka, I., Chatzistyli, K., Hickson, L., Manhertz, P., Miano, J., & Yamusah, S. (1996). *Risk perception and decision-making in interpersonal situations*. Paper presented at the Gatlinburg Conference on Research and Theory in Mental Retardation and Developmental Disabilities, Gatlinburg, TN.

Khemka, I., & Hickson, L. (in press). Decision making by adults with mental retardation in simulated situations of abuse. *Mental Retardation*.

Kishi, V., Teelucksingh, B., Zollers, N., Park-Lee, S., & Meyer, L. (1988). Daily decision-making in community residences: A social comparison of adults with and without mental retardation. *American Journal on Mental Retardation, 92*, 430–435.

Klayman, J. (1985). Children's decision strategies and their adaptation to task characteristics. *Organizational Behavior and Human Decision Processes, 35*, 179–201.

Koegel, R. L., Dyer, K., & Bell, L. K. (1987). The influence of child-preferred activities on autistic children's social behavior. *Journal of Applied Behavior Analysis, 20*, 243–252.

Koestner, R., Aube, J., Ruttner, J., & Breed, S. (1995). Theories of ability and the pursuit of challenge among adolescents with mild mental retardation. *Journal of Intellectual Disability Research, 39*, 57–65.

Kreitler, S., & Kreitler, H. (1988). The cognitive approach to motivation in retarded individuals. In N. R. Ellis & N. W. Bray (Eds.), *International review of research in mental retardation, Vol. 15*. Orlando, FL: Academic Press.

Kruglanski, A. W. (1996). A motivated gatekeeper of our minds. In R. M. Sorrentino & E. T. Higgins (Eds.), *Handbook of motivation and cognition*. New York: Guilford.

Kuhl, J. (1986). Motivation and information processing. In M. Sorrentino & E. T. Higgins (Eds.), *Handbook of motivation and cognition*. New York: Guilford.

Lefcourt, H. M. (1982). *Locus of control: Current trends in theory and research* (2nd Ed.). Hillsdale, NJ: Erlbaum.

Lent, R. W., & Hackett, G. (1987). Career self-efficacy: Empirical status and future directions. *Journal of Vocational Behavior, 30*, 347–382.

Mann, L., Harmoni, R., & Power, C. (1989). Adolescent decision-making: The development of competence. *Journal of Adolescence, 12*, 265–278.

Martella, R. C., Marchand-Martella, N. E., & Agran, M. (1993, July–September). Using a problem-solving strategy to teach adaptability skills to individuals with mental retardation. *Journal of Rehabilitation*, 55–60.

Maslow, A. H. (1962). *Toward a psychology of being*. Princeton, NJ: Nostrand.

Maule, A. J., & Mackie, P. (1990). A componential investigation of the effects of deadlines on individual decision-making. In K. Borcherding, O. I. Larichev, & D. M., Messick (Eds.), *Contemporary issues in decision making*. Amsterdam: North-Holland.

McGuire, W. J., & McGuire, C. V. (1991). The content, structure, and operation of thought systems. In Wyer, R. S., & Srull, T. K. (Eds.), *Advances in social cognition*, Vol. IV. Hillsdale, NJ: Erlbaum.

Miller, G. A. (1956). The magical number 7 + or − 2: Some limits on our capacity for information processing. *Psychological Review, 63*, 81–87.

Mithaug, D. E. (1993). *Self-regulation theory. How optimal adjustment maximizes gain*. Westport, CT: Praeger.

Morris, C. D., Niederbuhl, J. M., & Mahr, J. M. (1993). Determining the capability of individuals with mental retardation to give informed consent. *American Journal on Mental Retardation, 98*, 263–272.

Newell, A., & Simon, H. A. (1972). *Human problem solving*. Englewood Cliffs, NJ: Prentice-Hall.

Nezu, C. M., Nezu, A. M., & Arean, P. (1991). Assertiveness and problem-solving training for mildly mentally retarded persons with dual diagnosis. *Research in Developmental Disabilities, 12*, 371–386.

Oaksford, M., & Chater, N. (1993). Reasoning theories and bounded rationality. In K. I. Manktelow & D. E. Over (Ed.), *Psychological and philosophical perspectives*. New York: Routledge.

Ollendick, T. H., Greene, R. W., Francis, G., & Baum, C. G. (1991). Sociometric status: Its stability and validity among neglected, rejected and popular children. *Journal of Child Psychology and Psychiatry*, 525–534.

Park, H. S., & Gaylord-Ross, R. (1989). A problem-solving approach to social skills training in employment settings with mentally retarded youth. *Journal of Applied Behavior Analysis, 22*, 373–380.

Payne, J. W. (1976). Task complexity and contingent processing in decision-making: An information search and protocol analysis. *Organizational Behavior and Human Performance, 16*, 366–387.

Platt, J., & Spivack, G. (1989). *The MEPS procedure manual*. Philadelphia: Department of Mental Health Sciences, Hahnemann University.

Radford, M. H., Mann, L., Ohta, Y., & Nakane, Y. (1993). Differences between Australian and Japanese students in decisional self-esteem, decisional stress, and coping styles. *Journal of Cross-Cultural Psychology, 24*, 284–297.

Ross, D. M., & Ross, S. A. (1973). Cognitive training for the EMR child: Situational problem solving and planning. *American Journal of Mental Deficiency, 78*, 20–26.

Ross, D. M., & Ross, S. A. (1978). Cognitive training for EMR children: Choosing the best alternative. *American Journal of Mental Deficiency, 82*, 598–601.

Sands, D. J., & Kozleski, E. B. (1994). Quality of life differences between adults with and without disabilities. *Education and Training in Mental Retardation, 29*, 90–101.

Short, E. J., & Evans, S. W. (1990). Individual differences in cognitive and social problem-solving skills as a function of intelligence. In N. W. Bray (Ed.), *International review of research in mental retardation, Vol 16* (pp. 89–123). San Diego, CA: Academic Press.

Simon, H. A. (1957). *Administrative behavior* (2nd ed.). New York: Macmillan.

Simon, H. A. (1967). Motivational and emotional controls of cognition. *Psychological Review, 74*, 29–39.

Simon, H. A. (1974). How big is a chunk? *Science, 183*, 482–488.

Simon, H. A. (1985). Human nature in politics: The dialogue of psychology with political science. *American Political Science Review, 79*, 293–304.

Simon, H. A., Dantzig, G. B., Hogarth, B., Plott, C. R., Raiffa, H., Schelling, T. C., Shepsle, K. A., Thaler, R., Tversky, A., & Winter, S. (1986). *Decision making and problem solving. Report of the Research Briefing Panel on Decision Making and Problem Solving by the National Academy of Sciences*. Washington, DC: National Academy Press.

Smith, D. C. (1986). Interpersonal problem-solving skills of retarded and nonretarded children. *Applied Research in Mental Retardation, 7*, 431–442.

Sobsey, D. (1994). *Violence and abuse in the lives of people with disabilities: The end of silent acceptance*. Baltimore: Brookes.

Sobsey, D., & Doe, T. (1991). Patterns of sexual abuse and assault. *Journal of Sexuality and Disability, 9*, 243–259.

Spaulding, W. D. (1994). Introduction. In W. D. Spaulding (Ed.), *Integrative views of motivation, cognition, and emotion, Vol. 41 of the Nebraska Symposium on Motivation* (pp. ix–xii). Lincoln, NB: University of Nebraska Press.

Spitz, H. H., Webster, N. A., & Borys, S. V. (1982). Further studies of the tower of Hanoi problem-solving performance of retarded young adults and nonretarded children. *Developmental Psychology, 18*, 922–930.

Spivack, G., Platt, J. J., & Shure, M. B. (1976). *The problem-solving approach to adjustment*. San Francisco, CA: Jossey-Bass.

Strain, P. S., Cooke, T. P., & Appolloni, T. (1976). *Teaching exceptional children: Assessing and modifying social behavior*. New York: Academic Press.

Sundram, C. J., & Stavis, P. F. (1994). Sexuality and mental retardation: Unmet challenges. *Mental Retardation, 32*, 255–264.

Svenson, O. (1979). Process descriptions of decision making. *Organizational Behavior and Human Performance, 23*, 86–112.

Svenson, O., & Maule, A. J. (Eds.) (1993). *Time pressure and stress in human judgement and decision making*. New York: Plenum.

Switzky, H. N. (1997). Individual differences in personality and motivational systems in persons with mental retardation. In W. E. MacLean (Ed.), *Ellis' handbook of mental deficiency, psychological theory and research* (3rd ed.). Mahwah, NJ: Erlbaum.

Toda, M. (1980). Emotion in decision-making. *Acta Psychologica, 45*, 133–155.

Tustin, R. D., & Bond, M. J. (1991). Assessing the ability to give informed consent to medical and dental procedures. *Australia and New Zealand Journal of Developmental Disabilities, 17*, 35–47.

Tversky, A., & Kahneman, D. (1974). Judgment under uncertainty: Heuristics and biases. *Science, 185*, 1124–1131.

Tversky, A., & Kahneman, D. (1981). The framing of decisions and the psychology of choice. *Science, 211*, 453–458.

Tymchuk, A. J., Andron, L., & Rahbar, B. (1988). Effective decision-making/problem-solving training with mothers who have mental retardation. *American Journal on Mental Retardation, 92*, 510–516.

Tymchuk, A. J., Yokota, A., & Rahbar, B. (1990). Decision-making abilities of mothers with mental retardation. *Research in Developmental Disabilities, 11*, 97–109.

Vaughn, S. R., Ridley, C. A., & Cox, J. (1983). Evaluating the efficacy of an interpersonal training program with children who are mentally retarded. *Education and Training of the Mentally Retarded, 18*, 191–206.

Verplanken, B. (1993). Need for cognition and external information search: Responses to time pressure during decision-making. *Journal of Resarch in Personality, 27*, 238–252.

von Neumann, J., & Morgenstern, O. (1944). *Theory of games and economic behavior*. Princeton, NJ: Princeton University Press.

Ward, M. J. (1988). The many facets of self-determination. In NICHY National Information Center for Children and Youth with Disabilities, *Transition Summary, 5*, 2–3.

Wehmeyer, M. L. (1992). Self-determination and the education of students with mental retardation. *Education and Training in Mental Retardation, 27*, 302–314.

Wehmeyer, M. L. (1994). Perceptions of self-determination and psychological empowerment of adolescents with mental retardation. *Education and Training in Mental Retardation and Developmental Disabilities, 29*, 9–21.

Wehmeyer, M. L. (1996). Self-determination as an educational outcome. In D. J. Sands & M. L. Wehmeyer (Eds.), *Self-determination across the life span*. Baltimore: Brookes.

Wehmeyer, M. L. (1998). Self-determination and individuals with significant disabilities: Examining meanings and misinterpretations. *Journal of the Association for Persons with Severe Handicaps, 23*, 5–16.

Wehmeyer, M. L., & Kelchner, K. (1994). Interpersonal cognitive problem-solving skills of individuals with mental retardation. *Education and Training in Mental Retardation and Developmental Disabilities, 29*, 265–278.

Wehmeyer, M. L., & Palmer, S. B. (1997). Perceptions of control of students with and without cognitive disabilities. *Psychological Reports, 81*, 195–206.

Wicker, F. W., Wiehe, J. A., Hagen, A. S., & Brown, G. (1994). From wishing to intending: Differences in salience of positive versus negative consequences. *Journal of Personality, 62*, 347–368.

Wright, G. N. (1985). Organizational, group and individual decision making in cross-cultural perspective. In G. Wright (Ed.), *Behavioral decision making* (pp. 149–166). New York: Plenum.

Yates, J. F. (1990). *Judgment and decision making*. Englewood Cliffs, NJ: Prentice Hall.

Zajonc, R. B. (1980). Feeling and thinking: Preferences need no inferences. *American Psychologist*, *35*, 151–175.

Zey, M. (Ed.). (1992). *Decision-making: Alternatives to rational choice models*. Newbury Park, CA: Sage Publications.

"The Child That Was Meant?" or "Punishment for Sin?": Religion, Ethnicity, and Families with Children with Disabilities

LARAINE MASTERS GLIDDEN

DEPARTMENT OF PSYCHOLOGY
ST. MARY'S COLLEGE OF MARYLAND
ST. MARY'S CITY, MARYLAND

JEANNETTE ROGERS-DULAN

SCHOOL OF EDUCATION
LA SIERRA UNIVERSITY
RIVERSIDE, CALIFORNIA

AMY E. HILL

DEPARTMENT OF PSYCHOLOGY
ST. MARY'S COLLEGE OF MARYLAND
ST. MARY'S CITY, MARYLAND

I. INTRODUCTION

It has become commonplace to remark on the enormous changes in views towards families with children with disabilities (Byrne & Cunningham, 1985; Glidden, Kiphart, Willoughby, & Bush, 1993; Minnes, 1988; Ramey, Krauss, & Simeonsson, 1989). In the last decade, theorists and researchers began to move away from models that depicted, in a rather linear way, resulting burden and maladjustment when a child with disabilities entered the family (e.g., Hill, 1949,

INTERNATIONAL REVIEW OF RESEARCH IN
MENTAL RETARDATION, Vol. 22
0074-7750/99 $30.00

1958). In this recent work more complex models have been proposed, suggesting pluralistic influences on adjustment to the child (Crnic, Friedrich, & Greenberg, 1983; Glidden, 1989; McCubbin & Patterson, 1983; Wright, Granger, & Sameroff, 1984). These influences may reside within individual family members, including the child with disabilities. They may stem from characteristics of the family as a unit; or they may come from outside the family either proximally (e.g., neighborhood, local school system, friends) or distally (e.g., economic system, macrocultural values).

The recognition that adjustment is highly complex and is influenced by multiple factors has had a broadening influence on research about families with children with disabilities. Heretofore neglected topics are being explored, and investigations into the richness of family life are beginning to influence the field. Increasingly, researchers are coming to recognize the force that ethnicity and culture can exert on families who are rearing a child with disabilities. Culture and ethnicity generate and are reflective of many ways of being and knowing. Several of their manifestations—religious beliefs, values, and behavior—have been particularly fascinating to scholars over the centuries. However, in the study of families with members with disabilities, religion and religiousness have become the subject of scientific investigation only recently.

There are some exceptions to this historical neglect, and they assert the importance of religion in affecting adjustment to a child with disabilities. For example, two early studies by Zuk (1959) and Zuk, Miller, Bartram, and Kling (1961) are frequently cited. These studies explored the effects of religious affiliation—Catholic versus Protestant—using self-report techniques in a self-selected sample of clinic mothers. They concluded that Catholic mothers were slightly more accepting of their children with retardation than were Protestant mothers. The authors believed that this acceptance was mediated through religious beliefs, in that Catholic doctrine absolves parents from any guilt, and promotes the concept of the child as a gift from God. Our own research (Haworth, Hill, & Glidden, 1994, 1996) has reported similar findings, although not in the context of denominational affiliation. Several parents spoke of the child as "a blessing from God," or that "God just meant her to be ours."

Bernard Farber, often considered the father of research on families rearing children with disabilities, also studied religious affiliation and its effect on family adjustment. Based on extant sociological theory that the kind of social cohesion provided to active members of the Catholic church would relieve stress, Farber (1959) hypothesized that the marital integration of Catholic parents would not be lowered by keeping their retarded son at home. He also predicted that, regardless of religious affiliation, families with more frequent church attendance would have higher marital integration.

Farber tested these hypotheses in a sample of 240 married Caucasian families with at least one child with severe mental retardation. He found that marital integration was significantly higher among non-Catholics if the families had institutionalized their sons rather than reared them at home. In contrast, there were no significant differences in the way institutionalization influenced marital integration in Catholics. Institutionalization did not lead to improvements in the Catholic families in the sample, thus confirming the hypothesis that Farber had proposed. Farber's prediction about frequency of church attendance, however, was not upheld. There were no differences in marital integration among more versus less frequent church attenders.

More recent research has not found religious affiliation per se to be a variable influencing family adjustment. For example, in a study of religion and families who are rearing children with developmental delays, Weisner, Beizer, and Stolze (1991) found that denominational affiliation was not significantly related to variables of accommodation or well-being. Similarly, Dulan, Wild, and Blacher (1994) reported that neither parental stress nor placement outside of the home varied as a function of religious denomination in their sample of families raising children with severe disabilities. Perhaps the diversity within religious denominations in today's world makes this variable one that carries little discriminative value (Bauma, 1973). Moreover, these studies have tended to explore affiliation within Christian religions, all of which have substantial similarity in their belief systems. A broader look at religion and culture might find powerful influences.

Although the benefits of religiousness have been emphasized in much of the research, some investigators have claimed that the birth of a child with a disability may precipitate a religious crisis of faith, or confirm a parent's feelings of worthlessness, because some cultures view disability as a punishment for sin—a violation of divine dictate (Groce & Zola, 1993). For example, Stubblefield (1965) reported a case of a father who firmly believed that God had given him and his wife their son with retardation because they were not the kind of persons that He wanted them to be. This notion of the child as punishment for sin has been noted by a number of other writers (Robinson & Robinson, 1965; Smart & Smart, 1991; Zuniga, 1992).

Although not highly paradigmatic, some of the early work showed a sophisticated understanding of the multifaceted and intricately interconnected role that religion might play in influencing a family's adjustment to a child with a disability. Stubblefield (1965), for example, wrote the following:

> The role of religion in parental acceptance cannot be adequately appreciated apart from an understanding of the function of religion in the "life-economy" of persons and the theological teachings of the religious community to which they belong. Attention must be given to the belief systems which give meaning, order, and purpose to life and to the uses which these beliefs are put in meeting actual life situations. (p. 10)

Despite its wisdom, Stubblefield's recommendation was little heeded at the time.

Recent work, however, has begun to capture the diversity as well as the universality of these belief systems. One of the purposes of this chapter is to summarize briefly the most significant of that work. However, a second and more important objective is to place the study of religion and its influence on family adjustment to a child with disability in its cultural context, as Stubblefield recommended more than 30 years ago. Specifically, we propose that it is impossible to understand religiousness and its impact on family adjustment without also attending to cultural and ethnic group membership that shapes and reflects religions beliefs. As Weisner et al. (1991) have written: "To disentangle the more specific effects of religion, and fully understand the combined effects of religiosity, world view, and cultural differences, we would need diverse samples of families" (p. 660). Although we believe in the importance of examining religion within culture for all ethnicities, in this chapter we will focus only on African-American and Latino families, currently the two largest minority groups in the United States.

This focus is long overdue. Despite the disproportionate representation of ethnic minority children who are classified as mentally retarded or developmentally disabled (Hardman, Drew, & Egan, 1999, p. 47), most studies either utilize primarily Anglo-American samples, or they ignore ethnicity entirely in their description of their samples. For example, in 1989, the *American Journal on Mental Retardation* published a special issue on families. Of 12 articles reporting empirical work, only Flynt and Wood (1989) used a sample that was not predominantly of Anglo-European origin. Indeed, 50% of the articles in this special issue did not even mention the ethnic or cultural characteristics of the samples that were used. This scanty attention to the ecological context of the families being studied is counter to most of the models (e.g., Crnic et al., 1983) being proposed, and the recommendation of reviewers of research in the field (Keltner & Ramey, 1993).

In this chapter, then, we posit the importance of religion and religiousness, in general, for families rearing a child with disabilities, and describe how that importance is particularized for two different ethnic groups. We conclude with a model meant primarily as a heuristic tool for those interested in designing additional and much needed research in this area.

II. RELIGION AND DISABILITY

Writings on religion and disability have tended to dichotomize religiousness into categories of belief systems and support systems (Fewell, 1986; McIntosh, Silver, & Wortman, 1993). In general, religious belief systems are viewed as having a positive impact on family adjustment because they provide a way for family members to ascribe meaning to the disability (Friedrich, Wilturner, & Cohen, 1985; Krauss & Seltzer, 1993; Leyser, 1994). As Weisner et al. (1991) noted, "religious conviction plays an important role in parents' subjective experience of life with a child with developmental delays and in how they describe and interpret their situation" (p. 660).

In addition, religious organizations can provide direct support or help for a child with disabilities. The support may be instrumental, such as a congregation raising money so that a family can afford an expensive wheelchair. It may be emotional or social, as when the religious leader or co-worshipers share in the joys and sorrows of the parenting task. It may also be educational (e.g., adapting religious instruction for a child with mental retardation) or structural (e.g., including the child and family in the normal rites of religious passage such as baptism or bar mitzvah). Fewell (1986) wrote of these organizational activities, but found them less salient in the lives of families than the religious beliefs. Weisner et al. (1991) replicated that result, as did our own data described later in this chapter.

Assuming, then, that religiousness does play an important role in the adjustment of families to a child with disabilities, the question remains as to whether this role interacts with ethnicity to yield different effects for different groups. The next two sections examine this question for African-American families and Latino families.

III. RELIGION AND DISABILITY IN AFRICAN-AMERICAN FAMILIES

Historically, religion has been recognized as a major contributor to the cultural heritage and most basic values of the African-American family (Alston, McCowan, & Turner, 1994; Billingsley, 1992; Borchert, 1980; Boyd-Franklin, 1989; Hale-Benson, 1982; Rogers-Dulan, 1998b; Hill, 1993; Lincoln & Mamiya, 1990). Recent models and data have documented the positive impact of religions on family, parental, and child functioning (Brody, Stoneman, & Flor, 1996). Furthermore, investigators have emphasized the distinctive role of religion in the lives of African-Americans (Blaine & Crocker, 1995), with particular focus on the various functions of African-American churches. Religion not only influences spiritual aspects of African-Americans' worldviews, but with regard to churches, encompasses "family functions, social and economic activities, community services, and opportunities for self-expression and validation" (Brown, Ndubuisi, & Gary, 1990, p. 55). Yet, despite the acknowledged importance of religion in the lives of African-Americans, we know little of how it influences families rearing children with disabilities.

Most of what we do know about African-American families with children who have disabilities comes from comparative studies of ethnic families. For example, Mary's (1990) research informs us of initial reactions of African-American, Latino, and Anglo-Euro-American mothers to having a child with mental retardation. Her findings showed a common reaction of love and sorrow across ethnic groups and different levels of retardation. However, data from questionnaires and open-ended questions indicated that African-American mothers reported feeling less overwhelmed by having a child with disabilities than did mothers of other ethnicities. Flynt and Wood (1989), in a study of 90 mothers rearing children with moderate mental retardation reported similar results. African-American mothers had lower perceived family stress levels than did Anglo-Euro-American mothers. They also were more likely to use coping strategies that involved resources and social support within the family.

The ongoing work of Glidden and collaborators (see Glidden et al., 1993 for overview) also suggests the possibility of more favorable adjustment for African-American mothers than for Anglo-Euro-American mothers. *Project Parenting* is a longitudinal investigation of 249 families who are rearing either adopted or birth children with developmental disabilities. African-American mothers constitute 14.1% of the sample. Although most adjustment measures have not shown a relation to ethnicity for either adoptive or birth families, the few that do indicate better adjustment for African-American mothers. For example, correlational and regression analyses on a variety of individual and family adjustment measures indicated that African-American mothers perceived less of a personal burden in rearing their child with a disability than Anglo-Euro-American mothers did. They were more likely to answer true to items like *I rarely feel blue*, and false to items like *Sometimes I need to get away from the house*. Furthermore, African-American mothers, in contrast to Anglo-Euro-American mothers, were also likely to report more positive changes that had occurred in the family since the child had entered it. These findings were obtained despite the fact that African-American mothers were less well educated, had lower incomes and occupational status levels, and reported more financial stress than did the Anglo-Euro-American mothers. It is also true, however, that in this sample the African-American children had less severe disabilities than the Anglo-Euro-American children (Evans, Flaherty, & Glidden, 1999).

Finally, Rogers-Dulan's (1997) investigation of religion across cultures gives further credence to these findings. She investigated the relationship of religion to well-being for 338 families across three ethnic groups that included 114 Anglo, 63 African-American, and 161 Latino families who were rearing children with disabilities. The families were participants in the University of California, Riverside, Families Project. Responses to self-reported questions regarding degree of religiousness, church attendance, influence of religion in everyday feelings and actions, and religious beliefs as a source of encouragement were more highly correlated with well-being for African-American caregivers than for Anglo and Latino caregivers. Well-being was defined as reporting fewer symptoms of depression and less negative impact of the child with disabilities on the family. The findings suggest that religion is a contributor to greater well-being among African-American families.

Although the empirical evidence is still scanty, the current findings do provide support for the view that African-American families have strengths and resources that transcend the usual measures of socioeconomic status, and that these may facilitate the adjustment to rearing a child with disabilities. Many writers have suggested that one source of this strength is in the religiousness of the families (Alston et al., 1994; Billingsley, 1992; Brown & Gary, 1991; Hill, 1993; Willis, 1992).

Certainly, historically, the church served an exceptionally important role for African-American families. It was the principal channel by which the culture was transmitted. Within its structure, schools, banks, insurance companies, and low income housing were provided. The church was also an arena for political activities, and nurtured young talent for musical and artistic development (Lincoln & Mamiya, 1990). In addition to the traditional concerns of worship, moral behavior, education, and social control, the African-American church and its leaders involved itself in the development of secular organizations and institutions such as black college fraternities and sororities, The National Association for the Advancement of Colored People, and the National Urban League.

Thus, for African-Americans, the experiences of life in family functions, in cultural, social, and economic activities, and in community services, all were a part of the religious experience. This connectedness of religion to daily living in all domains, this manifestation of a "nation within a nation" (Frazier, 1974) has left its legacy. Even today, although religion may be less important than it once was (McAdoo, 1983), religious codes are integrated in the daily life of the believer. The influence of religion and its connectedness to all aspects of life is considered to be pervasive (Spencer, 1990) and can be found in various aspects of community life such as in the work of The Rev. George Clements, an African-American Roman-Catholic priest, and the recipient of a MacArthur Foundation grant. Reverend Clements is the founder of the "One Church–One Child" campaign for adopting black children, and has recently formulated a "One Church–One Addict" Program designed to catalyze religious organizations into helping addicts recover (Goodstein, 1994). His involvement in issues of social welfare is solidly in keeping with the African-American religious tradition. How might this pervasiveness of religion influence the adjustment of families to a child with disabilities? Because religion serves a multitude of roles for African-American families, influencing individuals in secular endeavors as well as in traditional religious ones, its effect may be stronger. This effect may be felt both in religious beliefs and spirituality, as well as in organized activities, including social support.

For example, the African-American church is often viewed as the conservator of morals and a bulwark of family life, as well as the final authority on right and wrong in daily activities (Staples, 1976). It may very well provide support for the family rearing a child with disabilities in that family members believe that a supreme being is in control and the family will ultimately triumph over suffering and hardships. In addition, the church teaches values of kindness and compassion, of offering help to those in distress (Willis, 1992). These values are relevant ones to the family struggling to overcome whatever burdens are entailed in rearing a child with disabilities.

Furthermore, attendance at church-related activities can reinforce the experience of group cohesiveness. The interactive style of worship and emphasis on a communal religious experience that are typical of African-American churches create an atmosphere wherein members relate to one another as extended family, offering social and material support in times of stress (Poole, 1990).

If religion is a particularly important life experience for African-Americans, and if religious beliefs and activities ease the task of rearing a child with disabilities, then religiousness may be one of the variables responsible for the more positive adjustment in African-American parents found by the few studies that have compared different ethnic groups (Flynt & Wood, 1989; Mary, 1990). The data of Glidden and her collaborators provide some support for this hypothesis. As already noted, Glidden's results provided some suggestion that African-American mothers experienced better outcomes in the rearing of their children with disabilities than did Anglo-Euro-American mothers. Research in *Project Parenting* also investigated the differences in religiousness between 35 African-American mothers and 204 Anglo-European-American mothers who were rearing children with developmental disabilities. Scores on a 12-item measure of religiousness (Fewell, 1986) were obtained during an interview that focused on adjustment to rearing a child with disabilities. These 12 items formed two separate 6-item scales, each one focusing on a different aspect of the role religion played in adjustment to a child with disabilities. One of the scales measures religious beliefs or spirituality, whereas the other measures participation in, and derived support from, organized religious activities. The mothers' scores on the Fewell scales were compared to determine if one ethnic group demonstrated more religion-based adjustment than the other. The results showed that African-American mothers scored significantly higher than Anglo-European-American mothers on both the spirituality and participation scales. Thus, religious beliefs and participation appeared to be a more important component of adjustment to rearing a child with disabilities for the African-American mothers than for the Anglo-European-American mothers.

Additional findings in the ongoing research of Rogers-Dulan and her collaborators (Dulan & Blacher, 1994; Rogers-Dulan, 1998b) confirm the importance of religion for African-American families rearing children with disabilities. Rogers-Dulan (1998b) reported the role of religion in adjustment to rearing a child with mental retardation for 52 African-American families. In a review of the literature she identified a range of religious experiences across five domains that included religion in personal and family life, religious socialization, media modes [e.g., radio, television], participation in organized religious groups, and support from religious groups. Her results indicated that the overall experience of religious connectedness among these families was significantly related to well-being as evidenced by reports of fewer depressive symptoms, stress, and less perceived negative impact of the child on the family. The two domains of (a) religion in personal and family life, and (b) support from organized religion were particularly relevant to these families as indicated by the significant relations across all measures of adjustment in the quantitative findings. Analyses of qualitative data in the form of comments in recorded field notes led to the same conclusion: spirituality and religious involvement are salient factors reflecting religious connectedness for these families.

Reported findings of religion and its impact on families generally reflect only maternal caregiver responses. However, Rogers-Dulan's (1998a) preliminary study of male and female caregivers' adjustment, found that the Likert scale responses of 33 male and female caregivers suggest that religion is equally important to adjustment for both. Their responses did not significantly differ. Although a slightly higher percentage of females (61%) than males (52%) indicated religious faith was a dominant theme, an approximately equal percentage of females (30%) and males (27%) indicated it was somewhat important to them. These indicants of the pervasive influence of religion were found even for those caregivers who were not church members, or who did not attend church regularly or at all. Thus, modes of expression of religiousness can take various forms, only one of which is formal participation.

In addition to showing an overall high level of religiousness, some of Dulan and Blacher's (1994) data suggested that religion played a role in ameliorating some of the difficulties associated with rearing children with disabilities. For example, respondents who scored high on a religious connectedness scale tended to be less depressed than other parents and perceived their child with disabilities as making fewer demands and causing less stress and strain. These parents also indicated that they would be less likely than others to place their child out of the home. Furthermore, these respondents seemed to have interpreted religion positively rather than negatively in adjusting to their child with disabilities. For example, 86% of the parents reported that religion was a positive force in their life, giving meaning to having a child with disabilities, and 91% indicated that their religious beliefs had remained strong or been strengthened after having a child with disabilities. In contrast, no respondents agreed that having a child with a handicap was a punishment by God (Dulan, Wild, & Blacher, 1994).

The Glidden and Rogers-Dulan data, of course, are quite suggestive, but they do have limitations. The Glidden data were collected without any plan or design to compare ethnic groups, and the African-American and Anglo-European-American mothers were not matched on a variety of measures that might be responsible for religiousness differences. It is not known how representative the families in the Rogers-Dulan sample might be of African-American families, in general, or of those raising children with disabilities, in particular. These two projects are not different from many others in their limitations, and these features pinpoint problems for the field. Clearly, research, from its inception, needs to consider ethnicity and culture and aim to identify the processes by which influences occur. In a later section of this chapter, we propose a model designed to represent the interrelationship between ethnicity and religion. This model is intended to be predominantly heuristic, posing questions and strategies that need to be explored in any research agenda that includes issues relating to families, ethnicity, and disability.

IV. RELIGION AND DISABILITY IN LATINO FAMILIES

One of the fastest growing minorities in the country, persons of Latino background are sometimes mistakenly seen as a single group, sharing a common cultural heritage. However, they are in some ways more diverse than similar. They come from different countries or regions (Mexico, Puerto Rico, Central and South America, Spain, Cuba), are varying acculturated, have different legal status, and may or may not be fluent in Spanish. Although the majority of Latinos are affiliated with the Roman Catholic church, even this similarity is far from universal, as other churches begin to convert individuals to their beliefs and organizations (Mardiros, 1989; Zuniga, 1992). The generalizations that follow, then, should be regarded only as starting points for promoting cultural understanding, rather than as definitive results to be applied stereotypically to members of an ethnic group. Indeed, it is essential to avoid stereotypes that might impede understanding of a given individual. We do not help people by labeling them as Latino, and then attributing to them a list of static characteristics deemed to be typical of their "group." Rather, as Lopez, Blacher, and Shapiro (1998) advise, we need to listen to the stories that our clients, patients, or subjects tell us, and use that cultural knowledge as context for understanding their interpretation of their experiences.

One example of the difficulty in forming generalizations, and then, using these generalizations to compare Latino with Anglo cultural norms, is in ascertaining the degree of religiousness in the two cultures. Certainly, many studies have found that Latinos are "more" religious than Anglos (Hood & Hall, 1977; Markides, 1983; Quirk et al., 1986; Heller, Markwardt, Rowitz, & Farber, 1994). Other research is contradictory, however. Using a sample of 137 Mexican-American women who had come to a community health center, Amaro (1988) investigated religion through personal interviews and questionnaires. The findings indicated that these Mexican-American women were only moderately religious, engaging in some type of religious activity just once a month, on average. The majority of women in this sample rated themselves as only somewhat or slightly religious, and reported fairly low church attendance. The results of this study contradict the common belief that Mexican-American women are extremely religious.

One explanation for differences in results, and also an important caveat for researchers and practitioners working with families with children with disabilities, is to understand the different manifestations that religious expression may take. Nuttall (1979) indicated that while 75% of a Puerto Rican single mother sample reported using prayer on a daily basis, only 11% belonged to a church or religious organization. Thus, spiritual beliefs may be very strong and provide a source of support, but church attendance and participation may not be highly valued. It is therefore critical to measure religiousness in a verity of ways, and to recognize that there may be some ethnic specificity to these different manifestations.

Work by Szalay, Ruiz, Strohl, Lopez, and Turbyville (1978) reinforces the importance of these varied manifestations. In comparing Latinos and Anglos, they concluded that the two ethnic groups differ in the way they interpret different aspects of religion and God. For example, Anglos appear to stress the importance of church and prayer, whereas Latinos emphasize religious faith and hope. Anglos also place more emphasis on Jesus and the teachings of the Bible than Latinos do. Anglos additionally tend to see God as a savior and father, emphasizing the human qualities and traits. Latinos, on the other hand, place more importance on the superhuman qualities of God, emphasizing his power and might, as well as his role as creator. God is conceptualized as a supreme and almighty being in the minds of Latinos, as well as a supernatural entity that encompasses all.

This conception of God as all-powerful and in control of events is relevant for understanding the reactions of Latino parents to the diagnosis of a child with disabilities, and the subsequent rearing of the child. Fitzpatrick (1981) notes the common usage of the phrase "*Si Dios quiere*" (If God wills it). This phrase denotes the acceptance of many life events as destined and inevitable, an attitude certainly applicable to the birth of a child with disabilities. Shapiro and Tittle (1986), in a study of the adjustment of low-income Mexican mothers to both disabled and nondisabled children, noted the high frequency with which the majority of their sample endorsed the concept of "God's will." The idea that God has a plan and that's what will be, can be a comfort to parents who have given birth to a child with disabilities. This *fatalismo*, or sense of destiny, exhibited by Latino families is sometimes interpreted as leading to acceptance of children with disabilities.

Several studies lend support to this interpretation. For example, Heller et al. (1994) found that Hispanics (almost all of either Mexican or Puerto Rican heritage) were more likely than non-Hispanics to endorse the statement, "Having a mentally retarded child is a test by God of [my] worthiness." Moreover, this greater sense of religious duty was related to the decreased burden of caregiving reported by Hispanic in comparison to non-Hispanic participants.

Additional confirming research was performed by Mardiros (1989) who investigated the response of Mexican-American parents to their child's disability. Findings indicated that a number of families employed the notion of "God's will" as a means of acceptance. One family in this study expressed this belief about their disabled child and said, "It's according to God's will that we should be her parents." Shapiro and Simonsen (1993) also discuss this tendency in their description and analysis of a support group for Latino families with children with Down syndrome. The common belief among these parents was that God wanted them to have these children, and that they had come to accept what had been given to them by God. These same authors cautioned, however, that many parents in this support group still displayed many of the symptoms of grief that are commonly associated with the diagnosis of a child with Down syndrome. Indeed, it is possible that although the religious tradition of acceptance may have facilitated adjustment in some families, it could actually impede it in others. For example, Mary (1990) refers to an Hispanic mother of a child with disabilities who was originally quite angry at God. If this anger is deemed "unacceptable" in the religious tradition, it could actually create more psychodynamic conflict, than if the anger is allowed free expression.

Some families who are highly religious may not be able to completely understand why they have been chosen by God to give birth to a child with disabilities. It may be true that more religious parents who have placed their faith in God are the ones who actually experience the negative feelings and effects of having a disabled child. Research has shown that it is common for parents to believe that God is punishing or testing them by giving them a disabled child. For example, Mardiros (1989) refers to a Latina mother who believed she must have done something for God to punish her by giving her a disabled child. Another parent made the comment, "My mind can't even begin to comprehend that God would sit there and send so and so this kind of child, because that's not God." These two parents were obviously looking to God for love, kindness, and support. They, and highly religious families like them, who place much faith and belief in God may be incapable of understanding why God has sent them a disabled child. Instead of viewing the child as an opportunity, the parents may see raising the child as a punishment or burden, and this may result in detrimental effects for both the child and the parents.

There are some aspects of Latino religious practices that are unique to the culture and may have an impact upon parents who have given birth to a disabled child. For example, Latinos place a strong emphasis on the mother of Jesus, or the Virgin of Guadalupe, as a very important patron saint (Liebman, 1976). Isasi-Diaz and Tarango (1992) organized various meetings of groups of Hispanic women to gather information about their lives and their religious experiences. A number of women mentioned the Virgin Mary and the impact this patron saint has had upon their lives. For example, one woman said, "The Virgin of Guadalupe comes the closest to giving my Christian womanhood the dignity that it needs." Another woman recalled how her grandparents made her pray the Hail Mary, and participate in the "Visits of the Virgin," in which a statue of the Virgin was brought to her house for a few days before being transferred to another home. A third woman noted that the first prayer she learned was the Hail Mary. From these findings, it becomes evident that the mother of Jesus has had an influence on the lives of Latina women. Additionally, the Virgin Mary may also affect Latino parents who have children with disabilities. For example, Zuniga (1992) noted that it is common for a Latino parent of a child with disabilities to ask or pray to the Virgin Mary to intercede and cure the child of the disability. Practices such as these contribute to the more unusual ways in which Latino families may use religion in coping with their disabled child.

Another example of the unique aspects of Latino religion includes the various types of folk medicine that may be utilized by Latino families as a means of explaining or coping with their child's disability. Fitzpatrick (1981) notes that folk religious practices and spiritism (in which one communicates with the spirit world) are fairly common and widespread among Latinos. In a study of Mexican-American families who had institutionalized a retarded child, Baca (1974) found that half of the families in the sample did use folk medicine. Additionally, a few of these families had superstitious beliefs about the etiology of the mental retardation, which could serve as a source of comfort to them in explaining why the disability occurred. Mardiros (1989) also noted the use of folk beliefs among Latinos in explaining the causation of disability. It is not uncommon for Latina mothers to believe that witchcraft, fright, or indigestion during pregnancy contributed to their child's disability. Other research has suggested that folk healers provide Latinos with a sense of reassurance that the power of God is involved in all situations (e.g., Schreiber & Homiak, 1981). This belief could serve as a source of comfort to families who have a child with disabilities.

However, folk beliefs and practices may not always serve as a positive source of support. For example, Leon, Mazur, Montalvo, and Rodrieguez (1984) described a Latina mother who had a child diagnosed with mental retardation. She attributed her son's behavior and actions to spiritualistic forces that she thought were determined to destroy her. Believing a child to be controlled by evil forces might lead to rejection or even abuse. Thus, folk medicine and practice may have a negative, as well as positive, effect on the adjustment of Latinos to their disabled children.

In sum, religiousness, in both its degree and manifestation, is part of a set of cultural values and context that helps to define the ecospace—the personal, social, and political contexts—inhabited by Latino families. To what extent these families and their adjustment to disability will be differentially affected by their religious values and actions is currently unknown. In the next and final section of this chapter, we describe a heuristic model, designed to provoke and guide research relevant to these issues.

V. A MODEL OF RELIGION, ETHNICITY, AND DISABILITY

The model of religion, ethnicity, and disability displayed in Figure 1 has been discussed in detail in Rogers-Dulan and Blacher (1995). It depicts key factors that interact to influence family adaptation and adjustment to rearing a child with disabilities. The model extends the contributions of ecological perspectives of family adaptation and adjustment to include religion as it interacts with the cultural context within which the family lives.

The mutual interaction of religion, family structure and functions, and ethnicity is critical to the understanding of the dynamic interplay implied in this model. As families interpret the meaning of having a child with disabilities, and marshal

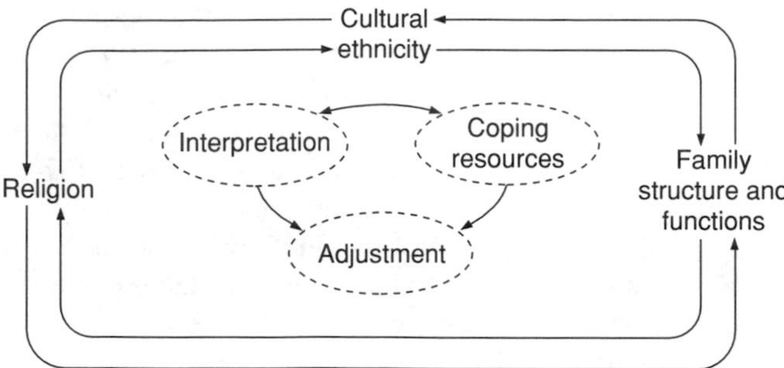

FIG. 1. A heuristic model for studying how religion and ethnicity interact to influence family adjustment to disability. (Reprinted from Rogers-Dulan & Blacher, 1995, with permission.)

their coping resources to deal with this life task, their adjustment and adaptation are influenced by their family characteristics, ethnicity, and religious beliefs and practices. This influence occurs both initially and over the course of the life span.

The model depicts two spheres of influence. The outer sphere of religion, family, and ethnicity influences in an enveloping, all-encompassing way, the link among elements in the inner sphere. The inner spheres of interpretation of the meaning of the event, coping resources and behaviors, and adjustment and adaptation are purposely drawn with broken lines to indicate their permeability. These inner spheres are more likely to change over time than are the more stable and macroecological features represented in the outer sphere.

How might this model be a heuristic tool? To illustrate the possibilities, we present two case studies that particularize the relations among elements in the outer and inner spheres of the model. As we have discussed earlier in this chapter, there is evidence that for some ethnic groups, religiousness is generally more pervasive, and therefore, exerts a greater influence on adaptation than it does for other ethnic groups. In these case studies, both of African-American families, we highlight different manifestations of religiousness. We also emphasize the variability of ethnic family structures, a variability that may reflect creative adaptations to situational and social problems. Figure 2 displays the detailed elements of the model that are described in these case studies. The elements displayed are only a subset of the various possibilities. The elements that are most important will be different for different families, and, more generally, for those with different ethnicities and degrees of religiousness.

A. Case Study 1: The McKenzie Family

Ellen and Jim McKenzie are a middle-aged couple who have been married for 28 years. They live in a stable and peaceful urban African-American neighborhood of modest, well-kept homes. Mr. McKenzie works as a nurse at a major medical

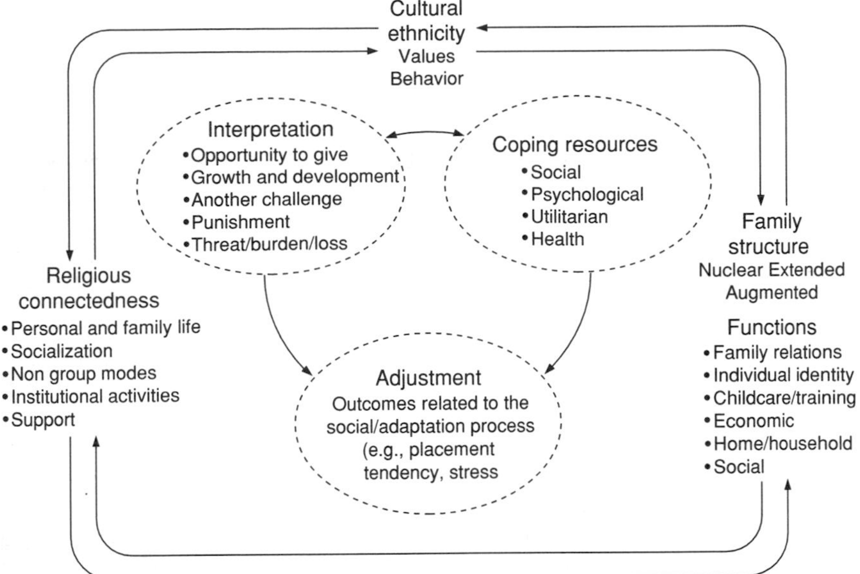

FIG. 2. A heuristic model for studying religion, ethnicity, and family adjustment to disability with case study examples. (Reprinted from Rogers-Dulan & Blacher, 1995, with permission.)

research center and Mrs. McKenzie manages custodial services for local businesses. Two adult children, both in school, live at home: Gregory, 25, is normally functioning, and Beth, 19, has severe mental retardation, the result of a chromosomal abnormality. She is nonambulatory, nonverbal, and needs assistance in feeding, grooming, dressing, and other daily living skills.

The McKenzies are a close-knit family and all share in the duties of Beth's care. Mr. McKenzie is actively involved on a daily basis. He takes her to medical and therapy appointments, attends all school planning meetings, and spends a great deal of time with her at home. Greg assumes primary responsibility when his parents go on vacation. In addition, the extended family participates in Beth's rearing, especially Mr. McKenzie's sister who is usually available and willing to assist with Beth. She initiates outings and birthday and other holiday celebrations for her.

The McKenzies are strongly religious. They attend church every week, and participate in community service activities organized via the church. Mrs. McKenzie believes that her religious faith has influenced her interpretation of Beth's disability and the family's positive adaptation to it. She describes her beliefs as a coping resource:

> Being a child of God helped me deal with situations we could not handle alone. I know the Lord better now. I know He does not wish bad situations on us. These things happen as part of life,

> but He gives us the strength to get through them. He doesn't always move the mountains in our lives—He certainly gives grace to climb them!

In addition to the strength derived from her belief in a supreme being, Mrs. McKenzie emphasized the religious connectedness she felt because of the instrumental support the family received from the congregation. She described one example:

> When we started carrying Beth to church, the church fixed up a special room for her. They purchased a special chair so she could be comfortable and provided things they thought would make her happy to be there.

Thus, at least in part because of the family's religious beliefs and practices, embedded within the specific African-American community, the interpretation of Beth's disability, and the coping resources of the family have all operated to keep the child within the family, and to adapt positively. The McKenzies exhibit a number of important family functions in rearing Beth. They are centered, in a cooperative way, around her. Their roles are adaptable, with all family members assuming the caretaking role, as needed. Also, it appears, on the basis of their sharing of this important life task, that kinship bonds, both nuclear and extended, are strengthened.

The family chosen for the second case study, the Jones, is quite different in its structure, yet for it as well, religious connectedness influences the interpretation, coping, and adjustment to a child with mental retardation.

B. Case Study 2: The Jones Family

Ruth Jones, a widow in her mid-50s, bore and raised six children. One of her daughters, Bonny, lived with and married an older man when she was only 14. The man was volatile and violent, often abusing Bonny. At the age of 15 and with no prenatal care, Bonny gave birth to the second of her three children, Denny. Now 14 years old, Denny displays retardation in the moderate range. The etiology of his disability is unknown, but it is likely that lack of prenatal care and generally inadequate living conditions were contributing factors. Indeed, because Bonny's living conditions were so poor, the court awarded custody of Denny and his two siblings to Mrs. Jones. She supports them with money received from social service as an in-home care provider.

Religion plays an important role in the adaptation of Mrs. Jones to rearing Denny. Her expression of her sense of religious connectedness is manifested in her personal and family life, in nongroup modes such as music, and in organized religious activities, as well as social/cultural events. Mrs. Jones explained during the interview that her religious beliefs and practices has helped her to adjust to rearing Denny:

> I knew almost from birth that something was wrong with Denny. I prayed to the Lord to help him. . . . I pray every morning for this kid. Having Denny is not the worse [sic] thing that could happen in my life. It is a good thing I have him. I love Denny and the Lord gives me the strength each day to do all I do for the kids.

Mrs. Jones accepts the diagnosis of Denny's mental retardation and her status as his legal guardian as one of many challenging events in her life. She faces his rearing not with resistance and despair, but with the understanding that life is synonymous with challenge, a challenge that she can meet adequately because of her belief in the Lord. Belief in a supreme being and daily prayer contribute to her positive interpretation of having a child with mental retardation.

Mrs. Jones derives support and personal validation from a variety of nongroup modes of religious expression. She listens to religious radio and watches religious television programs for several hours each week. She also plays religious music on her home organ. She talks about her playing of music as an important aspect of her adjustment: "I know I can sit here and play the organ and the music makes me feel better; the words remind me the Lord is always there for me."

In addition to these private modes of expression, Mrs. Jones attends church services as often as she can, averaging once a week. She works at the church shelter up to three times each week, preparing clothing for distribution to the needy. In addition to personal validation, she derives a sense of belonging, of being part of a social network from these activities: "Church members are happy when they see me and my grandsons coming to church. They want to do a lot for them, like take them places and do things."

In sum, Mrs. Jones's religiousness, in all its modes of manifestation, appears to filter through to all three internal spheres. She has a positive interpretation of Denny's mental retardation; her connection to God and her church lend emotional, psychological, and social support, all important coping resources. These characteristics, in turn, influence adaptation and adjustment.

With regard to family structure and function, a traditional view might identify Denny as a product of a dysfunctional home. However, it is important to recognize that interpreted within the cultural values of the African-American ethnicity, Denny exists within a functionally supportive extended family network. Although Mrs. Jones is technically a single female head of household, and not Denny's mother, she interacts daily with several of her children, who are involved and concerned with their mother and her grandsons. What might be interpreted as deviation and weakness can instead be understood as resourcefulness, resilience, and strength when cultural diversity and uniqueness are recognized. This understanding needs to be an integral part of our research questions and designs. Ultimately, it will aid us in predicting and understanding outcomes, and eventually in designing programs and interventions that are culturally sensitive and appropriate, as well as maximally effective.

This model is valuable in studying behavior both within a given cultural group and between cultural groups. By helping to summarize (but not stereotype) the basic cultural style of a given ethnic group, it should reveal that individual variation is usual, as typical as for any other complex variable. Successful summary should also expedite the study of differences between cultures. Once we understand what factors are important *within* a culture, it is possible to effectively design and conduct research that explores these factors *across* cultures, thereby beginning to assess the role of cultural differences in determining how those factors are influential. With more understanding of cultural style, investigators may be able to avoid some of the limitations and mistakes of earlier work, mistakes made because differences were frequently interpreted as deficits, and comparisons were made only with reference to the modal culture (Rogers-Dulan & Blacher, 1995).

VI. SUMMARY AND CONCLUSIONS

In this chapter, we have described how religion and religiousness can influence the way in which families adjust to rearing children with disabilities. Furthermore, we have underscored how this religiousness and its influence is firmly embedded in the cultural values and behaviors that are part of what defines any given ethnic group. Religious beliefs and activities are part of the worldview that individuals of a given ethnicity are likely to hold, and, as such, are essential to study. They give meaning to life, in general, and to rearing children with disabilities, in particular. They are, without doubt, important determinants of adjustment over the life span.

The model presented in this chapter is, at this point, heuristic. As investigators begin formally and systematically to incorporate religiousness and ethnicity into their designs and data begin to accumulate, the framework that we have provided will begin to be filled in more completely than we have done in our two case studies. Most importantly, we want to underscore the value of this enterprise. As others have also concluded (Lynch & Hanson, 1992; Mink, 1997) from both a practice and research perspective, the neglect of cultural and religious variables, often because of the difficulty of measuring and understanding them, is not benign. It has led, at times, to partial portraits and missed interpretations and, therefore, to incorrect conclusions. As we move toward more sophisticated methods that are capable of handling complex systems, religiousness and ethnicity should become usual and routine components of our investigations.

ACKNOWLEDGMENTS

This manuscript was written with the support of Grant No. HD 21993 from the National Institute of Child Health and Human Development to the first author, Grant No. HD 35202 to the second author, and Grant No. HD 21324 to Jan Blacher, with whom the second author worked as a postdoctoral research fellow.

REFERENCES

Alston, R. J., McCowan, C. J., & Turner, W. L. (1994). Family functioning as a correlate of disability adjustment for African Americans. *Rehabilitation Counseling Bulletin, 37,* 277–289.

Amaro, H. (1988). Women in the Mexican-American community: Religion, culture, and reproductive attitudes and experiences. *Journal of Community Psychology, 16,* 6–20.

Baca, G. M. (1974). Forty families: A comparative study of Mexican American and Anglo parents of an institutionalized retarded child (Doctoral dissertation, University of Denver, 1975). *Dissertation Abstracts International, 36,* 3128A. (University Microfilms No. 75-25-310).

Bauma, G. D. (1973). Beyond Lenski: A critical review of recent Protestant ethnic research. *Journal of the Scientific Study of Religion, 12,* 141–151.

Billingsley, A. (1992). *Climbing Jacob's ladder.* New York: Simon Schuster.

Blaine, B., & Crocker, J. (1995). Religiousness, race, and psychological well-being: Exploring social psychological mediators. *Personality and Social Psychology Bulletin, 21,* 1031–1041.

Borchert, J. (1980). *Alley life in Washington: Family, community, religion, and folklife in the city, 1850–1970.* Chicago: University of Illinois.

Boyd-Franklin, N. (1989). Five key factors in the treatment of black families. *Journal of Psychotherapy and the Family, 6,* 53–67.

Brody, G. H., Stoneman, Z., & Flor, D. (1996). Parental religiosity, family processes, and youth competence in rural, two parent African American families. *Developmental Psychology, 32,* 696–706.

Brown, D. R., & Gary, L. E. (1991). Religious socialization and educational attainment among African-Americans: An empirical assessment. *Journal of Negro Education, 60,* 411–426.

Brown, D. R., Ndubuisi, S. C., & Gary, L. E. (1990). Religiosity and psychological distress among Blacks. *Journal of Religion and Health, 29,* 55–68.

Byrne, E. A., & Cunningham, C. C. (1985). The effects of mentally handicapped children on families: A conceptual review. *Journal of Child Psychology and Psychiatry, 26,* 847–864.

Crnic, K. A., Friedrich, W. N., & Greenberg, M. T. (1983). Adaptation of families with mentally retarded children: A model of stress, coping, and family ecology. *American Journal of Mental Deficiency, 88,* 125–138.

Dulan, J., & Blacher, J. (1994, June). *The role of religion in African American families who have a child with disabilities.* Paper presented at the annual conference of the American Association on Mental Retardation, Boston, MA.

Dulan, J., Wild, M., & Blacher, J. (1994, March). *Impact of a child with disabilities on parents: The role of religion.* Paper presented at the Gatlinburg Conference on Research and Theory in Mental Retardation and Developmental Disabilities, Gatlinburg, TN.

Evans, J. N., Flaherty, E. M., & Glidden, L. M. (1999, March). *Family adjustment to rearing children with developmental disabilities: Does ethnicity make a difference?* Poster session presented at the annual meeting of the Gatlinburg Conference on Research in MR/DD, Charleston, SC.

Farber, B. (1959). Effects of a severely mentally retarded child on family integration. *Monographs of the Society for Research in Child Development,* 24 (2, Whole No. 71).

Fewell, R. R. (1986). Supports from religious organizations and personal beliefs. In R. R. Fewell &

P. F. Vadasy (Eds.), *Families of handicapped children: Needs and supports across the life span* (pp. 297–316). Austin, TX: Pro-Ed.

Fitzpatrick, J. (1981). The Puerto Rican family. In C. Mindel & R. Habenstein (Eds.), *Ethnic families in America* (pp. 189–214). New York: Elsevier.

Flynt, S. W., & Wood, T. A. (1989). Stress and coping of mothers of children with moderate mental retardation. *American Journal on Mental Retardation, 94*, 278–283.

Frazier, E. F. (1974). *The negro church in America: The black church since Frazier*. New York: Schocken.

Friedrich, W., Wilturner, L., & Cohen, D. (1985). Coping resources and parenting mentally retarded children. *American Journal of Mental Deficiency, 90*, 130–139.

Glidden, L. M. (1989). *Parents for children, children for parents*. Washington D. C.: American Association on Mental Retardation.

Glidden, L. M., Kiphart, M. J., Willoughby, J. C., & Bush, B. A. (1993). Family functioning when rearing children with developmental disabilities. In A. P. Turnbull, J. M. Patterson, S. K. Behr, D. L. Murphy, J. G. Marquis, & M. J. Blue-Banning (Eds.), *Cognitive coping, families, and disability* (pp. 183–194). Baltimore, MD: Paul H. Brookes.

Goodstein, L. (1994, February 23). Program calls on churches to 'adopt' addicts. *The Washington Post*, p. A6.

Groce, N. E., & Zola, I. K. (1993). Multiculturalism, chronic illness, and disability. *Pediatrics, 91*, 1048–1055.

Hale-Benson, J. E. (1982). *Black children*. Baltimore, MD: Johns Hopkins University.

Hardman, M. L., Drew, C. J., & Egan, M. W. (1999). *Human exceptionality* (6th ed.). Needham Heights, MD: Allyn and Bacon.

Haworth, A. M., Hill, A. E., & Glidden, L. M. (1994, March). *Religion and maternal adjustment to children with disabilities*. Paper presented at the Gatlinburg Conference on Research in Mental Retardation and Developmental Disabilities, Gatlinburg, TN.

Haworth, A. M., Hill, A. E., & Glidden, L. M. (1996). Measuring religiousness of parents of children with developmental disabilities. *Mental Retardation, 34*, 271–279.

Heller, T., Markwardt, R., Rowitz, L., & Farber, B. (1994). Adaptation of Hispanic families to a member with mental retardation. *American Journal on Mental Retardation, 99*, 289–300.

Hill, R. (1949). *Families under stress*. New York: Harper & Row.

Hill, R. (1958). Generic features of families under stress. *Social Casework, 39*, 139–150.

Hill, R. (1993). *Research on the African-American family*. Westport, CT: Auburn House.

Hood, R. W., & Hall, J. R. (1977). Comparison of reported religious experience in Caucasian, American Indian, and two Mexican American samples. *Psychological Reports, 41*, 657–658.

Isasi-Diaz, A. M., & Tarango, Y. (1992). *Hispanic women: Prophetic voice in the church*. Minneapolis: Fortress Press.

Keltner, B., & Ramey, S. L. (1993). Family issues. *Current Opinion in Psychiatry, 6*, 629–634.

Krauss, M. W., & Seltzer, M. M. (1993). Coping strategies among older mothers of adults with retardation: A lifespan development perspective. In A. P. Turnbull, J. M. Patterson, S. K. Behr, D. L. Murphy, J. G. Marquis, & M. J. Blue-Banning (Eds.). *Cognitive coping, families, and disabilities* (pp. 173–182). Baltimore: Brookes.

Leon, A. M., Mazur, R., Montalvo, E., & Rodrieguez, M. (1984). Self-help support groups for Hispanic mothers. *Child Welfare, 63*, 261–268.

Liebman, S. B. (1976). *Exploring the Latin American mind*. Chicago: Nelson-Hall.

Lincoln, C. E., & Mamiya, L. H. (1990). *The black church in the African-American experience*. Durham, NC: Duke University.

Lopez, S. R., Blacher, J. B., & Shapiro, J. (1998). *The interplay of culture and disability in Latino families*. Unpublished manuscript.

Lynch, E. W., & Hanson, M. J. (Eds.). (1992). *Developing cross-cultural competence: A guide for working with young children and their families*. Baltimore: Brookes.

McAdoo, H. P. (1983). Societal stress: The black family. In H. I. McCubbin & C. R. Figley (Eds.), *Stress and the family I: Coping with normative transitions* (pp. 178–187). New York: Brunner/Mazel.

McCubbin, H., & Patterson, J. (1983). Family stress adaptation to crises: A double ABCX model of family behavior. In H. McCubbin, M. Sussman, & J. Patterson (Eds.). *Social stresses and the family: Advances and developments in family stress theory and research.* New York: Haworth Press.

McIntosh, D. N., Silver, R. C., & Wortman, C. B. (1993). Religion's role in adjustment to a negative life event: Coping with the loss of a child. *Personality and Social Psychology, 65*, 812–821.

Mardiros, M. (1989). Conception of childhood disability among Mexican-American parents. *Medical Anthropology, 12*, 55–68.

Markides, K. S. (1983). Aging, religiosity, and adjustment: A longitudinal analysis. *Journal of Gerontology, 5*, 621–625.

Mary, N. L. (1990). Reactions of black, Hispanic, and white mothers to having a child with handicaps. *Mental Retardation, 28*, 1–5.

Mink, I. T. (1997). Studying culturally diverse families of children with mental retardation. In N. W. Bray (Ed.), *International review of research in mental retardation* (Vol. 20, pp. 75–98). San Diego, CA: Academic Press.

Minnes, P. M. (1988). Family stress associated with a developmentally handicapped child. In N. W. Bray (Ed.), *International review of research in mental retardation* (pp. 195–226). San Diego, CA: Academic Press.

Nuttall, E. V. (1979). The support system and coping patterns of the female Puerto Rican single parent. *Journal of Non-White Concerns in Personnel and Guidance, 7*, 128–137.

Poole, T. G. (1990). Black families and the black church: A sociohistorical perspective. In H. E. Cheatham & J. B. Stewart (Eds.), *Black families, interdisciplinary perspectives* (pp. 33–48). New Brunswick, NJ: Transaction.

Quirk, M., Ciottone, R., Minami, H., Wapner, S., Yamamoto, T., Ishii, S., Lucca-Irizarry, P., & Pacheco, A. (1986). Values mothers hold for handicapped and nonhandicapped preschool children in Japan, Puerto Rico, and the U. S. mainland. *International Journal of Psychology, 21*, 463–485.

Ramey, S. L., Krauss, M. W., & Simeonsson, R. J. (1989). Research on families: Current assessment and future opportunities. *American Journal on Mental Retardation, 94*, ii–vi.

Robinson, H. B., & Robinson, N. M. (1965). *The mentally retarded child: A psychological approach.* New York: McGraw-Hill.

Rogers-Dulan, J. (1997, March). Religion and well-being: Does culture make a difference? In J. Blacher (Chair), *Dimensions of family coping: Over time, across cultures.* Symposium conducted at the meeting of the Gatlinburg Conference on Research and Theory in Mental Retardation and Developmental Disabilities, Riverside, CA.

Rogers-Dulan, J. (1998a). *Perceptions of coping among African American mothers and fathers who have a child with mental retardation.* Manuscript in preparation.

Rogers-Dulan, J. (1998b). Religious connectedness among urban African American families who have a child with disabilities. *Mental Retardation, 36*, 94–103.

Rogers-Dulan, J., & Blacher, J. (1995). African-American families, religion, and disability: A conceptual framework. *Mental Retardation, 33*, 226–238.

Schreiber, J. M., & Homiak, J. P. (1981). Mexican Americans. In A. Harwood (Ed.), *Ethnicity and medical care.* Cambridge, MA: Harvard University Press.

Shapiro, J., & Simonsen, D. (1993). *An educational/support group for Latino families of children with Down syndrome: Observations and recommendations.* Unpublished manuscript, University of California, Irvine.

Shapiro, J., & Tittle, K. (1986). Psychosocial adjustment of poor Mexican mothers of disabled and nondisabled children. *American Journal of Orthopsychiatry, 56*, 289–302.

Smart, J. F., & Smart, D. W. (1991). Acceptance of disability and the Mexican American culture. *Rehabilitation Counseling Bulletin, 34*, 357–367.

Spencer, M. B. (1990). Parental values transmissions: Implications for the development of African-American children. In H. E. Cheatham & J. B. Stewart (Eds.), *Black families, interdisciplinary perspectives* (pp. 111–130). New Brunswick, NJ: Transaction.

Staples, R. (1976). *Introduction to Black sociology*. New York: McGraw-Hill.

Stubblefield, H. W. (1965). Religion, parents, and mental retardation. *Mental Retardation, 3*(4), 8–11.

Szalay, L. B., Ruiz, P., Strohl, J. B., Lopez, R., & Turbyville, L. (1978). *The Hispanic American cultural frame of reference: A communication guide for use in mental health, education, and training*. Washington, D. C.: Institute of Comparative Social and Cultural Studies, Inc.

Weisner, T. S., Beizer, L., & Stolze, L. (1991). Religion and families of children with developmental delays. *American Journal on Mental Retardation, 95*, 647–662.

Willis, W. (1992). Families with African-American roots. In E. W. Lynch & M. J. Hanson (Eds.), *Developing cross-cultural competence* (pp. 121–150). Baltimore: Brookes.

Wright, J. S., Granger, R. D., & Sameroff, A. J. (1984). Parental acceptance and developmental handicap. In J. Blacher (Ed.), *Severely handicapped young children and their families* (pp. 51–90). Orlando, FL: Academic Press.

Zuk, G. H. (1959). The religious factor and the role of guilt in parental acceptance of the retarded child. *American Journal of Mental Deficiency, 64*, 139–147.

Zuk, G. H., Miller, R. L., Bartram, J. B., & Kling, F. (1961). Maternal acceptance of retarded children: A questionnaire study of attitudes and religious background. *Child Development 32*, 525–540.

Zuniga, M. E. (1992). Families with Latino roots. In E. W. Lynch & M. J. Hanson (Eds.), *Developing cross-cultural competence: A guide for working with young children and their families* (pp. 151–179). Baltimore: Brookes.

Index

C

D

M

R

S

T

W

ISBN 0-12-366222-2

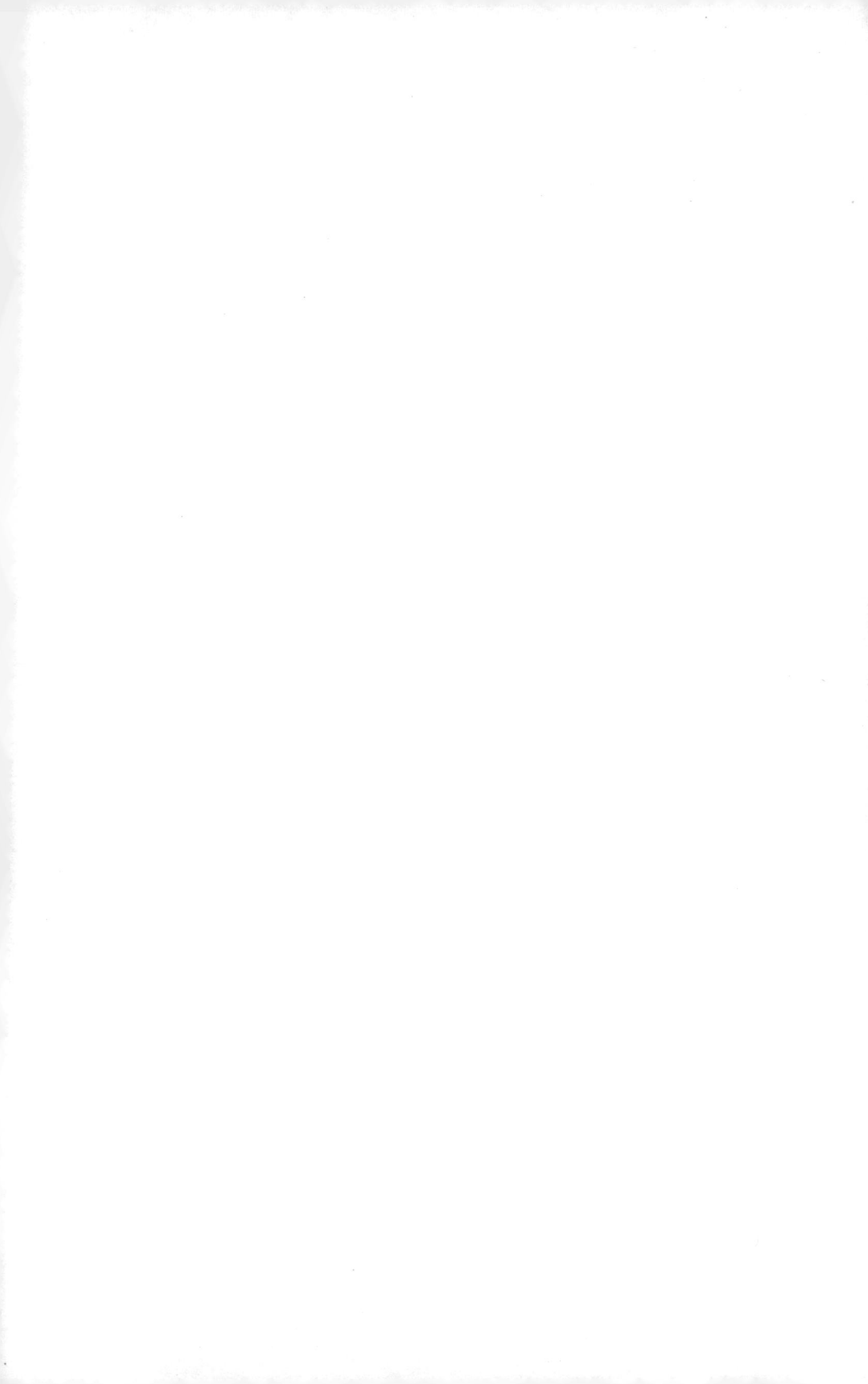